T0261068

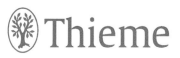

# Fluorescence-Guided Neurosurgery

**Neuro-oncology and Cerebrovascular Applications**

**Constantinos G. Hadjipanayis, MD, PhD**
Professor and Site Chair
Department of Neurosurgery
Mount Sinai Downtown Union Square/Beth Israel
Professor of Oncological Sciences
Icahn School of Medicine at Mount Sinai
Director of Neurosurgical Oncology
Mount Sinai Health System
New York, New York

**Walter Stummer, MD, PhD**
Professor and Chairman
Department of Neurosurgery
University of Münster
Münster, Germany

74 illustrations

Thieme
New York • Stuttgart • Delhi • Rio de Janeiro

Executive Editor: Timothy Y. Hiscock
Managing Editor: Sarah Landis
Director, Editorial Services: Mary Jo Casey
Production Editor: Naamah Schwartz
International Production Director: Andreas Schabert
Editorial Director: Sue Hodgson
International Marketing Director: Fiona Henderson
International Sales Director: Louisa Turrell
Director of Institutional Sales: Adam Bernacki
Senior Vice President and Chief Operating Officer: Sarah Vanderbilt
President: Brian D. Scanlan

**Library of Congress Cataloging-in-Publication Data**

Names: Hadjipanayis, Constantinos G., editor. | Stummer, Walter, editor.
Title: Fluorescence-guided neurosurgery : neuro-oncology and cerebrovascular applications / [edited by] Constantinos G. Hadjipanayis, Walter Stummer.
Description: New York : Thieme, [2019] | Includes bibliographical references.
Identifiers: LCCN 2018026854| ISBN 9781626237148 (print) | ISBN 9781626237155 (eISBN)
Subjects: | MESH: Neurosurgical Procedures–methods | Fluorescent Dyes | Brain Neoplasms–surgery | Cerebrovascular Disorders–surgery | Contrast Media | Brain Mapping–methods
Classification: LCC RD593 | NLM WL 368 | DDC 617.4/8–dc23 LC record available at https://lccn.loc.gov/2018026854

© 2019 Thieme Medical Publishers, Inc.

Thieme Publishers New York
333 Seventh Avenue, New York, NY 10001 USA
+1 800 782 3488, customerservice@thieme.com

Thieme Publishers Stuttgart
Rüdigerstrasse 14, 70469 Stuttgart, Germany
+49 [0]711 8931 421, customerservice@thieme.de

Thieme Publishers Delhi
A-12, Second Floor, Sector-2, Noida-201301
Uttar Pradesh, India
+91 120 45 566 00, customerservice@thieme.in

Thieme Publishers Rio de Janeiro, Thieme Publicações Ltda.
Edifício Rodolpho de Paoli, 25º andar
Av. Nilo Peçanha, 50 – Sala 2508
Rio de Janeiro 20020-906 Brasil
+55 21 3172-2297 / +55 21 3172-1896
www.thiemerevinter.com.br

Cover design: Thieme Publishing Group
Typesetting by Thomson Digital, India

Printed in The United States of America by King Printing Company, Inc.                5 4 3 2 1

ISBN 978-1-62623-714-8

Also available as an e-book:
eISBN 978-1-62623-715-5

**Important note:** Medicine is an ever-changing science undergoing continual development. Research and clinical experience are continually expanding our knowledge, in particular our knowledge of proper treatment and drug therapy. Insofar as this book mentions any dosage or application, readers may rest assured that the authors, editors, and publishers have made every effort to ensure that such references are in accordance with **the state of knowledge at the time of production of the book.**

Nevertheless, this does not involve, imply, or express any guarantee or responsibility on the part of the publishers in respect to any dosage instructions and forms of applications stated in the book. **Every user is requested to examine carefully** the manufacturers' leaflets accompanying each drug and to check, if necessary in consultation with a physician or specialist, whether the dosage schedules mentioned therein or the contraindications stated by the manufacturers differ from the statements made in the present book. Such examination is particularly important with drugs that are either rarely used or have been newly released on the market. Every dosage schedule or every form of application used is entirely at the user's own risk and responsibility. The authors and publishers request every user to report to the publishers any discrepancies or inaccuracies noticed. If errors in this work are found after publication, errata will be posted at www.thieme.com on the product description page.

Some of the product names, patents, and registered designs referred to in this book are in fact registered trademarks or proprietary names even though specific reference to this fact is not always made in the text. Therefore, the appearance of a name without designation as proprietary is not to be construed as a representation by the publisher that it is in the public domain.

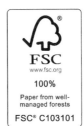

FSC
www.fsc.org
100%
Paper from well-managed forests
FSC® C103101

This book, including all parts thereof, is legally protected by copyright. Any use, exploitation, or commercialization outside the narrow limits set by copyright legislation, without the publisher's consent, is illegal and liable to prosecution. This applies in particular to photostat reproduction, copying, mimeographing, preparation of microfilms, and electronic data processing and storage.

This book is dedicated to my wife, Lorraine, who has always been there, and
my three children, Panikos, Athena, and Elias.

*- Constantinos G. Hadjipanayis*


Dedicated to the many patients that we have the privilege of treating.
May this book serve to improve what we do.

*- Walter Stummer*

# Contents

Contents

# Video Contents

**Video 4.1** Five-aminolevulinic acid (5-ALA) fluorescence-guided surgery for recurrent high-grade glioma resection. This video highlights the use of a wavelength-specific lighted suction device to aid in 5-ALA fluorescence-guided surgery.

**Video 5.1** Five-aminolevulinic acid (5-ALA) in suspected LGG.

**Video 8.1** An operative video of the case presented in **Fig. 8.2**. This is a 27-year-old woman who presented with neck and back pain. 5-aminolevulinic acid (5-ALA) fluorescence-guided resection was performed. Following the C3–C5 laminotomy, we encountered the swollen spinal cord. First, we opened the intratumoral cyst from the caudal pole. Next, we dissected the posterior median sulcus to expose the tumor, and started removal of it. The tumor had strong 5-ALA fluorescence. Along the sidewalls of the tumors, it was relatively easy to perform dissections to separate the tumor from the spinal cord. We continued dissection until we reached the ventral border. At the caudal end, a tumor on the edge was removed according to the red fluorescence. The yellowish tissues that did not exhibit fluorescence were left untouched. With 5-ALA fluorescence guidance, complete tumor resection was accomplished.

**Video 8.2** An operative video of the case presented in **Fig. 8.5**. This is a 57-year-old man who presented with hypersensation in his right lower extremity. Following a right C6 hemilaminectomy, the tumor was encountered. The relationships between the tumor and surrounding vasculatures were not clear. However, indocyanine green (ICG) videoangiography indicated the arterial feeders and helped surgeons to perform safe resection of this hypervascular tumor. A second ICG videoangiography confirmed no residual tumors. With ICG fluorescence guidance, complete tumor resection was accomplished.

**Video 10.1** Right interhemispheric craniotomy for resection of glioblastoma.

**Video 12.1** Resection of intraparenchymal metastasis with near-infrared fluorescence guidance.

**Video 19.1** The video demonstrates resection of a Spetzler–Martin grade 1 right temporal arteriovenous malformation (AVM) supplied by the right middle cerebral artery with superficial venous drainage to the superior sagittal sinus and transverse-sigmoid sinus. ICG angiography is performed prior to AVM resection to help identify the arteries, nidus, and veins of the AVM as well as normal arteries, veins, and capillaries adjacent to the AVM. The AVM was completely resected and confirmed with postoperative digital subtraction angiography.

**Video 20.1** ICG-VA for intraoperative confirmation of bypass patency in cerebral revascularization.

# Foreword

Neurosurgery has a long history of innovation and resourcefulness, incorporating through translation or new discovery novel, enabling technologies into its ever-challenging work. The operating microscope, electrocautery, stereotaxy and its offspring image-guidance, radiosurgery, intraoperative brainstem evoked responses and related neuromonitoring, and endovascular aneurysm repair (to name just a few) all have enhanced the ability of surgeons to better treat patients. Fluorescence-guidance for surgery has similarly developed and, having already generated Class 1 evidence for better surgery, has especially excited the neurosurgical community.

*Fluorescence-Guided Neurosurgery* is the definitive book on this subject. Edited by two of the foremost authorities on the topic, this volume encompasses the breadth of fluorescence technologies and applications. In Germany, Walter Stummer recognized early on the potential of 5-aminolevulinic acid (5-ALA)-induced protoporphyrin IX (PpIX) fluorescence in glioma surgery, steadfastly laying the groundwork for the landmark multi-institutional study of 2006, and he continues to advance our understanding of the capabilities of intraoperative fluorescence. On this side of the Atlantic, Constantinos Hadjipanayis resolutely led the effort to gain regulatory approval for the pro-drug in the United States and has continued to champion the technology for all of us. Together, they have carefully conceived and overseen the creation of this book with their expert knowledge of the subject and authoritative perspective on its role in neurosurgery.

Since Moore's 1947 report of using fluorescein for the identification of malignant tumor, only a small number of fluorescent agents have been available. The pro-drug 5-ALA, converted to the fluorophore PpIX and preferentially accumulating in tumor, vastly improved the diagnostic performance of other strategies in its selectivity. Fluorescein, established in ophthalmology and usable in the U.S. without the IND required of 5-ALA, was rediscovered for this neuro-oncologic purpose, and indocyanine green (ICG), in use for vascular indications, came to practice independently. All three of these drugs that underpin the technology are comprehensively presented here, in the context of clinical settings by experienced surgeons. Further, the intriguing development of potentially powerful new fluorophores, molecularly targeted specifically to tumor, are included here as well.

For 5-ALA and fluorescein, the initial neurosurgical application was for high-grade glioma, but not surprisingly, the potential utility of these agents in surgery for other tumors has been recognized and is being explored. Low-grade gliomas, meningiomas, metastatic tumors, spinal cord tumors, and pediatric tumors are appropriately covered in this text, as are both vascular and oncologic applications with ICG. Inclusion of other technologies such as confocal microscopy to help extend applicability, closely-related topics like Raman spectroscopy, and the important, practical topic of integrating fluorescence with other surgical adjuncts speak to the comprehensive nature of this resource.

With all that has been accomplished with fluorescence guidance, it is sometimes underappreciated just how early in its development and adoption this technology is. It is only in its infancy, and it has the potential to expand its applicability through new fluorophores and new imaging tools to a host of even broader applications. *Fluorescence-Guided Neurosurgery* presents and helps establish in a single accessible resource the current state-of-the-art in this most exciting field.

*David W. Roberts, MD*
*Professor, Active Emeritus*
*Department of Surgery (Neurosurgery)*
*Dartmouth-Hitchcock Medical Center*
*Lebanon, New Hampshire*

# Preface

Visualization and localization during any surgery is paramount to be able to delineate normal from abnormal structures. Neurosurgeons currently rely on visualization tools such as the operative microscope or endoscope for greater illumination and magnification during surgery. Dr. Theodore Kurze introduced the operative microscope into neurosurgery in 1967[1] and the neuro-endoscope by Dr. Victor Lespinasse arose in 1910.[2] While these tools were introduced into neurosurgery over 50 years ago, decades went by before they became mainstream tools routinely used by neurosurgeons as they are today. Another more recent advance in neurosurgery occurred with the introduction of frameless stereotactic neuronavigation in the early 1990s for localization of structures in the brain and image-guided neurosurgery.[3] Neuronavigation provided intra-operative localization of abnormal structures in the brain based on preoperative imaging (MRI or CT). The operative microscope, neuro-endoscope, and neuronavigation have led to scientific revolutions, or paradigm shifts, in neurosurgery.[4] Better visualization and localization has permitted the successful treatment of complex neurosurgical disorders while minimizing morbidity to the patient. Image-guided microscopic or endoscopic neurosurgery has become the standard of care for most cranial procedures performed by neurosurgeons worldwide.

We are now part of a new paradigm shift in neurosurgery with the addition of fluorescence-guided surgery (FGS). We can further delineate abnormal structures in real-time with agents that can permit direct fluorescence visualization in the brain. In 1947, Dr. G.E. Moore noticed that after intravenous administration of the ophthalmic agent fluorescein, a malignant brain tumor could be visualized by fluorescence in a patient during surgery.[5] Dr. Walter Stummer described for the first time in 1998 the use of 5-aminolevulinic acid (5-ALA) FGS of high-grade glioma (HGG) tumors in patients with use of a modified operative microscope.[6] In 2003, Dr. Andre Raabe initially described the use of the fluorescent agent indocyanine green (ICG) to visualize blood flow in vessels exposed in the surgical field.[7] The FGS technique, known as ICG videoangiography, would be used by neurosurgeons during aneurysm surgery for confirmation of proper surgical clip ligation.[8]

The approval of 5-ALA for resection of HGG tumors by the European Medicines Agency (EMA) in 2007 heralded the birth of fluorescence-guided neurosurgery globally. A landmark randomized Phase 3 clinical trial revealed how effective 5-ALA FGS was at almost doubling the amount of tumor neurosurgeons could remove due to the ability to better visualize the tumor in real time.[9,10] Ten years later in 2017, 5-ALA (Gleolan) would become approved by the Food and Drug Administration (FDA) in the United States as an imaging agent to facilitate the real-time detection and visualization of malignant tissue during glioma surgery.[11]

Two decades have now gone by since Dr. Stummer's initial description of 5-ALA FGS in a human patient. As with the operative microscope, neuro-endoscope, and neuronavigation, years pass before widespread adoption of new technologies in neurosurgery. We are now at a point in our specialty where fluorescence-guided neurosurgery will be adopted by most neurosurgeons throughout the world. In our book, we have brought together all the current applications of fluorescence-guided neurosurgery in both neuro-oncology and cerebrovascular surgery. We thank all the contributing authors who are experts in defining the new field of fluorescence-guided neurosurgery. A critical analysis of intraoperative tissue imaging is provided. In addition to 5-ALA, different fluorophores (e.g., fluorescein and ICG) and their applications are discussed in the book. Multiple tumor types (both adult and pediatric) and cerebrovascular applications for FGS are covered. The combination of FGS and intraoperative imaging (e.g., iMRI) is discussed. We include newer targeted fluorophores for FGS and other visualization technologies (e.g. confocal microscopy, Raman spectroscopy).

The future is bright with fluorescence-guided neurosurgery as newer visualization technologies and fluorophores will permit better visualization of tissue fluorescence in a more targeted manner. Other applications will be developed within neurosurgery as more neurosurgeons adopt the use of FGS.

*Constantinos G. Hadjipanayis, MD, PhD*
*Walter Stummer, MD, PhD*

# References

1. Kriss TC, Kriss VM. History of the operating microscope: from magnifying glass to microneurosurgery. Neurosurgery 1998;42(4):899–907, discussion 907–908 PubMed
2. Davis L. In: Neurological Surgery. Philadelphia: Lea and Febiger; 1936
3. Barnett GH, Kormos DW, Steiner CP, Weisenberger J. Use of a frameless, armless stereotactic wand for brain tumor localization with two-dimensional and three-dimensional neuroimaging. Neurosurgery 1993;33(4):674–678 PubMed
4. Kuhn T. The Structure of Scientific Revolutions. 2nd ed. Chicago: University of Chicago Press; 1962/1970a
5. Moore GE. Fluorescein as an Agent in the Differentiation of Normal and Malignant Tissues. Science 1947;106(2745):130–131 PubMed
6. Stummer W, Stocker S, Wagner S, et al. Intraoperative detection of malignant gliomas by 5-aminolevulinic acid-induced porphyrin fluorescence. Neurosurgery 1998;42(3):518–525, discussion 525–526 PubMed

7. Raabe A, Beck J, Gerlach R, Zimmermann M, Seifert V. Near-infrared indocyanine green video angiography: a new method for intraoperative assessment of vascular flow. Neurosurgery 2003;52(1):132–139, discussion 139 PubMed

8. Raabe A, Nakaji P, Beck J, et al. Prospective evaluation of surgical microscope-integrated intraoperative near-infrared indocyanine green videoangiography during aneurysm surgery. J Neurosurg 2005;103(6):982–989 PubMed

9. Stummer W, Pichlmeier U, Meinel T, Wiestler OD, Zanella F, Reulen HJ; ALA-Glioma Study Group. Fluorescence-guided surgery with 5-aminolevulinic acid for resection of malignant glioma: a randomised controlled multicentre phase III trial. Lancet Oncol 2006;7(5):392–401 PubMed

10. Stummer W, Reulen HJ, Meinel T, et al; ALA-Glioma Study Group. Extent of resection and survival in glioblastoma multiforme: identification of and adjustment for bias. Neurosurgery 2008;62(3):564–576, discussion 564–576 PubMed

11. https://www.fda.gov/downloads/AdvisoryCommittees/CommitteesMeeting Materials/Drugs/MedicalImagingDrugsAdvisoryCommittee/UCM557136.pdf

# Contributors

**Harish Babu, MD, PhD**
Resident Neurosurgeon
Department of Neurosurgery
Cedars-Sinai Medical Center
Los Angeles, California, USA

**Mitchel S. Berger, MD, FACS, FAANS**
Berthold and Belle N. Guggenhime Professor
Chairman, Department of Neurological Surgery
Director, Brain Tumor Center
University of California San Francisco
San Francisco, California, USA

**David Bervini, MD, MAdvSurg**
Attending Physician
Department of Neurosurgery
Bern University Hospital, Inselspital
University of Bern
Bern, Switzerland

**Jeffrey N. Bruce, MD**
Edgar M. Housepian Professor
Department of Neurological Surgery
Columbia University College of Physicians and Surgeons
New York, New York, USA

**Jan-Karl Burkhardt, MD**
Fellow
Department of Neurosurgery
NYU Langone Medical Center
New York, New York, USA

**Pramod Butte, MBBS, PhD**
Assistant Professor/Research Scientist I
Department of Neurosurgery
Cedars-Sinai Medical Center
Los Angeles, California, USA

**Paul A. Clark, PhD**
Associate Scientist
Department of Neurological Surgery
University of Wisconsin – Madison
Madison, Wisconsin, USA

**Jan Coburger, Priv. doz. Dr. med. habil.**
Oberarzt
Department of Neurosurgery
University of Ulm
Günzburg, Bavaria, Germany

**Jan Frederick Cornelius, MD**
Assistant Professor, Vice-Chairman
Klinik für Neurochirurgie
Universitätsklinikum Düsseldorf
Heinrich Heine Universität
Düsseldorf, Nordrhein-Westfalen, Germany

**Randy S. D'Amico, MD**
Resident
Department of Neurosurgery
Columbia University Medical Center
New York, New York, USA

**Ricardo Díez Valle, MD, PhD**
Consultant
Department of Neurosurgery
Clinica Universidad de Navarra
Pamplona, Spain

**Toshiki Endo, MD, PhD**
Deputy Director
Department of Neurosurgery
Kohnan Hospital
Sendai, Miyagi, Japan

**Joseph F. Georges, DO, PhD**
Resident Physician
Department of Neurosurgery
Philadelphia College of Osteopathic Medicine
Philadelphia, Pennsylvania, USA

**Isabelle M. Germano, MD, MBA**
Professor of Neurosurgery, Neurology, Oncological Sciences
Department of Neurosurgery
Icahn School of Medicine at Mount Sinai
New York, New York, USA

**Alexandra J. Golby, MD**
Professor of Neurosurgery
Professor of Radiology
Harvard Medical School
Haley Distinguished Chair in the Neurosciences
Associate Surgeon
Brigham and Women's Hospital
Department of Neurosurgery
Boston, Massachusetts, USA

**Constantinos G. Hadjipanayis, MD, PhD**
Professor and Site Chair
Department of Neurosurgery
Mount Sinai Downtown Union Square/Beth Israel
Professor of Oncological Sciences
Icahn School of Medicine at Mount Sinai
Director of Neurosurgical Oncology
Mount Sinai Health System
New York, New York, USA

**Seunggu Jude Han, MD**
Assistant Professor
Department of Neurological Surgery
Oregon Health and Sciences University
Portland, Oregon, USA

**Nils Hecht, MD**
Attending Neurosurgeon
Department of Neurosurgery
Charité - Universitätsmedizin Berlin
Berlin, Germany

**Todd C. Hollon, MD**
Neurosurgery Resident
Department of Neurosurgery
University of Michigan
Ann Arbor, Michigan, USA

**Tomoo Inoue, MD, PhD**
Department of Neurosurgery
Tohoku University Graduate School of Medicine
Sendai, Miyagi, Japan

**Steven N. Kalkanis, MD**
Chair and Professor
Department of Neurosurgery
Henry Ford Health System
Detroit, Michigan, USA

**Marcel A. Kamp, MD**
Consultant
Department of Neurosurgery
Heinrich-Heine-University
Düsseldorf, Germany

**Remi A. Kessler, BA**
Medical Student
Department of Neurosurgery
Icahn School of Medicine at Mount Sinai
New York, New York, USA

**Barbara Kiesel, MD**
Department of Neurosurgery
Medical University Vienna
Vienna, Austria

**David Scott Kittle, PhD**
Medical Device Engineer
Blaze Bioscience, Inc
Seattle, Washington, USA

**John S. Kuo, MD, PhD**
Inaugural Chair and Professor
Department of Neurosurgery
Surgical Director, Mulva Clinic for the Neurosciences
Dell Medical School
The University of Texas at Austin
Austin, Texas, USA

**Nikita Lakomkin, BA**
Research Associate
Department of Neurological Surgery
Icahn School of Medicine at Mount Sinai
New York, New York, USA

**Darryl Lau, MD**
Resident Physician
Department of Neurological Surgery
University of California, San Francisco
San Francisco, California, USA

**Michael T. Lawton, MD**
Professor & Chairman
Department of Neurosurgery
President & CEO
Chief of Vascular & Skull Base Neurosurgery
Robert F. Spetzler Endowed Chair in Neurosciences
Barrow Neurological Institute
Phoenix, Arizona, USA

**John Y.K. Lee, MD, MSCE**
Associate Professor
Department of Neurosurgery & Otolaryngology
Perelman School of Medicine
University of Pennsylvania
Philadelphia, Pennsylvania, USA

**Adam N. Mamelak, MD, FAANS**
Professor
Department of Neurosurgery
Cedars-Sinai Medical Center
Los Angeles, California, USA

**Justin R. Mascitelli, MD**
Cerebrovascular Fellow
Department of Neurosurgery
Barrow Neurological Institute
Phoenix, Arizona, USA

**Dennis M. Miller, PhD**
SVP Development
Blaze Bioscience, Inc
Seattle, Washington, USA

**Ramin A. Morshed, MD**
Resident Physician
Department of Neurosurgery
University of California San Francisco
San Francisco, California, USA

**Peter Nakaji, MD**
Professor of Neurological Surgery
Department of Neurological Surgery
Barrow Neurological Institute
Phoenix, Arizona, USA

**Justin A. Neira, MD**
Resident
Department of Neurological Surgery
Columbia University Medical Center
New York, New York, USA

**Daniel A. Orringer, MD**
Assistant Professor
Department of Neurosurgery
University of Michigan
Ann Arbor, Michigan, USA

**Julia E. Parrish-Novak, PhD**
Vice President of Research
Blaze Bioscience, Inc.
Seattle, Washington, USA

**Andreas Raabe, MD**
Professor and Chairman
Department of Neurosurgery
University of Bern
Bern, Switzerland

**Marion Rapp, MD**
Consultant
Department of Neurosurgery
University Hospital Heinrich Heine University
Düsseldorf, Germany

**David W. Roberts, MD**
Professor, Active Emeritus
Department of Surgery (Neurosurgery)
Dartmouth-Hitchcock Medical Center
Lebanon, New Hampshire, USA

**Michael Sabel, MD, PhD**
Professor
Department of Neurosurgery
University Hospital Duesseldorf
Düsseldorf, Germany

**Ryan D. Salinas, MD, MS**
Resident Physician
Department of Neurosurgery
University of Pennsylvania
Philadelphia, Pennsylvania, USA

**Nader Sanai, MD**
Professor
Department of Neurological Surgery
Barrow Neurological Institute
Phoenix, Arizona, USA

**Christina E. Sarris, MD**
Neurosurgery Resident
Department of Neurosurgery
Barrow Neurological Institute
Phoenix, Arizona, USA

**Philippe Schucht, MD**
Professor
Department of Neurosurgery
University Hospital Bern
Bern, Switzerland

**Sunil Singhal, MD**
Associate Professor of Surgery
Department of Surgery
University of Pennsylvania Perelman School of Medicine
Philadelphia, Pennsylvania, USA

**Hans-Jakob Steiger, MD, PhD**
Chairman and Director
Department of Neurosurgery
Heinrich-Heine-Universität
Düsseldorf, Germany

**Walter Stummer, MD, PhD**
Professor and Chairman
Department of Neurosurgery
University of Münster
Münster, Germany

**Teiji Tominaga, MD, PhD**
Professor and Chairman
Department of Neurosurgery
Tohoku University Graduate School of Medicine
Sendai, Miyagi, Japan

**Peter Vajkoczy, MD**
Full Professor and Chairman
Department of Neurosurgery
Charité - Universitätsmedizin Berlin
Berlin, Germany

**Pablo A. Valdes Quevedo, MD, PhD**
Neurosurgery Resident
Department of Neurosurgery
Harvard Medical School/Brigham and Women's Hospital
Boston, Massachusetts, USA

**Jamey P. Weichert, PhD**
Associate Professor
Department of Radiology
University of Wisconsin
Madison, Wisconsin, USA

**Lars Wessels, MD**
Department of Neurosurgery
Charité - Universitätsmedizin Berlin
Berlin, Germany

**Georg Widhalm, MD, PhD**
Associate Professor
Department of Neurosurgery
Medical University Vienna
Vienna, Austria
University of California, San Francisco
San Francisco, California, USA

**Johannes Wölfer, Priv.-Doz. Dr. med.**
Chief Physician
Department of Neurosurgery
Hufeland Klinikum GmbH
Mühlhausen, Thuringia, Germany

**Frank J. Yuk, MD**
Resident Physician
Department of Neurological Surgery
Mount Sinai Health System
New York, New York, USA

**Ryan D. Zeh, BS**
Medical Student
The Ohio State University College of Medicine
Columbus, Ohio, USA

**Ray R. Zhang, PhD**
Departments of Neurological Surgery and Radiology
University of Wisconsin – Madison
Madison, Wisconsin, USA

# 1 Current Fluorescence-Guided Neurosurgery and Moving Forward

*Remi A. Kessler, Frank J. Yuk, and Constantinos G. Hadjipanayis*

## Abstract

This introductory chapter provides a current overview of fluorescence-guided neurosurgery and includes future directions. The concepts of fluorescence and fluorescence-guided surgery (FGS) are introduced. Currently used fluorescent contrast agents in patients are summarized, including 5-aminolevulinic acid (5-ALA), fluorescein, and indocyanine green. Excitation light sources are discussed for each fluorescent contrast agent. Targeted fluorophores under clinical development for FGS are also introduced. Future directions in fluorescence-guided neurosurgery including handheld devices to better detect tumor fluorescence, dual fluorophore imaging, metabolic imaging in combination with FGS, and detection of the tumor margin will be discussed.

*Keywords:* fluorescence, near-infrared imaging, fluorescence-guided neurosurgery, fluorescence-guided surgery, fluorophore, fluorescein sodium, 5-ALA, indocyanine green, operative microscope

## 1.1 Fluorescence-Guided Surgery

The ability to delineate abnormal from normal structures is the hallmark of any surgical subspecialty. Enhanced visualization provides greater delineation of tissues, and as a result, the surgeon can perform better and safer surgery. While stains and dyes have long been used to identify biological structures and processes in tissue samples, real-time intraoperative detection of structures has relied on tissue magnification and illumination.[1] Fluorescence of abnormal tumor tissues or vascular blood flow has been introduced as a method to enhance visualization in the field of neurosurgery over the past two decades. Optical imaging of fluorescent contrast agents can permit sensitive and specific detection of tissues in the brain. The principle of fluorescence-guided surgery (FGS) relies on the use of optical imaging agents that are administered to patients prior to or during surgery that selectively accumulate in tumor tissues or vascular compartments. FGS provides real-time image guidance and improved intraoperative visualization of brain tumor tissue and vascular blood flow, independent of neuronavigation and brain shift.[2,3,4,5] In this introductory chapter, we will briefly discuss the currently used fluorescent agents in neurosurgery for neuro-oncology and cerebrovascular applications. We will also discuss the currently used operative microscopes that permit the visualization of fluorescence within the operative field and new technologies that will push FGS forward.

## 1.2 What Is Fluorescence?

Certain molecules have the capacity to absorb light energy, and this absorption causes an elevation to a higher energy state, termed the excited state. Once at this excited state, the energy absorbed decays over time, resulting in the emission of light energy known as fluorescence. A fluorophore is a molecule capable of fluorescence. In its low-energy ground state configuration, fluorophores do not fluoresce. When light from an external source illuminates the fluorophore, it can absorb the energy to reach an excited state; multiple excited states exist depending on the energy and wavelength of the light source. Since the fluorophore is unstable at this higher energy state, it will revert back to a lower energy state, and during this process emits light. This infinitesimally small amount of elapsed time is known as the excited lifetime. Each fluorescent agent has a maximal fluorescence, or a specific wavelength of light at which the largest number of fluorophores is excited (▶ Fig. 1.1). Nevertheless, there exists a spectrum of fluorescence excitation through which fluorophores can absorb and emit a wide range of wavelengths.[6] Photobleaching is the process by which fluorescence intensity can decay over time with continuous excitation of the fluorophore.[7]

### 1.2.1 Near-Infrared Fluorescence

Optical imaging technologies that utilize fluorescence can be further specialized to absorb and emit light in an optical spectrum of near-infrared (NIR), consisting of a wavelength range of 700 to 900 nm.[8,9] This is particularly useful when maximizing depth of tissue penetration is important. Fluorescent agents (e.g., protoporphyrin IX [PpIX], the fluorescent intracellular metabolite of 5-aminolevulinic acid [5-ALA], and fluorescein sodium) with excitation wavelengths below 700 nm typically possess a penetration depth of less than 1 cm and produce low tissue absorption. The light absorption of hemoglobin, lipid, melanin, and other tissues can result in autofluorescence in the visible light spectrum range up to 700 nm. An increase in wavelength causes a decrease in light scattering and light absorption. In the NIR spectrum, the interference of biomolecules and solvents is negligible and light can penetrate deeper into tissues. This provides for the detection of imaging signals at a depth of several centimeters. Of particular importance, NIR signals with emission of 700 nm and above maintain low-fluorescence background from blood absorption and tissue scattering, which can allow for optical detection of the exposed tumor.[10,11] A currently used NIR agent in neurosurgery is indocyanine green (ICG).

## 1.3 Fluorescent Contrast Agents Currently Used in Patients

### 1.3.1 5-Aminolevulinic Acid

5-ALA (brand name Gliolan or Gleolan) is a natural metabolite produced in the hemoglobin metabolic pathway. It is an orally administered pro-agent that can rapidly penetrate the blood–brain barrier (BBB) and accumulate within brain tumors.[4] After

# Fluorescence Emission Wavelengths

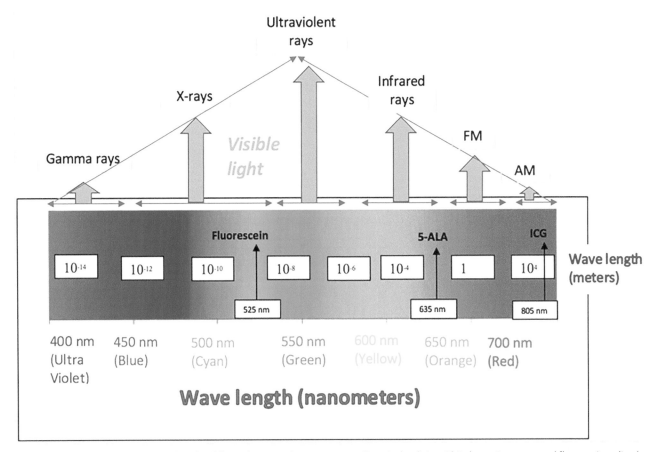

Fig. 1.1 Fluorescence emission wavelengths of fluorophores used in neurosurgery (5-aminolevulinic acid, indocyanine green, and fluorescein sodium).

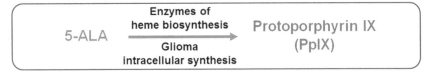

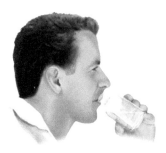

Fig. 1.2 Use of the operative microscope for excitation of the 5-aminolevulinic acid metabolite, PpIX, for intraoperative tumor fluorescence and real-time image-guided fluorescence-guided surgery.

uptake by glioma cells, 5-ALA is metabolized intracellularly into PpIX, its fluorescent metabolite (▶ Fig. 1.2).[12] Due to elevated PpIX levels within brain tumor cells, malignant tumor tissue can be visualized by violet–red fluorescence at 635 nm (smaller secondary peak at 704 nm) following excitation with 405 nm wavelength blue light.[13,14] The majority of high-grade glioma tumors will reveal solid red fluorescence, while a pink fluorescence will be visible at the tumor margin in which cancer cells infiltrate normal brain tissue. Tumor tissue fluorescence can persist for greater than 8 hours after oral administration. The mechanism for the accumulation of 5-ALA and its metabolite, PpIX, within glioma cells involves reduced levels of the enzyme, ferrochelatase, and impaired cellular clearance by an adenosine triphosphate (ATP)-binding cassette subfamily B member 6 (ABCB6) transporter.[15] Ferrochelatase is an enzyme that produces heme with the addition of iron (Fe) to PpIX. 5-ALA-induced fluorescence is also influenced by the vascularity of the tumor, BBB permeability, tumor cell proliferative activity, and cellular density.[4] 5-ALA is the only optical imaging agent approved by the U.S. Food and Drug Administration (FDA) and European Medicines Agency (EMA) for the real-time detection and visualization of malignant tissue during glioma surgery. 5-ALA is also the most extensively studied of all fluorescent agents available for FGS of central nervous system (CNS) tumors worldwide. Tissue fluorescence due to 5-ALA is correlated with high sensitivity, specificity, and positive predictive values (values over 90%) for the identification of malignant tumor tissue.[16,17,18,19,20,21,22,23] In particular, 5-ALA allows for intraoperative recognition of anaplastic foci and histopathologic diagnosis of gliomas with nonsignificant MRI contrast enhancement.[24] 5-ALA is essentially nontoxic, and can be used in resections of newly diagnosed (Chapter 3) and recurrent high-grade gliomas (Chapter 4), diffuse infiltrating gliomas with anaplastic foci (Chapter 5), low-grade gliomas (Chapter 5), meningiomas (Chapter 6), brain metastases (Chapter 7), ependymomas (Chapter 8), and other tumor types including pediatric tumors (Chapter 9).[2,25] A landmark randomized, controlled trial proved that the use of 5-ALA FGS results in a more complete resection of high-grade gliomas and better progression-free survival (PFS) in patients.[26]

### 1.3.2 Fluorescein Sodium

Fluorescein sodium is a small organic molecular salt that acts as a nonspecific extracellular fluorophore. It is currently FDA approved for retinal angiography and used off-label for brain tumor resections. Fluorescein is injected intravenously after intubation and prior to incision and relies on disruption of the BBB for accumulation in high-grade gliomas. Fluorescein sodium fluorescence of brain tumors appears as a yellow-green color under white light.[14] Fluorescein's peak excitation occurs at 480 nm (range 465–490 nm) with a fluorescence emission peak at 525 nm (range 500–530 nm).[14,27] Leakage and nonspecific tissue fluorescence can occur with fluorescein as the dura fluoresces in addition to the surrounding normal brain tissue if perturbed during surgery. The duration of fluorescein fluorescence is approximately 2 to 3 hours after systemic administration. Additionally, careful precautions should be taken when administering fluorescein as harmful side effects can result if injected too rapidly or in an excessive concentration.[28,29] Its utilization has primarily been described in high-grade gliomas (Chapters 10 and 11), but has been reported in other brain tumors (Chapter 10).[30,31,32,33]

### 1.3.3 Indocyanine Green

ICG is a small, water-soluble organic molecule that acts as a nonspecific extracellular fluorophore. ICG is an NIR fluorophore, which was approved by the U.S. FDA in 1956 for diagnostic use in disorders of cardiovascular and liver function. Supplemental U.S. FDA approval for ophthalmic angiography was granted in

1975. After intravenous bolus injection, ICG is bound within 1 to 2 seconds, mainly to globulins (α1-lipoproteins and albumin), and remains intravascular with normal vascular permeability. ICG flow lasts only approximately 15 seconds. Disruption of the BBB can permit accumulation of ICG in brain tumors. ICG maximum absorption or excitation occurs at 805 nm (range 700–850 nm) and fluorescence at 835 nm (range 780–950 nm). The fluorescence is recorded by a nonintensified video camera. An optical filter blocks both ambient and excitation light so that only ICG-induced fluorescence is visualized. Thus, arterial, capillary, and venous angiographic images can be observed on the video screen in real time. ICG videoangiography has become a useful way to allow real-time assessment of intraoperative vascular anatomy and analysis of flow dynamics. ICG is primarily used for intraoperative videoangiography during cerebrovascular surgery, specifically during surgical treatment for aneurysm ligation (Chapter 18), arteriovenous malformation (AVM) (Chapter 19), and extracranial intracranial (EC-IC) bypass (Chapter 20).[34,35,36] Recently, ICG has been used to detect brain tumors based on disruption of the BBB. Coined "second window" ICG (SWIG) in order to distinguish it from traditional videoangiography procedures that visualize the molecule within minutes of injection, this method relies on visualization 24 hours following high-dose intravenous infusion (Chapter 12).[37]

## 1.4 Excitation Light Source

Currently, the most commonly used excitation light source in neurosurgery procedures is the surgical operative microscope adapted with a filter set that permits visualization of fluorescence excitation in a specific wavelength range (▶ Fig. 1.3). The adaptation includes a standard white light emission source and a combination of excitation and observation low- and high-pass optical filters, with slightly overlapping transmission integrated into their optical configuration. The proposed filter set is

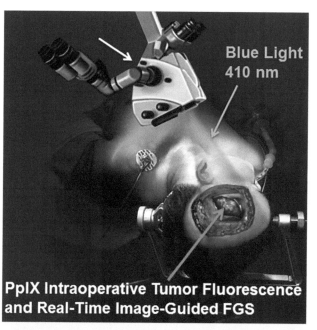

**Blue Light 410 nm**

**PpIX Intraoperative Tumor Fluorescence and Real-Time Image-Guided FGS**

Fig. 1.3 Conversion of 5-aminolevulinic acid to intracellular fluorescent metabolite, protoporphyrin IX, after oral administration.

commercially available. For PpIX fluorescence visualization, two xenon light sources are utilized with the operative microscope. Blue light (405 nm) is emitted from the microscope, which excites the PpIX, emitting fluorescence in the 480 to 730 nm range. Since blue light has a short wavelength, brain and tumor tissue depth penetration is limited. The red fluorescence emitted does not contain as much energy as the blue excitation light. Therefore, in order for the surgeon to visualize 100% of the red tumor fluorescence, a filter aimed at blocking 90% of the blue light must be applied. Only 90% of the blue light is blocked as the surgeon still requires some light to complete the resection. Fluorescein imaging is possible with an operative microscope that is equipped with dedicated filter sets for fluorescein imaging. The microscope offers blue-light excitation and 540 to 690 nm emission filters for visualizing fluorescein.

For NIR fluorescence visualization (e.g. ICG), a motorized wheel within the light source changes the filters to increase the light visible to the surgeon from 700 to 800 nm. This supplemental NIR energy is key for the mechanism by which injected ICG undergoes excitation and subsequently fluoresces. The ability to visualize ICG fluorescence is dependent on a specialized black and white high-sensitive NIR camera and an 820 to 860 nm filter. This must be utilized to illuminate the fluorescence that is invisible to the surgeon's eye. The addition of recording software to the operative microscope is critical as blood flow is a dynamic process and ICG flow lasts only approximately 15 seconds. As such, it is essential for the surgeon to have the capacity to rewind images and play them again in slow motion. In the fluorescent operative microscope, the vascular fluorescent loop can be played back with a touch of a button.[38]

## 1.5 Targeted Fluorophores under Clinical Development

### 1.5.1 Fluorescent Alkylphosphocholine Analogs 1501 and 1502

Alkylphosphocholines (APCs) are small phospholipid molecules capable of antineoplastic activity. Fluorescent APC analogs are a new development for the intraoperative identification of tumor margins in combination with imaging modalities (Chapter 13). Fluorescent APCs can be used with positron emission tomography (PET) imaging for noninvasive localization, cancer staging, and in radiation therapy.[39,40] The same APC backbone can be linked to two distinct fluorophores (1501 and 1502), with 1502 developed specifically for FGS and involving NIR fluorescence. APC 1502 was validated in preclinical rodent models for FGS, and other forms of APC analogs are currently in clinical development.[41]

### 1.5.2 Tozuleristide

Tozuleristide is an NIR molecule with the capability to target brain tumors (Chapter 14). Its composition consists of chlorotoxin, a tumor-targeting peptide, and ICG.[42] It has been tested in several phase I clinical trials, and no toxicity or harmful side effects have been shown.[43] Further clinical trial testing is currently underway to determine tozuleristide's capabilities for glioma FGS. A Scanning Infrared Imaging System (SIRIS) is

necessary to detect the NIR light produced from tozuleristide in tumor tissue, and its ability to accurately differentiate normal brain tissue from tumor tissue has been shown.[44]

## 1.6 Future Handheld Technologies

Current operative microscope fluorescence technologies have limited detection sensitivity and identification accuracy and are unable to detect visible fluorescence in the majority of low-grade or diffuse infiltrating gliomas.[4] Future handheld technologies are in development to provide enhanced visualization and increased sensitivity of fluorophores in tumor tissue. A handheld spectroscopic device that is capable of ultrasensitive detection of PpIX fluorescence has been recently described.[5] Intraoperative spectroscopy was reported to be at least three orders of magnitude more sensitive than the current operative microscope allowing ultrasensitive detection of as few as 1,000 tumor cells. For detection specificity, intraoperative spectroscopy allowed the differentiation of brain tumor cells from normal brain cells with a contrast signal ratio over 100. It was recently demonstrated that quantitative measurements of PpIX with a fiberoptic probe can be used intraoperatively to visualize nonfluorescing low-grade gliomas.[45] Confocal microscopy is also a promising novel technology to amplify intraoperative detection of low-grade gliomas.[46] It can be used with a specific handheld probe, which also offers a close working distance as compared to the standard microscope that is located much further away from the operative field. The advent of handheld devices with increased sensitivity to capture fluorescent signals will allow for greater visualization of PpIX in tumor tissue that is presently not detectable with current operative microscope technologies.

## 1.7 Dual Fluorophore Labeling and Fluorescence-Guided Surgery

A new method to capitalize on the benefits of multiple fluorophores is dual labeling for FGS. One group has begun investigations into the coadministration of 5-ALA with fluorescein in patients with high-grade gliomas. The combination of agents results in 5-ALA distinguishing tumor and fluorescein providing tissue fluorescence of adjacent brain tissue. In a pilot study of six patients, dual labeling provided superior background information that facilitated 5-ALA-guided tumor discrimination and resection of pathologic tissue during FGS.[47]

## 1.8 Combination of Metabolic Imaging and Fluorescence-Guided Surgery

Gliomas are highly infiltrative tumors that are characterized by infiltrating tumor cells that extend centimeters away from the tumor bulk. Currently, contrast-enhanced MRI is used to define primary treatment volumes for surgery. However, contrast enhancement does not identify the tumor entirely, resulting in limited local tumor control. Whole-brain spectroscopic MRI (sMRI) is a preoperative imaging technique that allows for

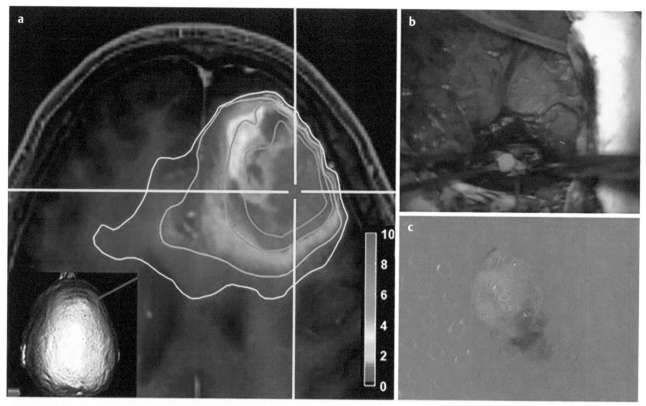

**Fig. 1.4** Spectroscopic MRI and 5-aminolevulinic acid (5-ALA) fluorescence-guided surgery (FGS). **(a)** View of anatomical and metabolic data with neuronavigation including choline/N-acetylaspartate (Chol/NAA) ratio contours in a high-grade glioma patient (yellow, 1.5-fold; green, twofold; orange, fivefold; red, 10-fold increases in Chol/NAA over normal contralateral white matter). **(b)** The region of metabolic abnormality was identified with neuronavigation and 5-ALA-induced tissue fluorescence utilizing the operative microscope. **(c)** 5-ALA FGS tissue sample. (Reproduced with permission from Cordova et al.[48])

identification of brain regions with tumor infiltration based on metabolic perturbations (choline [Cho], N-acetylaspartate [NAA]).[2] Whole-brain metabolic maps based on sMRI can be overlaid on intraoperative neuronavigation for surgical planning (▶ Fig. 1.4). The combination of high-resolution sMRI with 5-ALA FGS in high-grade glioma patients may permit more complete resection of tumors.[48] A feasibility study has been completed in high-grade glioma patients in which sMRI permitted identification of tumor infiltrated regions that directed 5-ALA FGS to regions of the tumor that appeared normal on conventional contrast-enhanced MRI.[48]

## 1.9 Fluorescence-Guided Surgery and Tumor Margin

Use of FGS has permitted the identification of the infiltrative tumor margin in high-grade gliomas. In particular, 5-ALA FGS is able to differentiate the tumor bulk from the margin by the intensity of fluorescence visualized with the operative microscope.[23] Areas of strong, red–violet 5-ALA fluorescence intensity and intraoperative spectroscopic signal correspond to high-density, proliferating brain tumor cells, while weaker pink fluorescence intensity and intraoperative spectroscopic signal correspond to infiltrative tumor tissue.[49] These features permit the real-time intraoperative distinction of the tumor margin.

Selective sampling of the tumor margin can permit a better understanding of the genomic and proteomic changes that could represent targets of therapy since almost all high-grade glioma recurrences are local.[50]

## References

[1] Alturkistani HA, Tashkandi FM, Mohammedsaleh ZM. Histological stains: a literature review and case study. Glob J Health Sci. 2015; 8(3):72–79

[2] Hadjipanayis CG, Jiang H, Roberts DW, Yang L. Current and future clinical applications for optical imaging of cancer: from intraoperative surgical guidance to cancer screening. Semin Oncol. 2011; 38(1):109–118

[3] Hadjipanayis C. Current applications and advances in fluorescence-guided neurosurgery. Lecture presented at: AANS NREF Webinar; September 14, 2016

[4] Hadjipanayis CG, Widhalm G, Stummer W. What is the surgical benefit of utilizing 5-aminolevulinic acid for fluorescence-guided surgery of malignant gliomas? Neurosurgery. 2015; 77(5):663–673

[5] Kairdolf BA, Bouras A, Kaluzova M, et al. Intraoperative spectroscopy with ultrahigh sensitivity for image-guided surgery of malignant brain tumors. Anal Chem. 2016; 88(1):858–867

[6] Fluorescence Tutorials. Invitrogen. Thermo Fisher Scientific. Available at: https://www.thermofisher.com/us/en/home/support/tutorials.html. Accessed January 24, 2018

[7] Diaspro A, Chirico G, Usai C, Ramoino P, Dobrucki J. Photobleaching. In: Pawley J, ed. Handbook of Biological Confocal Microscopy. Boston, MA: Springer; 2006:690–699

[8] Hawrysz DJ, Sevick-Muraca EM. Developments toward diagnostic breast cancer imaging using near-infrared optical measurements and fluorescent contrast agents. Neoplasia. 2000; 2(5):388–417

[9] Jiang H, Ramesh S, Bartlett M. Combined optical and fluorescence imaging for breast cancer detection and diagnosis. Crit Rev Biomed Eng. 2000; 28(3–4): 371–375

[10] Liebert A, Wabnitz H, Obrig H, et al. Non-invasive detection of fluorescence from exogenous chromophores in the adult human brain. Neuroimage. 2006; 31(2):600–608

[11] Troyan SL, Kianzad V, Gibbs-Strauss SL, et al. The FLARE intraoperative near-infrared fluorescence imaging system: a first-in-human clinical trial in breast cancer sentinel lymph node mapping. Ann Surg Oncol. 2009; 16(10):2943–2952

[12] Ferraro N, Barbarite E, Albert TR, et al. The role of 5-aminolevulinic acid in brain tumor surgery: a systematic review. Neurosurg Rev. 2016; 39(4):545–555

[13] Stummer W, Stocker S, Wagner S, et al. Intraoperative detection of malignant gliomas by 5-aminolevulinic acid-induced porphyrin fluorescence. Neurosurgery. 1998; 42(3):518–525, discussion 525–526

[14] Pogue BW, Gibbs-Strauss S, Valdés PA, Samkoe K, Roberts DW, Paulsen KD. Review of neurosurgical fluorescence imaging methodologies. IEEE J Sel Top Quantum Electron. 2010; 16(3):493–505

[15] Matsumoto K, Hagiya Y, Endo Y, et al. Effects of plasma membrane ABCB6 on 5-aminolevulinic acid (ALA)-induced porphyrin accumulation in vitro: tumor cell response to hypoxia. Photodiagn Photodyn Ther. 2015; 12(1):45–51

[16] Lau D, Hervey-Jumper SL, Chang S, et al. A prospective phase II clinical trial of 5-aminolevulinic acid to assess the correlation of intraoperative fluorescence intensity and degree of histologic cellularity during resection of high-grade gliomas. J Neurosurg. 2016; 124(5):1300–1309

[17] Stummer W, Novotny A, Stepp H, Goetz C, Bise K, Reulen HJ. Fluorescence-guided resection of glioblastoma multiforme by using 5-aminolevulinic acid-induced porphyrins: a prospective study in 52 consecutive patients. J Neurosurg. 2000; 93(6):1003–1013

[18] Coburger J, Engelke J, Scheuerle A, et al. Tumor detection with 5-aminolevulinic acid fluorescence and Gd-DTPA-enhanced intraoperative MRI at the border of contrast-enhancing lesions: a prospective study based on histopathological assessment. Neurosurg Focus. 2014; 36(2):E3

[19] Díez Valle R, Tejada Solis S, Idoate Gastearena MA, García de Eulate R, Domínguez Echávarri P, Aristu Mendiroz J. Surgery guided by 5-aminolevulinic fluorescence in glioblastoma: volumetric analysis of extent of resection in single-center experience. J Neurooncol. 2011; 102(1):105–113

[20] Ewelt C, Nemes A, Senner V, et al. Fluorescence in neurosurgery: its diagnostic and therapeutic use. Review of the literature. J Photochem Photobiol B. 2015; 148:302–309

[21] Idoate MA, Díez Valle R, Echeveste J, Tejada S. Pathological characterization of the glioblastoma border as shown during surgery using 5-aminolevulinic acid-induced fluorescence. Neuropathology. 2011; 31(6):575–582

[22] Hauser SB, Kockro RA, Actor B, Sarnthein J, Bernays RL. Combining 5-aminolevulinic acid fluorescence and intraoperative magnetic resonance imaging in glioblastoma surgery: a histology-based evaluation. Neurosurgery. 2016; 78(4):475–483

[23] Roberts DW, Valdés PA, Harris BT, et al. Coregistered fluorescence-enhanced tumor resection of malignant glioma: relationships between δ-aminolevulinic acid-induced protoporphyrin IX fluorescence, magnetic resonance imaging enhancement, and neuropathological parameters. Clinical article. J Neurosurg. 2011; 114(3):595–603

[24] Widhalm G, Kiesel B, Woehrer A, et al. 5-Aminolevulinic acid induced fluorescence is a powerful intraoperative marker for precise histopathological grading of gliomas with non-significant contrast-enhancement. PLoS One. 2013; 8(10):e76988

[25] Cordova JS, Gurbani SS, Holder CA, et al. Semi-automated volumetric and morphological assessment of glioblastoma resection with fluorescence-guided surgery. Mol Imaging Biol. 2016; 18(3):454–462

[26] Stummer W, Pichlmeier U, Meinel T, Wiestler OD, Zanella F, Reulen HJ, ALA-Glioma Study Group. Fluorescence-guided surgery with 5-aminolevulinic acid for resection of malignant glioma: a randomised controlled multicentre phase III trial. Lancet Oncol. 2006; 7(5):392–401

[27] Sjöback R, Nygren J, Kubista M. Absorption and fluorescence properties of fluorescein. Spectrochim Acta A Mol Biomol Spectrosc. 1995; 51(6):L7–L21

[28] Dilek O, Ihsan A, Tulay H. Anaphylactic reaction after fluorescein sodium administration during intracranial surgery. J Clin Neurosci. 2011; 18(3):430–431

[29] Tanahashi S, Iida H, Dohi S. An anaphylactoid reaction after administration of fluorescein sodium during neurosurgery. Anesth Analg. 2006; 103(2):503

[30] da Silva CE, da Silva JL, da Silva VD. Use of sodium fluorescein in skull base tumors. Surg Neurol Int. 2010; 1:70

[31] Höhne J, Hohenberger C, Proescholdt M, et al. Fluorescein sodium-guided resection of cerebral metastases-an update. Acta Neurochir (Wien). 2017; 159(2):363–367

[32] Acerbi F, Broggi M, Schebesch KM, et al. Fluorescein-guided surgery for resection of high-grade gliomas: a multicentric prospective phase II study (FLUOGLIO). Clin Cancer Res. 2018; 24(1):52–61

[33] Neira JA, Ung TH, Sims JS, et al. Aggressive resection at the infiltrative margins of glioblastoma facilitated by intraoperative fluorescein guidance. J Neurosurg. 2017; 127(1):111–122

[34] Balamurugan S, Agrawal A, Kato Y, Sano H. Intra operative indocyanine green video-angiography in cerebrovascular surgery: an overview with review of literature. Asian J Neurosurg. 2011; 6(2):88–93

[35] Raabe A, Beck J, Gerlach R, Zimmermann M, Seifert V. Near-infrared indocyanine green video angiography: a new method for intraoperative assessment of vascular flow. Neurosurgery. 2003; 52(1):132–139, discussion 139

[36] Raabe A, Nakaji P, Beck J, et al. Prospective evaluation of surgical microscope-integrated intraoperative near-infrared indocyanine green videoangiography during aneurysm surgery. J Neurosurg. 2005; 103(6):982–989

[37] Lee JY, Thawani JP, Pierce J, et al. Intraoperative near-infrared optical imaging can localize gadolinium-enhancing gliomas during surgery. Neurosurgery. 2016; 79(6):856–871

[38] Sturgis M. Design and use of the surgical microscope in fluorescence-guided surgery. In: Rosenthal E, Zinn K, eds. Optical Imaging of Cancer: Clinical Applications. New York, NY: Springer; 2010:49–58

[39] Swanson KI, Clark PA, Zhang RR, et al. Fluorescent cancer-selective alkylphosphocholine analogs for intraoperative glioma detection. Neurosurgery. 2015; 76(2):115–123, discussion 123–124

[40] Zhang RR, Swanson KI, Hall LT, Weichert JP, Kuo JS. Diapeutic cancer-targeting alkylphosphocholine analogs may advance management of brain malignancies. CNS Oncol. 2016; 5(4):223–231

[41] Zhang RR, Schroeder AB, Grudzinski JJ, et al. Beyond the margins: real-time detection of cancer using targeted fluorophores. Nat Rev Clin Oncol. 2017; 14(6):347–364

[42] Parrish-Novak J, Byrnes-Blake K, Lalayeva N, et al. Nonclinical Profile of BLZ-100, a Tumor-Targeting Fluorescent Imaging Agent. Int J Toxicol. 2017; 36(2): 104–112

[43] Miller D, Patil C, Walker D, et al. Phase 1 safety study of BLZ-100 for fluorescence-guided resection of glioma in adult subjects. Neuro-oncol. 2016; 18 suppl 6:vi12–vi13

[44] Butte PV, Mamelak A, Parrish-Novak J, et al. Near-infrared imaging of brain tumors using the Tumor Paint BLZ-100 to achieve near-complete resection of brain tumors. Neurosurg Focus. 2014; 36(2):E1

[45] Valdés PA, Leblond F, Kim A, et al. Quantitative fluorescence in intracranial tumor: implications for ALA-induced PpIX as an intraoperative biomarker. J Neurosurg. 2011; 115(1):11–17

[46] Sanai N, Snyder LA, Honea NJ, et al. Intraoperative confocal microscopy in the visualization of 5-aminolevulinic acid fluorescence in low-grade gliomas. J Neurosurg. 2011; 115(4):740–748

[47] Suero Molina E, Wölfer J, Ewelt C, Ehrhardt A, Brokinkel B, Stummer W. Dual-labeling with 5-aminolevulinic acid and fluorescein for fluorescence-guided resection of high-grade gliomas: technical note. J Neurosurg. 2018; 128(2): 399–405

[48] Cordova JS, Shu HK, Liang Z, et al. Whole-brain spectroscopic MRI biomarkers identify infiltrating margins in glioblastoma patients. Neuro-oncol. 2016; 18 (8):1180–1189

[49] Stummer W, Tonn JC, Goetz C, et al. 5-Aminolevulinic acid-derived tumor fluorescence: the diagnostic accuracy of visible fluorescence qualities as corroborated by spectrometry and histology and postoperative imaging. Neurosurgery. 2014; 74(3):310–319, discussion 319–320

[50] Ross JL, Cooper LAD, Kong J, et al. 5-Aminolevulinic acid guided sampling of glioblastoma microenvironments identifies pro-survival signaling at infiltrative margins. Sci Rep. 2017; 7(1):15593

# 2 Designing and Reporting Studies on Intraoperative Tissue Imaging in the Brain

*Walter Stummer*

## Abstract

Intraoperative optical tissue imaging for identifying tumor-infiltrated brain is a rapidly expanding field. Clinically, intraoperative tissue fluorescence is the most commonly used method clinically at present, but other methods are in the pipeline or translating into clinical medicine. Due to the expanding role of intraoperative tissue imaging, harmonized and consented methods for evaluating and comparing the performance of these methods are urgently needed. This chapter attempts to shed light on the background, confounders, and pitfalls potentially involved in studies for testing the accuracy and clinical benefit of methods for intraoperative tissue imaging, and discusses aspects that should be reported to ensure transparency, reproducibility, and comparability.

*Keywords:* fluorescence, intraoperative tissue diagnosis, diagnostic accuracy, sensitivity, specificity

## 2.1 Introduction

Surgery for gliomas has changed considerably during the past two decades. The value of safe maximal resection in all types of gliomas is well established[1,2,3] as reflected by neuro-oncological guidelines.[4,5] Methods of intraoperative mapping and monitoring are more and more being employed to ensure maximal safety.[6] However, regarding the process of resection, it is commonly acknowledged that the surgeon's visual perception of tumor-infiltrated brain, affording at best subtle variations of color and texture compared to normal brain, and the haptic impression of infiltrated brain are limited in their utility for identifying tumor[7] even when using the surgical microscope. Due to inevitable neurologic morbidity, operating with a safety margin within the brain is seldom an option. Exact identification of tissue dignity is of utmost importance for improving oncological outcome, whereas neurological function has to remain intact.

This realization has spawned methods for intraoperative identification of residual tumor, such as the intraoperative MRI,[8,9,10] ultrasound,[11,12,13] or neuronavigation.[14,15,16] All of these techniques have inherent limitations, such as the price for MRI or brain shift for navigation, and none of these methods are truly real time. All require interrupting surgery to collect more or less accurate information on where infiltrated brain might be located. This information then needs to be transposed into the surgical cavity before the surgeon can resume surgery. Highly precise methods such as intraoperative histology from frozen sections, or newer methods such as confocal microscopy,[17,18] autofluorescence spectroscopy,[19,20] or Raman spectroscopy[21,22,23] have a high resolution and exact spatial allocation. However, only small regions of the cavity can be assessed at one time, making these techniques useful for "near-time" intraoperative biopsies but limiting their usefulness for real-time resection in a macroscopic environment.

Due to these limitations, it is clear that the new and expanding field of intraoperative optical tissue diagnosis is attractive to neurosurgeons. Optimally, techniques of this type would allow direct visualization of tissue under the surgical microscope.

The advantages offered by optical tissue imaging are many (▶ Table 2.1). Information on tissue dignity can be obtained in real time, and surgical decisions can be made immediately, without having to interrupt surgery, since the surgeon is seeing the signal (e.g., fluorescence) through the microscope in the tissue while he or she is operating. Tissue manipulation and tumor resection are possible while utilizing the additional optical information at the accustomed magnification. Brain shift, a confounder in neuronavigation, is not a worry with visual methods, and the optical technology is integrated into the operating microscope and does not require additional equipment in already overfilled operating rooms. Furthermore, using the adapted surgical microscope, the surgeon is operating with his or her familiar magnification on the visual aid he or she feels comfortable with after years of training.

There are several potential drawbacks however. Restricting the optical signal coming from the tissue might also result in *loss* of visual information. This is particularly true for fluorescence. Since only selected wavelengths of excitation light are employed, the background is generally not nearly as strongly illuminated as accustomed. While this problem can be partially mitigated by toggling between conventional and fluorescence illumination, it still hinders unimpaired surgery. Furthermore, methods of intraoperative tissue diagnosis will typically offer only surface information in a two-dimensional fashion, and the tissue signal might be obscured by blood or hemostatic agents, such as Surgicel. Strong light might lead to bleaching of signal in case of dyes that are used,[24,25] and surgical disruption of the blood–brain barrier might result in extravasation of agents carried by blood.[26,27]

Table 2.1 Potential advantages and disadvantages of intraoperative optical tissue imaging

*Advantages*

- Real time
- Accustomed magnification
- Brain shift is no concern
- Full integration into the surgical microscope

*Disadvantages*

- To a certain extent, loss of normal optical information while using the optical imaging strategy
- Time dependency of selected methods
- Regulatory issues regarding drugs, devices
- Two-dimensional representation
- Signal often obscured during surgery (blood, hemostatic agents)
- Signal alteration by surgical manipulation

In its present form, intraoperative tissue diagnosis was spawned by the introduction of porphyrins induced in tumor tissue by 5-aminolevulinic acid[25,28] (5-ALA), which can be visualized with appropriate excitation light and filter systems incorporated into the microscope. 5-ALA remains the only approved agent for the purpose of intraoperative tissue imaging. After approval of 5-ALA in Europe by the European Medicines Agency in 2007 and by the Food and Drug Administration (FDA) in 2017,[29] this field has gained further momentum. ALA, as approved for brain surgery, is thus the only regulatory precedent at present. However, many new methods are being explored using different fluorochromes, which are either non-targeted or targeted to malignant tumor tissue.[30]

## 2.2 Regulatory Perspective

From the FDA perspective,[31] approval of an agent is principally linked to two aspects: safety and benefit to the patient. Endpoints that simply correlate a tissue signal, for example, fluorescence, with the location of a known tumor may not be considered sufficient for approval. Furthermore, for approval, cost-effectiveness is primarily not an issue, as the responsibilities of FDA when evaluating technologies and agents do not initially focus on costs. This is an issue for the Centers for Medicare & Medicaid Services (CMS) at a later stage of the introduction of an agent.

Regulatory issues also pertain to the hardware side of technologies for intraoperative imaging. Approved devices might be tested in conjunction with new agents, or new devices might have to be tested with known agents, with the intent of improving imaging from the hardware side using the known agent. This chapter does not cover possible requirements for marketing application of device clearance by the FDA nor how such devices might be tested in detail or compared.

An agent for which approval might be considered will have to demonstrate a benefit to patients. Benefit could be based on the additional identification of diseased tissue after standard surgical resection. This, however, assumes that a more complete removal of malignant tissue is directly correlated with survival or other clinical benefits, such as a reduced need for reoperation. A correlation between histologically clear margins and survival is already well established for many types of cancer. The same may be true for debulking surgery. For example, if prior evidence indicates that debulking correlates to better outcomes, it may be sufficient to show that the optical technique improves the surgical safety and effectiveness of debulking procedures.[31] In the context of gliomas, regulatory bodies have principally questioned these points. This aspect was a central point of discussion with the FDA in the process of gaining approval for 5-ALA, the reason being the paucity of randomized studies in neurosurgery addressing these issues, despite the conviction of the neuro-oncological community.

One major issue during the conduct of imaging studies is the minimization of bias.[31] Randomization might be a solution; however, blinding the operating surgeon is obviously not an option. Intraoperative controlled studies might be another option, that is, using one method (conventional illumination), and then the new method in a controlled way. Again, such an approach would also have to be well designed to diminish biases, which are inherent to any optical method.

**Table 2.2** Development steps for brain intraoperative imaging agents or technologies

- Toxicology and pharmacokinetics
- Diagnostic accuracy based on histology
- Diagnostic measures PPV, NPV, sensitivity, specificity
- Sensitivity relative to tumor cell density
- Relationship of highlighted tissue to the specific MRI sequences
- Relationship of new method to established methods
- Benefit to patients

Abbreviations: MRI, magnetic resonance imaging; NPV, negative predictive value; PPV, positive predictive value.

## 2.3 Practical Approach

### 2.3.1 Developmental Steps

The first obvious step in assessment of a method—after establishing toxicological safety and pharmacokinetics—would be to verify the diagnostic performance of that method. Does the method truly show tumor and to what extent it is capable of showing tumor-infiltrated brain (▶ Table 2.2)? Such data might first be generated by animal experiments and subsequently in patients.

Later steps might be to determine how the tissue signal relates to the tumor as depicted on the MRI or to establish methods of preoperative tumor imaging. In this context, it must be remembered that gliomas are diffusely and extensively infiltrating lesions. Expecting a method to find every single tumor cell would not be feasible in the context of glioma surgery. Typically, the extent of visualizing low-grade glioma would be the MRI fluid-attenuated inversion recovery (FLAIR) anomaly, and in high-grade gliomas the gadolinium-enhancing portion of the tumor.

Finally, it would be convincing to demonstrate that the use of these agents will translate into improved clinical outcomes, such as enhanced, safe resections or prolonged progression-free and overall survival, the ultimate goal of surgical oncology. On a bynote, the FDA does not specifically require survival as an endpoint for demonstrating the effects of an intraoperative imaging technique.[31]

Importantly, given the plethora of agents and procedures for intraoperative tissue imaging that are being developed, the fundamental question will arise on how these methods perform when they are directly compared. Methods might compete based on price and utility, but ultimately patient safety and efficacy will prevail as the most important factors characterizing an agent and and lead to its preference over others.

For this reason, it is clear that the community requires standards for assessing intraoperative imaging methods. Little precedent is available so far, and to our knowledge the FDA offers no guidance regarding this new field.

The last part of this chapter will discuss aspects related to the assessment of the diagnostic performance. In particular, this chapter will give an overview of perceptions and possible misconceptions regarding the assessment and reporting of intraoperative methods of imaging. Since this is an emerging field without detailed regulatory precedent, the academic community should help in defining possible approaches to these issues as soon as possible.

## 2.3.2 Possible Variables and Pitfalls Related to Assessments of Diagnostic Accuracy in Intraoperative Imaging

When reporting on intraoperative diagnostic methods, there are several issues that may require being addressed as described in the following:

- *The way the signal is detected and used for resection is the way the signal should be tested.* For example, if a method relies on visual discrimination, then that method should be tested by visual discrimination, since this is what later will be used for treating patients. Using, for example, spectrometry or determining the brightness of the signal as returned by a camera for assessing diagnostic accuracy may not reflect the true performance of that agent during surgery, since the surgeon will not be able to consciously determine thresholds during surgery based on his visual perception.

- *Thresholds and their influence on diagnostic accuracy.* Some methods will also highlight normal tissue to a certain degree. This would be expected for methods that rely on intrinsic signals, for example, autofluorescence[19,20] and would also be expected for technologies that use agents for highlighting tumors that circulate in the vessels after being administered intravascularly, for example, fluorescein.[26,27,32,33] These compounds will highlight all brain tissue to a certain extent, despite having higher concentrations in tumor tissue. Especially low signal-to-noise ratio methods will require some form of threshold definition, above which a sample is considered positive. This threshold will have to be clearly described. Increasing the threshold will lead to fewer false negatives, while lowering the threshold will lead to more false positives. Thus, defining a threshold will directly affect diagnostic accuracy. Optimally, receiver operating curves[34] should be employed to relate all thresholds to their respective diagnostic accuracies. Again, it is important that thresholding will only play a role with methods that rely on imaging processing. With visual methods, defining thresholds will not be an option. Human visual cognition is too flexible and adaptable to allow objective thresholding.

- *Changes in intraoperative signal over time.* Researchers should be mindful that during a neurosurgical procedure lasting several hours, the signals induced in tissue will change over time. This is the case for ALA-induced porphyrins with a maximum at about 8 hours.[35] With intraoperative dyes such as fluorescein, the situation is somewhat more complex.[27,36,37]

While fluorescein has no specific affinity to tumor cells, concentrations are at first high in perfused tissue and are later extravasated in tumor, leading to pseudoselectivity. However, there is some concern about unspecific propagation with edema.[38] Reporting timing here is essential.[39] With "intelligent" fluorophores, they are selectively retained in tumors, for example, alkylphosphocholine (APC) analogs,[40] fluorochromes conjugated with chlorotoxin,[41,42] or fluorochromes targeting integrin receptors.[43] These will first be in the plasma and will enter the tumor via a breached blood–brain barrier, but will selectively be retained due to the specific interaction or binding of the fluorochrome to the tumor cells. Unspecifically, extravasated surplus dye molecules will be washed out of the brain interstitial space and dye will be cleared from plasma with time. The results on diagnostic accuracy will thus have to be reported in conjunction with the time after application of a compound.

- *Truth standards.* In order to determine the diagnostic accuracy of an agent for correctly identifying the dignity of tissue, generally acknowledged comparators need to be defined on which to base this assessment. The most obvious comparator is histology. However, especially in diffusely growing tumors it may not always be possible for neuropathologists to correctly identify single tumor cells. Molecular markers, such as isocitrate dehydrogenase 1 (IDH1) mutations, Ki-67/MIB-1, or p53 might increase the sensitivity of actually finding tumor cells as opposed to simple hematoxylin and eosin (H&E) staining. Since the sensitivity of detecting tumor cells will directly influence the reported diagnostic performance of a method, the methods used need to be reported exactly.

Established methods might serve as comparators or truth standards. For the randomized 5-ALA study, the comparators were resection rates using conventional microsurgery with white light. Future studies might require resection rates using 5-ALA fluorescence-guided resection to be a comparator. Another possible truth standard might be MRI, since our assessments of the completeness of resection and disease status are based on this modality. Using MR as a truth standard would imply an exact correlation between intraoperative signal and MRI, for example, by neuronavigation. Resolution issues and brain shift may be distinct confounders that need to be accounted for. ▶ Table 2.3 compiles several truth standards, the type of study they might be used in, and possible confounders related to such truth standards.

**Table 2.3** Possible comparators or truth standards

| Comparator or truth standard | Possible study type | Confounders |
|---|---|---|
| Assessment based on histology | • Single arm<br>• Randomized | Differing results based on differing methodology, e.g., including molecular markers (IDH1, Ki-67, p53) or simple H&E |
| Comparison to established optical imaging method | • Sequentially randomized<br>• Randomized | Bias resulting from open label, nonblindable optical assessments |
| Comparison based on MRI resection rates | • Case control<br>• Preferably randomized | Case selection in individual study confound single-arm assessments and comparability.<br>Which MR sequence should be used? |
| PFS, OS | • Case control<br>• Preferably randomized | Case selection in one-armed studies confound interpretation; effects on resection difficult to grasp since not intraoperative detection but resection rates are driving outcomes |
| Safety | • Single arm<br>• Preferably randomized | Toxicological safety; procedural safety related to surgery |

Abbreviations: H&E, hematoxylin and eosin; IDH1, isocitrate dehydrogenase 1; MRI, magnetic resonance imaging; OS, overall survival; PFS, progression-free survival.

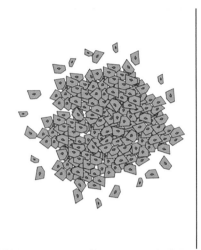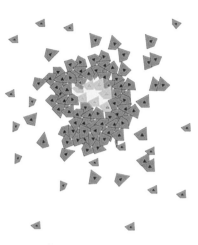

**Fig. 2.1** This scheme illustrates the differences in infiltration zones between metastasis (*left*) and gliomas (*right*). Whereas intraoperative imaging methods would be expected to show all tumor cells in metastasis, enabling a histologically complete resection, this is not the goal in surgery for a glioma. Gliomas are extensively infiltrative and, for functional reasons, resection will be restricted to those parts of the tumor with a higher degree of cell densities, approximating the fluid-attenuated inversion recovery (FLAIR) anomaly on MRI for low-grade gliomas and the enhancing tumor in high-grade gliomas (*circle*).

### 2.3.3 Using Accustomed Parameters for Diagnostic Accuracy

*Complete tumor removal versus cytoreduction:* In general surgical oncology, margins that are completely clear of tumor are the goal of surgery (▶ Fig. 2.1). In glioma surgery, this aim is virtually unachievable due to the infiltrative biology of tumors. It is well accepted that extensive cytoreduction is the aim of surgery, trying to diminish residual tumor cell burden as much as possible. Despite optimal resection results on the MRI (complete resection of the contrast enhancing tumor), residual infiltrating cells will be acceptable and expected in glioblastoma (GBM) tumors even centimeters away from contrast-enhancing lesions on the MR. In non–central nervous system (CNS) cancers, intraoperative imaging techniques will have to correctly identify all tumor cells. For such cancers, a dichotomous approach in determining diagnostic accuracy will be appropriate (tumor yes/no). In infiltrating CNS malignancies, on the other hand, the technique will have to demonstrate visualization down to a certain cell density. The principle that sufficient cytoreduction is of value is difficult to grasp for the general oncologist, and has resulted in intense discussions during the approval process for 5-ALA with the FDA. The accustomed measures specificity, sensitivity, positive predictive value (PPV), and negative predictive values (NPV) appear inadequate when accepting reasonable cytoreduction. Visualizing the tumor burden down to a cell density of 10% infiltrating cells may be sufficient in the context of a glioma, as this density can be found beyond contrast-enhancing tumor, the removal of which has always been the aim of surgery. When using a dichotomous definition of tumor (tumor yes/no), even a highly effective optimal imaging method down to a tumor cell density of 10% would not appear to perform well due to a high number of falsely negative biopsies.

Therefore, accepting the aim of surgery to be cytoreduction to a certain degree, descriptors such as "sensitivity" or "specificity" that utilize a dichotomous approach may oversimplify the requirements for assessing the diagnostic accuracy for intraoperative tissue diagnosis in infiltrating brain tumors. It is for this reason that it would make sense for tests to state to what cell densities tumor cells might be visualized by an intraoperative optical method.

If investigators nevertheless wish to adopt these classical measures of diagnostic accuracy, multiple confounders and biases need to be accounted for and require transparent reporting.

Ideally, with intraoperative imaging, the fluorescent agent would be expected to highlight *only* gross tumor or infiltrated tissue to the surgeon, whereas normal tissue would be negative for the fluorescing agent.

If asked to determine diagnostic accuracy, the neurosurgeon would be inclined to collect biopsies from tissue in order to determine the following:
- All samples with tumor and fluorescence (true positives).
- All samples with tumor without fluorescence (false negatives).
- All samples with normal tissue showing fluorescence (false positives).
- All samples with normal tissue correctly devoid of fluorescence (true negatives).

The neurosurgeon would then use calculations and terminology he is familiar with, such as sensitivity, specificity, and positive and negative predictive values (▶ Table 2.4). This approach appears straightforward; however, the use of these calculations and terms for evaluating intraoperative imaging methods may not be that simple.

First, these measures were developed for diagnostic purposes in which one sample is taken from one patient, such as in the determination of prostate-specific antigen (PSA).[44] In the brain, typically, the perception would be to take as many samples as

**Table 2.4** Diagnostic decision matrix

| | | True disease state | |
|---|---|---|---|
| | | **Present** | **Absent** |
| Test result | Positive | True positive (TP) | False positive (FP) |
| | Negative | False negative (FN) | True negative (TN) |

Notes: sensitivity = TP/(TP + FN).
Specificity = TN/(TN + FP).
Positive predictive value (PPV) = TP/(TP + FP).
Negative predictive value (NPV) = TN/(TN + FN).

possible for the calculated sensitivities and specificities to be as highly accurate as possible. It is exactly this perception that renders all attempts at determining sensitivity and specificity of an agent in the brain as highly prone to biases and misinterpretations. Multiple tissue samples, typically collected for the assessment of intraoperative imaging methods, require special statistical considerations and exact definitions of frequencies and locations at which samples are collected.

For example, sensitivity and specificity will depend on the number of samples taken in fluorescent or nonfluorescent areas. Taking three instead of one nonfluorescing sample might completely change calculated sensitivities and specificities. Similarly, taking 10 instead of 2 samples in correctly fluorescing areas will also give different values for the same patients.

Values such as sensitivity and specificity will directly depend on where in infiltrating tumor biopsies are taken. If they are taken close to the main tumor mass, infiltrating cells are likely to be found and NPV, sensitivity, and specificity will appear low due to many false-negative biopsies. If samples are taken far from the main mass, the number of false negatives will be low, and the specificity, sensitivity, and NPV will be high.

Too few biopsies would not account for the inter- and intratumoral heterogeneity characteristics for gliomas.

Nevertheless, sensitivity, specificity, PPV, and NPV may be acceptable descriptors, provided the method of collecting samples is absolutely transparent and reproducible and multiple biopsies are accounted for statistically.

## 2.4 Conclusion

In the rapidly expanding field of intraoperative tissue imaging, the neurosurgical community needs to develop reporting standards in order to ensure reproducibility, transparency, and comparability of methods. The authors of future papers in this field are encouraged to reflect on some of the biases and confounders discussed in this chapter.

## References

[1] Sanai N, Polley M-Y, McDermott MW, Parsa AT, Berger MS. An extent of resection threshold for newly diagnosed glioblastomas. J Neurosurg. 2011; 115(1):3–8

[2] Sanai N, Berger MS. Glioma extent of resection and its impact on patient outcome. Neurosurgery. 2008; 62(4):753–764, discussion 264–266

[3] Stummer W, Reulen HJ, Meinel T, et al. ALA-Glioma Study Group. Extent of resection and survival in glioblastoma multiforme: identification of and adjustment for bias. Neurosurgery. 2008; 62(3):564–576, discussion 564–576

[4] Weller M, van den Bent M, Tonn JC, et al. European Association for Neuro-Oncology (EANO) Task Force on Gliomas. European Association for Neuro-Oncology (EANO) guideline on the diagnosis and treatment of adult astrocytic and oligodendroglial gliomas. Lancet Oncol. 2017; 18(6):e315–e329

[5] Stupp R, Brada M, van den Bent MJ, Tonn JC, Pentheroudakis G, ESMO Guidelines Working Group. High-grade glioma: ESMO Clinical Practice Guidelines for diagnosis, treatment and follow-up. Ann Oncol. 2014; 25 suppl 3:iii93–iii101

[6] De Witt Hamer PC, Robles SG, Zwinderman AH, Duffau H, Berger MS. Impact of intraoperative stimulation brain mapping on glioma surgery outcome: a meta-analysis. J Clin Oncol. 2012; 30(20):2559–2565

[7] Albert FK, Forsting M, Sartor K, Adams HP, Kunze S. Early postoperative magnetic resonance imaging after resection of malignant glioma: objective evaluation of residual tumor and its influence on regrowth and prognosis. Neurosurgery. 1994; 34(1):45–60, discussion 60–61

[8] Kubben PL, ter Meulen KJ, Schijns OEMG, ter Laak-Poort MP, van Overbeeke JJ, van Santbrink H. Intraoperative MRI-guided resection of glioblastoma multiforme: a systematic review. Lancet Oncol. 2011; 12(11):1062–1070

[9] Senft C, Bink A, Franz K, Vatter H, Gasser T, Seifert V. Intraoperative MRI guidance and extent of resection in glioma surgery: a randomised, controlled trial. Lancet Oncol. 2011; 12(11):997–1003

[10] Schneider JP, Trantakis C, Rubach M, et al. Intraoperative MRI to guide the resection of primary supratentorial glioblastoma multiforme–a quantitative radiological analysis. Neuroradiology. 2005; 47(7):489–500

[11] Prada F, Mattei L, Del Bene M, et al. Intraoperative cerebral glioma characterization with contrast enhanced ultrasound. BioMed Res Int. 2014; 2014:484261

[12] Šteňo A, Karlík M, Mendel P, Čík M, Šteňo J. Navigated three-dimensional intraoperative ultrasound-guided awake resection of low-grade glioma partially infiltrating optic radiation. Acta Neurochir (Wien). 2012; 154(7): 1255–1262

[13] Lindner D, Trantakis C, Renner C, et al. Application of intraoperative 3D ultrasound during navigated tumor resection. Minim Invasive Neurosurg. 2006; 49(4):197–202

[14] Wirtz CR, Albert FK, Schwaderer M, et al. The benefit of neuronavigation for neurosurgery analyzed by its impact on glioblastoma surgery. Neurol Res. 2000; 22(4):354–360

[15] Mikuni N, Okada T, Enatsu R, et al. Clinical impact of integrated functional neuronavigation and subcortical electrical stimulation to preserve motor function during resection of brain tumors. J Neurosurg. 2007; 106(4):593–598

[16] Suess O, Picht T, Kuehn B, Mularski S, Brock M, Kombos T. Neuronavigation without rigid pin fixation of the head in left frontotemporal tumor surgery with intraoperative speech mapping. Neurosurgery. 2007; 60(4) Suppl 2: 330–338, discussion 338

[17] Sanai N, Eschbacher J, Hattendorf G, et al. Intraoperative confocal microscopy for brain tumors: a feasibility analysis in humans. Neurosurgery. 2011; 68(2) suppl operative:282–290, discussion 290

[18] Foersch S, Heimann A, Ayyad A, et al. Confocal laser endomicroscopy for diagnosis and histomorphologic imaging of brain tumors in vivo. PLoS One. 2012; 7(7):e41760

[19] Croce AC, Fiorani S, Locatelli D, et al. Diagnostic potential of autofluorescence for an assisted intraoperative delineation of glioblastoma resection margins. Photochem Photobiol. 2003; 77(3):309–318

[20] Poon WS, Schomacker KT, Deutsch TF, Martuza RL. Laser-induced fluorescence: experimental intraoperative delineation of tumor resection margins. J Neurosurg. 1992; 76(4):679–686

[21] Tanahashi K, Natsume A, Ohka F, et al. Assessment of tumor cells in a mouse model of diffuse infiltrative glioma by Raman spectroscopy. BioMed Res Int. 2014; 2014:860241

[22] Jermyn M, Mok K, Mercier J, et al. Intraoperative brain cancer detection with Raman spectroscopy in humans. Sci Transl Med. 2015; 7(274):274ra19

[23] Kast R, Auner G, Yurgelevic S, et al. Identification of regions of normal grey matter and white matter from pathologic glioblastoma and necrosis in frozen sections using Raman imaging. J Neurooncol. 2015; 125(2):287–295

[24] Song L, Hennink EJ, Young IT, Tanke HJ. Photobleaching kinetics of fluorescein in quantitative fluorescence microscopy. Biophys J. 1995; 68(6): 2588–2600

[25] Stummer W, Stocker S, Wagner S, et al. Intraoperative detection of malignant gliomas by 5-aminolevulinic acid-induced porphyrin fluorescence. Neurosurgery. 1998; 42(3):518–525, discussion 525–526

[26] Suero Molina E, Wölfer J, Ewelt C, Ehrhardt A, Brokinkel B, Stummer W. Dual-labeling with 5-aminolevulinic acid and fluorescein for fluorescence-guided resection of high-grade gliomas: technical note. J Neurosurg. 2017(March): 1–7

[27] Stummer W. Factors confounding fluorescein-guided malignant glioma resections: edema bulk flow, dose, timing, and now: imaging hardware? Acta Neurochir (Wien). 2016; 158(2):327–328

[28] Stummer W, Novotny A, Stepp H, Goetz C, Bise K, Reulen HJ. Fluorescence-guided resection of glioblastoma multiforme utilizing 5-ALA-induced porphyrins: a prospective study in 52 consecutive patients. J Neurosurg. 2000; 93(6):1003–1013

[29] U.S. Food & Drug Administration. Approved drugs: aminolevulinic acid hydrochloride, known as ALA HCl (Gleolan, NX Development Corp.) as an optical imaging agent indicated in patients with gliomas. Available at: https://www.fda.gov/Drugs/InformationOnDrugs/ApprovedDrugs/ucm562645.htm. Accessed September 10, 2017

[30] Senders JT, Muskens IS, Schnoor R, et al. Agents for fluorescence-guided glioma surgery: a systematic review of preclinical and clinical results. Acta Neurochir (Wien). 2017; 159(1):151–167

[31] Tummers WS, Warram JM, Tipirneni KE, et al. Regulatory aspects of optical methods and exogenous targets for cancer detection. Cancer Res. 2017; 77 (9):2197–2206

[32] Lovato RM, Vitorino Araujo JL, Esteves Veiga JC. Low-cost device for fluorescein-guided surgery in malignant brain tumor. World Neurosurg. 2017; 104:61–67

[33] Chen B, Wang H, Ge P, et al. Gross total resection of glioma with the intraoperative fluorescence-guidance of fluorescein sodium. Int J Med Sci. 2012; 9(8):708–714

[34] Florkowski CM. Sensitivity, specificity, receiver-operating characteristic (ROC) curves and likelihood ratios: communicating the performance of diagnostic tests. Clin Biochem Rev. 2008; 29(suppl 1):S83–S87

[35] Stummer W, Stepp H, Wiestler OD, Pichlmeier U. Randomized, prospective double-blinded study comparing 3 different doses of 5-aminolevulinic acid for fluorescence-guided resections of malignant gliomas. Neurosurgery. 2017; 81(2):230–239

[36] Schwake M, Stummer W, Suero Molina EJ, Wölfer J. Simultaneous fluorescein sodium and 5-ALA in fluorescence-guided glioma surgery. Acta Neurochir (Wien). 2015; 157(5):877–879

[37] Roberts DW, Olson J. Fluorescein guidance in glioblastoma resection. N Engl J Med. 2017; 376(18):e36

[38] Stummer W, Götz C, Hassan A, Heimann A, Kempski O. Kinetics of photofrin II in perifocal brain edema. Neurosurgery. 1993; 33(6):1075–1081– discussion 1081––108–2

[39] Diaz RJ, Dios RR, Hattab EM, et al. Study of the biodistribution of fluorescein in glioma-infiltrated mouse brain and histopathological correlation of intraoperative findings in high-grade gliomas resected under fluorescein fluorescence guidance. J Neurosurg. 2015; 122(6):1360–1369

[40] Swanson KI, Clark PA, Zhang RR, et al. Fluorescent cancer-selective alkylphosphocholine analogs for intraoperative glioma detection. Neurosurgery. 2015; 76(2):115–123, discussion 123–124

[41] Butte PV, Mamelak A, Parrish-Novak J, et al. Near-infrared imaging of brain tumors using the Tumor Paint BLZ-100 to achieve near-complete resection of brain tumors. Neurosurg Focus. 2014; 36(2):E1

[42] Akcan M, Stroud MR, Hansen SJ, et al. Chemical re-engineering of chlorotoxin improves bioconjugation properties for tumor imaging and targeted therapy. J Med Chem. 2011; 54(3):782–787

[43] Moore SJ, Hayden Gephart MG, Bergen JM, et al. Engineered knottin peptide enables noninvasive optical imaging of intracranial medulloblastoma. Proc Natl Acad Sci U S A. 2013; 110(36):14598–14603

[44] Heidenreich A, Abrahamsson P-A, Artibani W, et al. European Association of Urology. Early detection of prostate cancer: European Association of Urology recommendation. Eur Urol. 2013; 64(3):347–354

# 3 5-Aminolevulinic Acid and High-Grade Gliomas

*Ricardo Díez Valle and Walter Stummer*

## Abstract

5-aminolevulinic acid (5-ALA) is a compound used for fluorescence-guided tumor resection in neurosurgery. It was the first drug to be developed specifically for this purpose and is presently the only agent approved by the European Medicines Agency and the Food and Drug Administration for intraoperative tissue imaging. This chapter reviews the experimental and clinical background of this drug for its use in malignant glioma surgery.

*Keywords:* malignant glioma, fluorescence, ALA, porphyrins, fluorescence-guided resection, glioblastoma

## 3.1 Background

### 3.1.1 High-Grade Gliomas

High-grade gliomas (HGGs) are diffuse tumors that extensively infiltrate the brain and seldom have a histologically distinct border. In most cases, these tumors consist of a core of solidly proliferating tumor cells surrounded by brain containing invading cells, but little information is available about the amount, characteristics of invasive cells, and the distance of invasion. Serial biopsy studies performed in the past suggested that enhancing areas on CT and MRI corresponded mostly to solid tumor, while hypointense or surrounding T2 abnormal areas contained variable amounts of invasive cells.[1] After these early studies, little relevant information has been acquired on this topic, and, importantly, there is no standard method to quantify and report the degree of invasion in specific areas of the brain.

### 3.1.2 Role of Resection in High-Grade Gliomas

Given the diffuse nature of malignant glial tumors, surgery is never curative, and the benefit of surgery has been a matter of discussion. There is no level 1 evidence from appropriate randomized trials on this subject. One randomized trial found resection superior to biopsy.[2] However, the conclusions from this study were limited by the inclusion of only elderly patients, small patient numbers, a combination of WHO grade III and IV cases, and a lack of standardized adjuvant therapies. Other available studies are retrospective in nature. Nevertheless, a plethora of data suggest that resection of HGG has a favorable impact on overall survival (OS).[3] When the degree of resection is measured by postoperative MRI, a strong positive correlation can be observed between extent of resection (EOR) and longer OS. This correlation was initially shown with the resection of glioblastoma (GBM) and postoperative MRI,[4] and confirmed in successive, larger series,[5,6] so that the contrast-enhancing tumor has become the target of resection.

For GBM, the study with the best evidence[7] is a cohort study that provides level 2b evidence that survival depends on complete resection of enhancing tumor (CRET) in GBM. A larger retrospective series, with detailed volumetric analysis over 721 patients, found a continuous, nonlinear relationship between OS and extent of resection, supporting a maximal safe resection approach to GBM.[8] For other types of HGG, series are smaller, and there are less high-quality data, mostly supporting the same philosophy. Given the available data, it is highly improbable that a randomized trial will be performed for resection versus nonresection of a GBM, since available data prevent equipoise.

### 3.1.3 Results of Resection

Due to the diffuse, infiltrative nature of HGGs, neurosurgeons have understood that resection should be restricted to tissue areas that are visualized by MRI contrast enhancement. Thus, CRET has been the surgical paradigm in most neurosurgical centers. However, multiple reports indicate that this aim is seldom actually achieved. Rates of around 30% or less have been reported in leading institutions of the world, as reviewed by Sanai and Berger.[9] There are several reasons why the resection of contrast-enhancing tumor is not always complete. As surgery is not curative, it is important to perform a safe resection, strictly avoiding neurological deficits. Intentional sparing of assumed eloquent regions invaded by tumor is one reason for incomplete resections. However, safety does not seem to be the main reason. At least two studies have compared the visual impression of the surgeon at the end of surgery to the actual resection as verified by postcontrast MRI. The first study from 1994 found that surgeons expected complete resections in 54% of the cases based on their visual impression of the resection cavity. MRI disproved them, showing that the intraoperative impression was true for only 18% (one-third of cases).[4] A similar study published in 2012, more than 20 years later, found that resection was complete in only 30% of cases in which the surgeon had expected resections to be complete.[10] The authors of this particular study also identified 17 cases in which complete resections were considered safe by expert panel review. Only 24.5% of these patients were subject to a complete resection. Such results show very clearly that the contrast-enhancing limit of the tumor is not reliably identified by the surgeon during standard surgery based on the visual impression and haptic information only.

## 3.2 Preclinical Data of 5-Aminolevulinic Acid Fluorescence

### 3.2.1 Physiopathology

5-aminolevulinic acid (5-ALA) is the first committed precursor of heme synthesis, situated in the metabolic pathway just beyond the controlling step. External, excess supply of the compound to cells increases porphyrin synthesis, ending in protoheme. 5-ALA is not a fluorophore, but some of the dependent metabolites in the heme synthesis are. Prior work found that administration of 5-ALA could produce a chemical model of porphyria, as some of its metabolites are phototoxic. This observation later spawned the idea of using 5-ALA for photodynamic therapy (PDT). This therapeutic concept exploits the accumulation of photosensitizing molecules at a high enough concentration to eliminate tumor cells with light exposure and creation of toxic reactive oxygen species (ROS). A number of in vitro and animal experiments completed in the past showed that accumulation of fluorescent porphyrin compounds, especially protoporphyrin IX (PpIX), was indeed much higher in certain tumors (skin, bladder, and gastrointestinal tumors) than in normal tissue. PDT has a number of challenges, as it requires the delivery of light to cells in sufficient amounts, subsequent formation of enough toxic metabolites (ROS) to kill cells, and a wide distribution in the tumor to be effective.

Visualization of fluorescence as guidance for resection emerged as a more straightforward application of 5-ALA and its PpIX metabolite. PpIX is readily excited by light in the blue/violet range of the spectrum around 400 nm, and it is fluorescent with two emission peaks, at 635 and at 704 nm, which is observed by the human eye as red light. The differential concentration between malignant tumor cells and normal cells is enough for differential fluorescence visualization of tumors.

As 5-ALA is readily absorbed within the intestine and rapidly passes into the bloodstream (within 1 hour), it is administered orally and needs to be given prior to general anesthesia. Once 5-ALA reaches the plasma, viable glioma cells start to accumulate PpIX minutes later, in an active metabolic process through the heme biosynthesis pathway. Most of the synthesized PpIX remains intracellular. 5-ALA is a small, polar molecule that does not readily cross the intact blood–brain barrier (BBB).[11] However, due to its size (131.131 g/mol), only minor perturbations of the BBB function are needed for 5-ALA to reach tumor cells, even in areas that do not accumulate MR contrast (gadolinium). The tumor cell targeting of 5-ALA, the number of viable tumor cells, and their intrinsic metabolic activity will impact the generation of PpIX and fluorescence emission. Necrotic tumor regions do not produce visible 5-ALA-induced fluorescence, as PpIX accumulation requires intact tumor cell metabolism.

5-ALA fluorescence will not be present in vascular compartment, or tissues that do not actively synthetize porphyrins in great quantity. However, the administration of oral 5-ALA does produce an increase in porphyrin synthesis in organs such as the skin and liver. 5-ALA administration can lead to transient skin phototoxicity or transiently (but not critically) elevated liver enzymes.

## 3.2.2 Experimental Data In Vitro and In Vivo

The first experimental results utilizing 5-ALA in glioma cells were published in 1998.[12] 5-ALA was shown to induce fluorescence in incubated C6 rat glioma cells, and in orthotopic syngeneic tumors derived from the intracranial implantation of C6 cells in rats. After intraperitoneal administration of 5-ALA, at a dose of 100 mg/kg, tumors were visualized as intensely fluorescent, while faint fluorescence could be seen in some areas of normal tissue, pia, choroid plexus, and surrounding white matter tracts. In the same year, another group published similar results utilizing C6 and also 9 L glioma models with a higher dose of 5-ALA (200 mg/kg). Tumor fluorescence was visualized

between 2 and 8 hours after 5-ALA administration and disappeared by 22 hours. After using this dose, the group noted fluorescence in the ependyma, and also slight fluorescence in the normal brain.[13]

In subsequent experiments with multiple different cell lines, differences in 5-ALA-induced fluorescence intensities were found. However, tumor fluorescence was still sufficient for differentiating tumor cells from normal neuronal cell lines and cultured astrocytes at an incubation time of 120 minutes.[14] No malignant glioma cell line has been reported to be negative for 5-ALA-induced fluorescence. PpIX fluorescence is also present in GBM cancer stem cells in vitro in concentrations that have been demonstrated to be sufficient for cell killing by PDT.[15]

The amount of PpIX accumulation in tumor cells and visible fluorescence can be modified, at least in vitro, by a number of substances that affect porphyrin metabolism. Iron chelation with deferoxamine increases fluorescence in the glioma xenograft U251 model,[16] and also in cancer stem cells.[17] On the other hand, antiepileptic drugs, such as phenytoin and valproic acid, can diminish accumulation of PpIX. The most commonly used antiepileptic in brain tumor patients, levetiracetam, shows no effect.[18] In the same experimental series, the addition of dexamethasone to the other drugs appeared to further diminish the amount of PpIX produced, while increasing the retention inside the cells. Dexamethasone and phenytoin together have been shown to lower intracellular accumulation of PpIX.[18]

# 3.3 Clinical Application

## 3.3.1 Early Clinical Experience

The first clinical use of fluorescence-guided surgery (FGS) with 5-ALA for gliomas was reported in 1998.[19] In a cohort of nine HGG patients, utilizing an oral dose of 10 mg/kg, the authors used a violet–blue (375- to 440-nm) xenon excitation light and a 455-nm long-pass filter adapted to an operating microscope. A specifically developed 455-nm long-pass filter allowed red light emitted by the PpIX to reach the observer along with a small fraction of the excitation light, the latter necessary for allowing background illumination with red porphyrin fluorescence observable on a blue rather than black background (▶ Fig. 3.1). This allowed blue field surgery to be possible even under the fluorescence mode of the microscope.

In this first trial, 89 tissue biopsies of specimens with or without 5-ALA-induced fluorescence were analyzed. A calculated sensitivity of 85% and a specificity of 100% for the detection of malignant tissue were found in this study. Chapter 2 in this book deals with the problem of evaluating intraoperative diagnostic methods, and how the use of traditional descriptors of diagnostic accuracy, such as sensitivity and specificity in this setting, is difficult to determine amidst a number of biases and confounders. Nevertheless, the first results confirmed the potential utility of 5-ALA for detection of tumor in HGGs, as all the fluorescent samples contained tumor, and most of the non-fluorescent samples did not. For seven of nine patients, visible 5-ALA-induced fluorescence led to additional resection of tumor. The authors also closely assessed the effect of photobleaching (porphyrin degeneration due to standard operating white light illumination) as a potential problem. Under operating light conditions, fluorescence decayed to 36% in 25 minutes

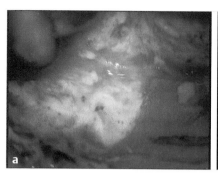
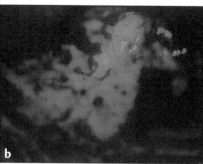

**Fig. 3.1** Border of resection of a glioblastoma showing an area with normal aspect under white light **(a)** where fluorescence with 5-ALA shows residual tumor **(b)**.

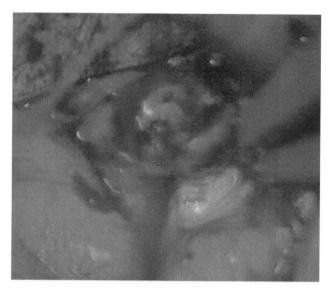

**Fig. 3.2** Image showing the different quality of intense, red fluorescence versus pale, pink fluorescence.

for violet–blue light using intensities comparable to those obtained during surgery, and in 87 minutes for white light. This study also contained the first description of a seemingly nonenhancing glioma with an anaplastic focus, which was detected by fluorescence after 5-ALA administration.

Two years later, the same group published the results of surgery utilizing 5-ALA fluorescence guidance in 52 HGG patients.[20] In this phase II trial, 5-ALA was administered at an oral dose of 20 mg/kg of body weight, which has now become the standard dose administered to patients. The same combination of excitation light and long-pass filter coupled to the surgical microscope was used. Fluorescence was useful for guiding the resection in all cases, and two discernible fluorescence qualities were observed: a strong solid red fluorescence in viable solid tumor, surrounded by a transition zone with less intense, pink fluorescence in the region of the infiltrating tumor margin (▶ Fig. 3.2). Necrotic tumor tissue was not fluorescent but could be differentiated under normal light. Selective biopsies with different fluorescence qualities were taken and analyzed for the presence of tumor. Solid fluorescence was usually characterized by solid, coalescent tumor, with PpIX fluorescence in the cytoplasm of the cells, while vague or weaker pink fluorescence usually featured infiltrating tumor of medium to high density.

This trial compared the results of the FGS to the postoperative contrast MRI, the standard for resection control in GBM, and the effect of residual fluorescence on OS. CRET was achieved in 33 patients (63%). Resection was mostly limited due to functional considerations. The resection cavity had collapsed and fluorescence was not visualized in only one patient with a cystic lesion. Complete resection of the contrast-enhancing tumor was achieved in 16 of 17 patients. Complete resection of fluorescent tissue was achieved in 9 of 12 cases with resection of all areas with intense fluorescence. Only in 8 of 23 patients was intense tissue fluorescence left behind. There was a significant correlation between any kind of residual fluorescence and residual enhancing tumor on MRI, and an even stronger correlation between residual solid fluorescence and residual enhancing tumor on the MRI. The Kaplan–Meier analysis revealed survival was longer in patients with CRET than in those without CRET (no enhancement, 103 ± 11 weeks; residual enhancement, 54 ± 5 weeks), and similarly, resection of fluorescent tissue was superior to leaving fluorescing tissue behind (no fluorescence, 101 ± 15 weeks; vague fluorescence, 79 ± 6 weeks; solid fluorescence, 51 ± 3 weeks). The difference was significant only for residual solid, intense fluorescence. In summary, this work confirmed the association between removal of 5-ALA-induced tumor fluorescence and more extensive tumor resections with improved outcomes in OS. Increasing the rate of CRET was better achieved with 5-ALA FGS in comparison to historical studies of HGG tumor resection at that time.

## 3.3.2 Randomized Clinical Trial

For approval of 5-ALA by the European Medicines Agency (EMA), a randomized multicenter clinical trial was designed to validate the prior early phase II results of 5-ALA FGS. This would be the first-ever randomized study utilizing an optical imaging agent for FGS in HGGs. Newly diagnosed HGG patients were recruited into the phase III study if they were considered by the treating neurosurgeon as candidates for complete resection of the contrast-enhancing portion of their tumor. Patients were randomized to undergo administration of 5-ALA and FGS or conventional microsurgery without 5-ALA administration. Patients were allocated according to the covariables of the following: age (younger or older than 55 years); the Karnofsky performance scale (KPS; better than 80, or not better); eloquent brain tumor location; and study surgeon. The primary endpoints of the study were the proportion of patients with histologically confirmed malignant glioma on central neuropathological review without residual contrast-enhancing tumor on postoperative MRI and progression-free survival at 6 months (PFS-6). Treating neurosurgeons were not blinded or could not be blinded to the treatment arm, which is not feasible for this kind of optical method. However, both neuropathology and neuroradiological assessors were unaware of study group allocation. The first endpoint was to evaluate the utility of 5-ALA FGS for its intended purpose: complete resection of HGG tumors. The second was to correlate this with a clinical benefit for the patients of PFS-6. It is of interest to note how the trial defined the absence of residual contrast-enhancing tumor (CRET in current terminology), as this is sometimes a subject of misunderstanding. Residual enhancement was defined as MR contrast enhancement with a volume larger than 0.175 cm$^3$. The endpoint of complete resection could be misinterpreted to indicate "subtotal" resection if the residual MR contrast enhancement was larger than 0.175 cm$^3$. Rather, the volume of 0.175 cm$^3$ corresponded to 1 voxel on MRI at the time of the study and was actually the limit of spatial resolution of MRI. By contrast, most studies fail to define CRET regarding the interpretation of tiny residual points, smaller than 1 voxel. Just to be put in perspective, 0.175 cm$^3$ residual contrast enhancement (tumor) would be 0.4% of the volume of a typical 40-mL tumor.

The predetermined interim analysis showed both primary endpoints were met with 270 patients analyzed, and the study was terminated prematurely and published.[21] Contrast-enhancing tumor was resected completely in 65% of patients assigned to the 5-ALA group compared with 36% of those assigned to the conventional surgery white light group (difference between groups 29% [95% confidence interval (CI): 17–40]; $p < 0.0001$). Patients allocated to 5-ALA had higher PFS-6 than those allocated to white light (41.0% [32.8–49.2] vs. 21.1% [14.0–28.2]; $p = 0.0003$, Z-test).

The phase III randomized trial with 5-ALA was designed before the chemotherapy agent temozolomide became standard of care in combination with radiotherapy (Stupp protocol) for HGGs.[22] All the patients received only radiotherapy upfront, resulting in a PFS-6 significantly better for 5-ALA group, but still comparably low in either study group in both (41 vs. 21%). A recent 5-ALA multicenter retrospective study completed in Spain analyzed HGG patients treated with the Stupp protocol who underwent tumor resection with or without 5-ALA and found similar differences, with higher PFS-6 rates in both groups (69 vs. 48%; $p = 0.002$).[23]

Both groups did not differ in the frequency of severe adverse events or adverse events in any organ system class reported within 7 days after surgery. This landmark study led to 5-ALA being approved in Europe in 2007 for guidance during malignant glioma surgery and was instrumental for FDA approval of 5-ALA in 2017.

### 3.3.3 Fluorescence and Pathological Morphology

FGS is a tool for guiding resection, so precise identification of tumor by fluorescence is essential. However, trying to measure and express this accuracy is complex. In the special situation of surgical guidance to a tumor, there are many biases and confounders involved in using specificity and sensitivity as measures of diagnostic accuracy, and for calculating the positive (positive predictive value [PPV], fluorescent tumor samples/all fluorescing samples) and negative predictive value (NPV; tumor negative, nonfluorescent samples/all nonfluorescing samples). Chapter 2 in this book is dedicated to this issue (evaluating intraoperative diagnostic methods). However, there are two important nonstatistical issues about glioma pathology and the use of 5-ALA that should be considered.

On the one hand, HGGs are diffuse and heterogeneous tumors, which include regions of necrosis, solid viable tumor, and brain parenchyma with variable degrees of tumor infiltration. There are no uniform criteria to define HGG tumor invasion, so histopathology should be the "gold standard," but it is not perfect. Also, pathology in recurrent GBM is different from pathology in newly diagnosed GBM. Fluorescence and recurrent GBM are considered in Chapter 4 and, principally, the results obtained with newly diagnosed and recurrent HGG cases should not be pooled together.

In addition, 5-ALA tumor fluorescence is heterogeneous, with red, bright fluorescence visible in viable central tumor areas bordered by a gradient of fluorescence intensity toward infiltrative margin of these invasive tumors. It is for this reason that pathological correlations should be considered separately for different fluorescent qualities. The paradigm used for selecting samples will also influence the results. There is little difficulty in selecting a bright red sample from the center of the tumor bulk. However, vaguely fluorescent areas toward the infiltrative border have a fluorescence intensity gradient. Nonfluorescent, negative samples can be harvested immediately next to fluorescing tumor or, very remotely, away from the tumor in the unaffected brain.

Different trials addressing the relationship between fluorescence and histology have utilized different approaches with biopsies of different tumor regions and quantification of the fluorescence signal emitted by the PpIX.

Bright red fluorescence corresponds to the pathology of malignant tumor in most of the analyzed samples of GBM or HGGs, and the PPV reported for solid tumor has been 100% ($n = 72$),[24] 100% ($n = 90$),[25] 100% ($n = 84$),[26] 95.3% ($n = 86$),[27] 97.4% ($n = 38$),[28] and 94% ($n = 99$),[29] this latter group not using the same modified microscope described previously.

When vague fluorescence is considered, the PPV can be different depending on the intensity of the vaguely fluorescent tissue selected and on the pathological definition of true positives. Many samples will have solid tumor, and many will have infiltrative tumor to a varying extent. Completely normal tissue results are quite uncommon. In the first description by Stummer et al, most samples revealed infiltrating tumor (78%, 18/23); the rest revealed solid tumor. In another report, 72 weakly fluorescent samples were collected just at the limit of the fluorescent tissue. The PPV for the presence of tumor tissue was 97%. Only in 6.9% of the samples was a GBM diagnosis possible, while 90.3% of samples had hypercellularity and atypical cells, and 2.8% were defined as being normal.[30] In another detailed analysis, the overall PPV for any kind of tumor tissue in vague fluorescence was 92.2%. Again, more samples revealed infiltration rather than solid tumor.[25] Similar results were obtained by Coburger et al in over 12 vaguely fluorescent samples. One failed to show tumor, 7 were infiltrating, and 4 were solid tumor, with a PPV of 92%.[26]

NPV has been reported as being low in most series but varies with the types of staining by the pathologist, and the distance from the fluorescent tissue to the point where the samples were taken. This is quite understandable, as HGGs are diffuse infiltrating tumors that will invade beyond surgical and radiological limits. Infiltrating glioma cells extend variable distances away from the main tumor mass. Due to the extensive infiltration of these tumor cells even to the contralateral brain, not a single biopsy of the brain may be truly negative in a patient with an HGG.

Different authors have reported detailed results regarding nonfluorescent biopsies. In over 52 biopsies, Stummer et al found solid tumor in 10%, invasive tumor in 40%, and no tumor in 50% of samples[20]; Díez et al ($n = 36$) found solid tumor in 0%, infiltration in 33%, and no tumor in 66%[30]; and Coburger et al ($n = 18$) found solid tumor in 33%, infiltration in 44%, and no tumor in 22% of biopsies.[26] The NPV in other studies with different modes of analysis give varying results, that is, 26%,[27] 37%,[28] and 69%.[29]

In this context, it is important to realize that the majority of nonfluorescent biopsies contain low densities of tumor cells compared to visibly fluorescing tissue. These cells still appear to contain PpIX, which cannot be observed using the unaided eye. Such fluorescence can still be detected by spectrometry[25,31,32] and it has been proposed that spectrometry might be used to increase the sensitivity for detecting tumor infiltration.

Necrosis also fails to reveal fluorescence since it contains no metabolically active tissue. Such biopsies sometimes cause confusion when analyzing nonfluorescent biopsies, as they represent parts of the tumor. However, we do not consider the failure of grossly necrotic tumor to fluoresce as a confounder since necrosis is readily distinguished under white light.

In a different approach, the correlation between fluorescence and pathology has been addressed by using quantitative or semiquantitative scales. The intensity of fluorescence can be quantified using spectrometry, or, on a semi quantitative level, a level of fluorescence intensity can be assigned, typically given as 3 or 4 degrees of intensity. Pathology has been qualitatively graded based on the presence of tumor features or cellularity, and the mitotic index can also be measured and quantified. All the trials to date have found strong correlations between histological features of malignancy and 5-ALA-induced fluorescence.

The intensity of fluorescence qualities perceived by the surgeon has been shown to have a strong association to spectrometry and cell density.[25] Roberts et al published a detailed analysis of the relationship between fluorescence and histopathology, finding a correlation coefficient of 0.51 ($p < 0.001$) for fluorescence and histopathological score, and 0.49 ($p < 0.001$) for fluorescence and tumor burden (Spearman rank).[27]

There also appears to be a relationship between fluorescence intensity and the Ki-67/MIB-1 index, used as an indirect quantifier of tumor cells. Idoate et al found a Ki-67/MIB-1 index of 23.9% (95% CI: 15.2–32.7) in central areas, 6.4% (95% CI: 3.7–9.1) in weakly fluorescing biopsies, and 1.7% (95% CI: 0.9–2.5) in nonfluorescent samples.[24] These differences between areas of peripheral, weak fluorescence, and nonfluorescent biopsies appear particularly relevant, considering that in this study samples were taken in immediate proximity to one another.

The Ki-67/MIB-1 index has also been shown to be higher in fluorescing grade III gliomas than in nonfluorescing tumors.[33]

Fluorescence of the ventricular wall represents a special situation in FGS with 5-ALA. Ventricular wall fluorescence has been observed frequently in surgery for HGG reaching the ventricle, sometimes limited to the area where the tumor reaches the ventricle and sometimes extending significantly further, without clear tumor extensions being visible under white light microscopy or with MRI. This phenomenon is not yet clearly understood. A preliminary report suggested ventricular fluorescence to imply tumor ependymal dissemination with a corresponding high risk of hydrocephalus.[34] This interpretation was not supported by later reports from larger cohorts.[35,36] Biopsies from the ependymal surface have been positive for tumor in around half the cases (5 of 8 in one review[35] and 5 of 11 in the other).[36] Prognosis was worse for all the cases where tumor reached the ventricle, but similar in the cases where the ventricular wall was fluorescent, or not fluorescent.[35]

### 3.3.4 Association between Fluorescence and Radiological Parameters

FGS has been confirmed to be clinically helpful to neurosurgeons for achieving their goal of maximal safe resection in HGG surgery, that is, CRET. However, as stated before, GBM is a diffuse tumor with no real border with the normal brain. However, the MRI T1Gd contrast volume is only a surrogate marker of tumor. Solid 5-ALA fluorescence corresponds mostly to T1Gd, while vague fluorescence appears to exceed this margin.[25,27] When surgeons achieve a complete resection of solidly fluorescing tissue, most patients have a complete resection on T1Gd, even when vague residual fluorescence is left unresected.[20] Initial comparisons of fluorescence quality of the tissue to MRI were achieved using navigation, which is subject to error due to brain shift. The same has been verified recently using intraoperative MRI, with 5-ALA being found to be superior to intraoperative MRI (iMRI) for identification of pathological tissue outside the T1Gd contrast areas.[26,29]

Comparisons between tumor size by 5-ALA-induced fluorescence using MRI-based neuronavigation showed newly diagnosed GBM to have a larger fluorescing volume than expected from T1Gd imaging (average diameter 29 vs. 23 mm),[37] corresponding to a factor of 2 regarding volume. Another group, comparing the tissue resected in cases with complete resection of fluorescent tissue to the tumor volume on T1Gd, found the resected volume was on average a little greater than double the T1Gd volume.[38]

### 3.3.5 Other Clinical Results

Many trials have reported single center experiences with 5-ALA since the randomized phase 3 study. The results are difficult to compare, as the case mix of each center and surgical techniques are different, but CRET rates of around 80% have been reported by multiple authors.[30,39,40,41] Two meta-analyses found 5-ALA FGS increases the rate of resection,[42,43] with the second study reporting a mean CRET rate of 75.4% (95% CI: 67.4–83.5; $p < 0.001$). These rates of CRET are well above the classical value of 30% or less. Thus, the conventional observation of the neurosurgeon missing residual tumor in the majority of cases has now changed. Still, FGS is only a tool that permits visualization of tumor tissue on the surface. In some situations, residual tumor can remain unseen due to overhanging tissue, a deep, narrow surgical corridor, a suboptimal illumination angle, photobleaching, isolated small nodules, or intervening tumor necrosis. Schucht et al prospectively analyzed GBM cases with unintentional incomplete GBM resection using FGS. They found unintentional incomplete resections in 9 out of 151 (6%) patients, a figure much different from earlier figures.[44]

Other groups have published results with lower rates of CRET, below 50%. In this context, it should be remembered that 5-ALA is only a tool for identification of the tumor in the surgical field. It is the responsibility of the surgeon to use this information judiciously. Thus, even with visible tumor intraoperatively, such tumor will not always be resected due to involvement of eloquent brain.[45,46]

As of February 2017, more than 37,000 patients have been operated upon with 5-ALA (data courtesy of Medac, excluding the United States, Japan, Canada, and Korea). 5-ALA FGS appears to work in all GBM cases. No case with GBM pathology has been reported to not have tumor fluorescence after 5-ALA administration. Vague fluorescence has been reported for some GBM cases with atypical MRI (patchy contrast enhancement). Even in this situation, pockets of strong fluorescence were more common.[33]

FGS seems to be also useful in all MR contrast-enhancing grade III gliomas. In tumors without typical radiological features of GBM, 5-ALA appears to highlight the enhancing areas and most malignant regions of tumor.[11,47] In the largest published series, 166 glioma cases without typical radiological features of GBM were operated on using 5-ALA. In this series, contrast enhancement and tumor volume predicted fluorescence. In all, 77.6% of grade III tumors were fluorescent. Fluorescence was correlated with WHO grade ($p < 0.001$) and Ki-67/MIB-1 index ($p < 0.001$), but not with the methyl guanine methyltransferase (MGMT) promoter methylation status, IDH1 mutation status, or 1p19q co-deletion status. The Ki-67/MIB-1 index in fluorescing grade III gliomas was higher than that in nonfluorescing tumors.[33]

### 3.3.6 Adverse Events

Photosensitivity of the skin is a potential adverse event of 5-ALA. Recommendations for the use of 5-ALA include the avoidance of intense light, especially direct sun exposure over a period of 24 hours after 5-ALA administration. Skin erythema has been rarely observed and no serious burns have been reported.

The administration of 5-ALA leads to transient liver enzyme elevation (about twofold over that induced by surgery itself), but no cases of clinically significant liver damage were found in two reviews that included over 300 patients.[48,49] Anemia and thrombocytopenia are mentioned as adverse events in the official approval of the product by EMA, but were more related to surgery rather than the administration of 5-ALA. A review that included 200 cases found no difference to control surgery without 5-ALA.[48]

Surgery with 5-ALA offers the ability for more extensive tumor resection. However, surgical resection of HGGs alone without 5-ALA can lead to neurological deterioration. Not only is it difficult to justify a loss in quality of life for patients with a short life expectancy, but it has also been reported that patients with new motor or language deficits from surgery even had shorter survival.[50] The 5-ALA randomized trial found a nonsignificant but small increase in the number of aphasias reported as severe adverse events in the 5-ALA group. All these patients already had speech impairment before surgery, even after steroid pretreatment. This finding, together with the knowledge that vague fluorescence can be found in infiltrating parts of the tumor, allows the conclusion that functional areas in these patients were already invaded, but were still functional. This observation has led to the recommendation of using intraoperative neurophysiologic monitoring/mapping techniques in combination with FGS if the tumor involves an eloquent area. If a maximal resection is planned, it should be remembered that vague fluorescence could extend beyond MR contrast enhancement regions, and reach eloquent areas beyond the T1Gd limit. Excellent results have been reported with the combination of FGS and neurophysiological monitoring.[39,40,51]

### 3.3.7 Extended Resection

The concept of performing a resection surpassing the MRI T1Gd volume, provided it is safe, has been proposed using different methods (e.g., fluid-attenuated inversion recovery [FLAIR]). However, there is little evidence for this concept as yet.

In a larger, retrospective series, 876 patients with CRET were analyzed, and OS was longer for patients that had a resection surpassing 53% of the abnormal volume on FLAIR imaging.[52] Utilizing FLAIR imaging for resection purposes can be challenging in most cases. Yan et al defined a more selective target to use such as diffusion tensor imaging (DTI). They reported longer OS in patients in whom resection included a volume exceeding the DTI volume of tumor that extended beyond the T1Gd-enhancing tumor.[53]

Amino acid PET is assumed to image a larger volume of brain involved by a GBM tumor than the T1Gd image,[54,55] and better OS has been reported in patients with no residual tumor on postoperative PET in a single-center review.[56] More recently in a multicenter review, OS was longer for patients with less tumor burden on PET before starting radiotherapy.[57] Tissue areas with abnormal signals using PET can be incorporated into neuronavigation for surgical planning, but cannot be updated for resection and brain shift in the intraoperative setting. There is a partial correlation between 5-ALA fluorescence and AA-PET abnormal areas,[33,58] which could be interesting as resection of fluorescence tissue increases the resection of PET abnormal tissue, while abnormal areas in PET would help in predicting the extent of fluorescent tissue.

As has been discussed, vaguely fluorescent tissue reveals brain tissue with tumor infiltration beyond T1Gd positive areas. There is little information on the benefit gained from an additional resection of all fluorescent tissue. In the first publication to observe this difference,[20] patients with some residual vague fluorescence lived 79 weeks versus 101 weeks for the cases without any residual fluorescence. Possibly due to the small sample, this difference was not significant, with only 12 with vague fluorescence compared to 17 patients without any fluorescence. In another study, 52 patients with newly diagnosed GBM and CRET were compared based on the presence of residual fluorescence or not; 25 patients who had no residual fluorescence tissue lived much longer than the 27 with some residual fluorescence tissue (27.0 [22.4–31.6] vs. 17.5 months [12.5–22.5]; $p = 0.015$). The influence of residual fluorescence was maintained in the multivariate analysis with all relevant covariables, with a hazard ratio of 2.5 ($p = 0.041$).[59] Another group has also reported longer OS with FGS supramarginal resection, using a slightly different technique.[60]

Of all the proposed techniques for supramarginal resections, FGS is the easiest to implement as it shows the tissue in real time in the surgical field. Image-based concepts are subject to the brain shift problem, or require time-consuming iMRI. However, the benefit of supramarginal resection remains unclear, and the risk of resecting invading functional brain tissue needs to be carefully considered in every case.

# References

[1] Earnest F, IV, Kelly PJ, Scheithauer BW, et al. Cerebral astrocytomas: histopathologic correlation of MR and CT contrast enhancement with stereotactic biopsy. Radiology. 1988; 166(3):823–827

[2] Vuorinen V, Hinkka S, Färkkilä M, Jääskeläinen J. Debulking or biopsy of malignant glioma in elderly people: a randomised study. Acta Neurochir (Wien). 2003; 145(1):5–10

[3] Brown TJ, Brennan MC, Li M, et al. Association of the extent of resection with survival in glioblastoma: a systematic review and meta-analysis. JAMA Oncol. 2016; 2(11):1460–1469

[4] Albert FKMD, Forsting M, Sartor K, Adams HP, Kunze S. Early postoperative magnetic resonance imaging after resection of malignant glioma: objective evaluation of residual tumor and its influence on regrowth and prognosis. Neurosurgery. 1994; 34(1):45–60, discussion 60–61

[5] Lacroix M, Abi-Said D, Fourney DR, et al. A multivariate analysis of 416 patients with glioblastoma multiforme: prognosis, extent of resection, and survival. J Neurosurg. 2001; 95(2):190–198

[6] Sanai N, Polley MY, McDermott MW, Parsa AT, Berger MS. An extent of resection threshold for newly diagnosed glioblastomas. J Neurosurg. 2011; 115(1):3–8

[7] Stummer W, Reulen HJ, Meinel T, et al. ALA-Glioma Study Group. Extent of resection and survival in glioblastoma multiforme: identification of and adjustment for bias. Neurosurgery. 2008; 62(3):564–576, discussion 564–576

[8] Marko NF, Weil RJ, Schroeder JL, Lang FF, Suki D, Sawaya RE. Extent of resection of glioblastoma revisited: personalized survival modeling facilitates more accurate survival prediction and supports a maximum-safe-resection approach to surgery. J Clin Oncol. 2014; 32(8):774–782

[9] Sanai N, Berger MS. Glioma extent of resection and its impact on patient outcome. Neurosurgery. 2008; 62(4):753–764, discussion 264–266

[10] Orringer D, Lau D, Khatri S, et al. Extent of resection in patients with glioblastoma: limiting factors, perception of resectability, and effect on survival. J Neurosurg. 2012; 117(5):851–859

[11] Widhalm G, Wolfsberger S, Minchev G, et al. 5-Aminolevulinic acid is a promising marker for detection of anaplastic foci in diffusely infiltrating gliomas with nonsignificant contrast enhancement. Cancer. 2010; 116(6): 1545–1552

[12] Stummer W, Stocker S, Novotny A, et al. In vitro and in vivo porphyrin accumulation by C6 glioma cells after exposure to 5-aminolevulinic acid. J Photochem Photobiol B. 1998; 45(2)(3):160–169

[13] Hebeda KM, Saarnak AE, Olivo M, Sterenborg HJ, Wolbers JG. 5-Aminolevulinic acid induced endogenous porphyrin fluorescence in 9L and C6 brain tumours and in the normal rat brain. Acta Neurochir (Wien). 1998; 140(5):503–512, discussion 512–513

[14] Duffner F, Ritz R, Freudenstein D, Weller M, Dietz K, Wessels J. Specific intensity imaging for glioblastoma and neural cell cultures with 5-aminolevulinic acid-derived protoporphyrin IX. J Neurooncol. 2005; 71(2):107–111

[15] Schimanski A, Ebbert L, Sabel MC, et al. Human glioblastoma stem-like cells accumulate protoporphyrin IX when subjected to exogenous 5-aminolaevulinic acid, rendering them sensitive to photodynamic treatment. J Photochem Photobiol B. 2016; 163:203–210

[16] Valdés PA, Samkoe K, O'Hara JA, Roberts DW, Paulsen KD, Pogue BW. Deferoxamine iron chelation increases delta-aminolevulinic acid induced protoporphyrin IX in xenograft glioma model. Photochem Photobiol. 2010; 86(2):471–475

[17] Wang W, Tabu K, Hagiya Y, et al. Enhancement of 5-aminolevulinic acid-based fluorescence detection of side population-defined glioma stem cells by iron chelation. Sci Rep. 2017; 7:42070

[18] Lawrence JE, Steele CJ, Rovin RA, Belton RJ, Jr, Winn RJ. Dexamethasone alone and in combination with desipramine, phenytoin, valproic acid or levetiracetam interferes with 5-ALA-mediated PpIX production and cellular retention in glioblastoma cells. J Neurooncol. 2016; 127(1):15–21

[19] Stummer W, Stocker S, Wagner S, et al. Intraoperative detection of malignant gliomas by 5-aminolevulinic acid-induced porphyrin fluorescence. Neurosurgery. 1998; 42(3):518–525, discussion 525–526

[20] Stummer W, Novotny A, Stepp H, Goetz C, Bise K, Reulen HJ. Fluorescence-guided resection of glioblastoma multiforme by using 5-aminolevulinic acid-induced porphyrins: a prospective study in 52 consecutive patients. J Neurosurg. 2000; 93(6):1003–1013

[21] Stummer W, Pichlmeier U, Meinel T, Wiestler OD, Zanella F, Reulen HJ, ALA-Glioma Study Group. Fluorescence-guided surgery with 5-aminolevulinic acid for resection of malignant glioma: a randomised controlled multicentre phase III trial. Lancet Oncol. 2006; 7(5):392–401

[22] Stupp R, Mason WP, van den Bent MJ, et al. European Organisation for Research and Treatment of Cancer Brain Tumor and Radiotherapy Groups, National Cancer Institute of Canada Clinical Trials Group. Radiotherapy plus concomitant and adjuvant temozolomide for glioblastoma. N Engl J Med. 2005; 352(10):987–996

[23] Díez Valle R, Slof J, Galván J, Arza C, Romariz C, Vidal C, VISIONA study researchers. Observational, retrospective study of the effectiveness of 5-aminolevulinic acid in malignant glioma surgery in Spain (The VISIONA study). Neurologia. 2014; 29(3):131–138

[24] Idoate MA, Díez Valle R, Echeveste J, Tejada S. Pathological characterization of the glioblastoma border as shown during surgery using 5-aminolevulinic acid-induced fluorescence. Neuropathology. 2011; 31(6):575–582

[25] Stummer W, Tonn JC, Goetz C, et al. 5-aminolevulinic acid-derived tumor fluorescence: the diagnostic accuracy of visible fluorescence qualities as corroborated by spectrometry and histology and postoperative imaging. Neurosurgery. 2014; 74(3):310–319, discussion 319–320

[26] Coburger J, Engelke J, Scheuerle A, et al. Tumor detection with 5-aminolevulinic acid fluorescence and Gd-DTPA-enhanced intraoperative MRI at the border of contrast-enhancing lesions: a prospective study based on histopathological assessment. Neurosurg Focus. 2014; 36(2):E3

[27] Roberts DW, Valdés PA, Harris BT, et al. Coregistered fluorescence-enhanced tumor resection of malignant glioma: relationships between δ-aminolevulinic acid-induced protoporphyrin IX fluorescence, magnetic resonance imaging enhancement, and neuropathological parameters. Clinical article. J Neurosurg. 2011; 114(3):595–603

[28] Lau D, Hervey-Jumper SL, Chang S, et al. A prospective phase II clinical trial of 5-aminolevulinic acid to assess the correlation of intraoperative fluorescence intensity and degree of histologic cellularity during resection of high-grade gliomas. J Neurosurg. 201 6; 124(5):1:300–1–3–0–9

[29] Yamada S, Muragaki Y, Maruyama T, Komori T, Okada Y. Role of neurochemical navigation with 5-aminolevulinic acid during intraoperative MRI-guided resection of intracranial malignant gliomas. Clin Neurol Neurosurg. 2015; 130:134–139

[30] Díez Valle R, Tejada Solis S, Idoate Gastearena MA, García de Eulate R, Domínguez Echávarri P, Aristu Mendiroz J. Surgery guided by 5-aminolevulinic fluorescence in glioblastoma: volumetric analysis of extent of resection in single-center experience. J Neurooncol. 2011; 102(1):105–113

[31] Utsuki S, Oka H, Sato S, et al. Possibility of using laser spectroscopy for the intraoperative detection of nonfluorescing brain tumors and the boundaries of brain tumor infiltrates. Technical note. J Neurosurg. 2006; 104(4):618–620

[32] Valdés PA, Kim A, Brantsch M, et al. δ-aminolevulinic acid-induced protoporphyrin IX concentration correlates with histopathologic markers of malignancy in human gliomas: the need for quantitative fluorescence-guided resection to identify regions of increasing malignancy. Neuro-oncol. 2011; 13 (8):846–856

[33] Jaber M, Wölfer J, Ewelt C, et al. The value of 5-aminolevulinic acid in low-grade gliomas and high-grade gliomas lacking glioblastoma imaging features: an analysis based on fluorescence, magnetic resonance imaging, 18F-fluoroethyl tyrosine positron emission tomography, and tumor molecular factors. Neurosurgery. 2016; 78(3):401–411, discussion 411

[34] Hayashi Y, Nakada M, Tanaka S, et al. Implication of 5-aminolevulinic acid fluorescence of the ventricular wall for postoperative communicating hydrocephalus associated with cerebrospinal fluid dissemination in patients with glioblastoma multiforme: a report of 7 cases. J Neurosurg. 2010; 112(5): 1015–1019

[35] Tejada-Solís S, Aldave-Orzaiz G, Pay-Valverde E, Marigil-Sánchez M, Idoate-Gastearena MA, Díez-Valle R. Prognostic value of ventricular wall fluorescence

during 5-aminolevulinic-guided surgery for glioblastoma. Acta Neurochir (Wien). 2012; 154(11):1997–2002, discussion 2002

[36] Moon JH, Kim SH, Shim JK, et al. Histopathological implications of ventricle wall 5-aminolevulinic acid-induced fluorescence in the absence of tumor involvement on magnetic resonance images. Oncol Rep. 2016; 36(2):837–844

[37] Eljamel S, Petersen M, Valentine R, et al. Comparison of intraoperative fluorescence and MRI image guided neuronavigation in malignant brain tumours, a prospective controlled study. Photodiagn Photodyn Ther. 2013; 10 (4):356–361

[38] Schucht P, Knittel S, Slotboom J, et al. 5-ALA complete resections go beyond MR contrast enhancement: shift corrected volumetric analysis of the extent of resection in surgery for glioblastoma. Acta Neurochir (Wien). 2014; 156 (2):305–312, discussion 312

[39] Schucht P, Beck J, Abu-Isa J, et al. Gross total resection rates in contemporary glioblastoma surgery: results of an institutional protocol combining 5-aminolevulinic acid intraoperative fluorescence imaging and brain mapping. Neurosurgery. 2012; 71(5):927–935, discussion 935–936

[40] Della Puppa A, De Pellegrin S, d'Avella E, et al. 5-aminolevulinic acid (5-ALA) fluorescence guided surgery of high-grade gliomas in eloquent areas assisted by functional mapping. Our experience and review of the literature. Acta Neurochir (Wien). 2013; 155(6):965–972, discussion 972

[41] Schucht P, Seidel K, Beck J, et al. Intraoperative monopolar mapping during 5-ALA-guided resections of glioblastomas adjacent to motor eloquent areas: evaluation of resection rates and neurological outcome. Neurosurg Focus. 2014; 37(6):E16

[42] Zhao S, Wu J, Wang C, et al. Intraoperative fluorescence-guided resection of high-grade malignant gliomas using 5-aminolevulinic acid-induced porphyrins: a systematic review and meta-analysis of prospective studies. PLoS One. 2013; 8(5):e63682

[43] Eljamel S. 5-ALA fluorescence image guided resection of glioblastoma multiforme: a meta-analysis of the literature. Int J Mol Sci. 2015; 16(5): 10443–10456

[44] Schucht P, Murek M, Jilch A, et al. Early re-do surgery for glioblastoma is a feasible and safe strategy to achieve complete resection of enhancing tumor. PLoS One. 2013; 8(11):e79846

[45] Roder C, Bisdas S, Ebner FH, et al. Maximizing the extent of resection and survival benefit of patients in glioblastoma surgery: high-field iMRI versus conventional and 5-ALA-assisted surgery. Eur J Surg Oncol. 2014; 40(3): 297–304

[46] Teixidor P, Arráez MA, Villalba G, et al. Safety and efficacy of 5-aminolevulinic acid for high grade glioma in usual clinical practice: a prospective cohort study. PLoS One. 2016; 11(2):e0149244

[47] Widhalm G, Kiesel B, Woehrer A, et al. 5-aminolevulinic acid induced fluorescence is a powerful intraoperative marker for precise histopathological grading of gliomas with non-significant contrast-enhancement. PLoS One. 2013; 8(10):e76988

[48] Honorato-Cia C, Martinez-Simón A, Cacho-Asenjo E, Guillén-Grima F, Tejada-Solís S, Diez-Valle R. Safety profile of 5-aminolevulinic acid as a surgical adjunct in clinical practice: a review of 207 cases from 2008 to 2013. J Neurosurg Anesthesiol. 2015; 27(4):304–309

[49] Offersen CM, Skjoeth-Rasmussen J. Evaluation of the risk of liver damage from the use of 5-aminolevulinic acid for intra-operative identification and resection in patients with malignant gliomas. Acta Neurochir (Wien). 2017; 159(1):145–150

[50] McGirt MJ, Mukherjee D, Chaichana KL, Than KD, Weingart JD, Quinones-Hinojosa A. Association of surgically acquired motor and language deficits on overall survival after resection of glioblastoma multiforme. Neurosurgery. 2009; 65(3):463–469, discussion 469–470

[51] Feigl G, Ritz R, Moraes M, et al. Resection of malignant brain tumors in eloquent cortical areas: a new multimodal approach combining 5-aminolevulinic acid and intraoperative monitoring. J Neurosurg. 20 1 0; 113 (2):352–357

[52] Li YM, Suki D, Hess K, Sawaya R. The influence of maximum safe resection of glioblastoma on survival in 1229 patients: can we do better than gross-total resection? J Neurosurg. 2016; 124(4):977–988

[53] Yan JL, van der Hoorn A, Larkin TJ, Boonzaier NR, Matys T, Price SJ. Extent of resection of peritumoral diffusion tensor imaging-detected abnormality as a predictor of survival in adult glioblastoma patients. J Neurosurg. 201 7(1): 234–241

[54] Miwa K, Shinoda J, Yano H, et al. Discrepancy between lesion distributions on methionine PET and MR images in patients with glioblastoma multiforme: insight from a PET and MR fusion image study. J Neurol Neurosurg Psychiatry. 2004; 75(10):1457–1462

[55] Arbizu J, Tejada S, Marti-Climent JM, et al. Quantitative volumetric analysis of gliomas with sequential MRI and 11C-methionine PET assessment: patterns of integration in therapy planning. Eur J Nucl Med Mol Imaging. 2012; 39(5): 771–781

[56] Pirotte BJ, Levivier M, Goldman S, et al. Positron emission tomography-guided volumetric resection of supratentorial high-grade gliomas: a survival analysis in 66 consecutive patients. Neurosurgery. 2009; 64(3):471–481, discussion 481

[57] Suchorska B, Jansen NL, Linn J, et al. German Glioma Network. Biological tumor volume in 18FET-PET before radiochemotherapy correlates with survival in GBM. Neurology. 2015; 84(7):710–719

[58] Floeth FW, Sabel M, Ewelt C, et al. Comparison of (18)F-FET PET and 5-ALA fluorescence in cerebral gliomas. Eur J Nucl Med Mol Imaging. 2011; 38(4): 731–741

[59] Aldave G, Tejada S, Pay E, et al. Prognostic value of residual fluorescent tissue in glioblastoma patients after gross total resection in 5-aminolevulinic Acid-guided surgery. Neurosurgery. 2013; 72(6):915–920, discussion 920–921

[60] Eyüpoglu IY, Hore N, Merkel A, Buslei R, Buchfelder M, Savaskan N. Supra-complete surgery via dual intraoperative visualization approach (DiVA) prolongs patient survival in glioblastoma. Oncotarget. 2016; 7(18):25755–25768

# 4 5-Aminolevulinic Acid and Recurrent High-Grade Gliomas

*Ramin A. Morshed, Darryl Lau, Seunggu Jude Han, Barbara Kiesel, and Mitchel S. Berger*

**Abstract**

Greater extent of resection has an impact on clinical outcomes in the setting of recurrent malignant gliomas. However, achieving this goal in cases with invasive tumor is difficult even with the use of neuronavigation. Furthermore, in the context of recurrence, there are other unique challenges including identification of tumor versus pseudoprogression on preoperative imaging and the impact of treatment-related tissue changes on intraoperative identification of true tumor tissue. 5-aminolevulinic acid (5-ALA) fluorescence-guided surgery offers an aide to identify tumor tissue intraoperatively and has been associated with greater extent of resection and improved outcomes for patients with newly diagnosed high-grade gliomas. Evidence of this intraoperative technique in the context of recurrent gliomas is less robust but still encouraging. In this chapter, we review the impact that 5-ALA fluorescence-guided surgery has on extent of resection as well as morbidity and mortality. Furthermore, we discuss how fluorescence may be affected in the context of recurrent lesions and the correlation between fluorescence and histological evidence of tumor tissue.

*Keywords:* 5-ALA, recurrent glioma, correlation of fluorescence and histology, extent of resection

## 4.1 Introduction

Evidence continues to demonstrate that greater extent of surgical resection affects both progression-free survival (PFS) and overall survival (OS) in the context of high-grade gliomas.[1,2,3,4] Even a subtotal resection (STR) of at least 78% of the contrast-enhancing portion of tumor in patients with newly diagnosed glioblastoma (GBM) has led to survival benefits.[5] For recurrent glioma, surgery can be multipurpose: to aid in diagnosis of recurrent tumor, to debulk tumor adjacent to eloquent cortex to maintain quality of life, and to achieve further cytological reduction to improve survival. As evidence of the latter, there are several reports demonstrating that complete extent of resection (EOR) of the contrast-enhancing portion of tumor leads to greater survival for patients with recurrent high-grade glioma.[6,7,8] Furthermore, complete resection at first recurrence has even been found to compensate for an incomplete tumor removal at the initial surgery in terms of impact on survival.[6] Therefore, while the goal of reoperation for patients with possible recurrence may vary, for many the purpose is still to achieve the greatest EOR possible without compromising neurological function.

Yet, achieving a high-degree of resection, or gross total resection (GTR), is challenging for many reasons. Across the board, in practice, GTR of the contrast-enhancing tumor is achieved in only 20 to 30% of patients.[1,2,3,4,9,10] Even in patients amenable to GTR based on preoperative imaging, it is achieved in only 24% despite the use of neuronavigation.[10] Sometimes a complete resection of the tumor is not feasible due to the presence of functional tissue. As one approaches the invasive tumor border in cases of high-grade malignant glioma, the distinction between pathologic and normal tissue can be almost impossible to make based solely on gross visualization and tactile feedback without the aid of other tools and technologies. Thus, fluorescence-guided techniques were introduced to brain tumor resections to aide a surgeon's ability to achieve an extensive resection when possible.

5-aminolevulinic acid (5-ALA) is a compound that has been used to improve the intraoperative visualization of malignant glioma tissue. European data on 5-ALA have shown promising results demonstrating greater EOR and improved 6-month PFS and OS in the context of newly diagnosed, untreated grade III and IV malignant gliomas.[11] However, class I evidence of the use of 5-ALA in the context of recurrent high-grade gliomas is not available, and ongoing work is still required to determine its utility in this disease context. Here, we review clinical outcome data and considerations for the use of 5-ALA for recurrent high-grade gliomas. Topics covered include its impact on EOR, correlation with tumor pathology, and the influence of adjuvant therapies on fluorescence.

## 4.2 Considerations for the Use of 5-Aminolevulinic Acid

There are many considerations when selecting patients with recurrent gliomas for 5-ALA fluorescence-guided surgery (FGS). As with an initial surgery with 5-ALA, preoperative labs are acquired to rule out organ and marrow dysfunction. This involves ensuring that the leukocyte count is greater than 3,000/µL, the absolute neutrophil count is greater than 1,500/µL, the platelet count is greater than 100,000 µL, the total bilirubin level is within normal limits, aspartate aminotransferase (AST)/alanine aminotransferase (ALT) are less than 2.4 times the upper normal limit, and creatinine is within normal limits with a creatinine clearance greater than 60 mL/min/1.73m$^2$. Adjuvant therapies may lead to abnormalities within these values preventing a patient from being a candidate for this approach. For example, temozolomide has led to 7% of patients developing leukopenia, 7% developing neutropenia, 12% developing thrombocytopenia, and 1% developing anemia.[12] Exclusion criteria for the use of 5-ALA usually include patients who report a history of allergy to compounds of similar chemical or biological composition to 5-ALA, personal or family history of porphyria, pregnancy, and hypotension.

Prior to surgery, a single administration of ALA (20 mg/kg body weight) is given orally 3 hours before anesthesia. After administration, light precautions are undertaken to protect the patient from the effects of skin photosensitivity during surgery and the postoperative period. Fortunately, the complication rate associated with 5-ALA is low. Lau et al found a 5-ALA attributable complication rate of 3.4% with patients developing intraoperative hypotension and a rash across the torso that responded to low oral doses of diphenhydramine.[13] Stummer et al reported minor elevations in GGT and AST/ALT at 24 hours but otherwise did not see a difference in adverse events between the 5-ALA group and the control group.[11]

## 4.3 Impact on Extent of Resection

The primary purpose of 5-ALA FGS is to provide better visualization of pathological tissue in order to achieve a greater EOR. Limitations to a more extensive resection include invasion into eloquent cortex and inability to identify pathological tissue. Typically, the goal for high-grade gliomas is to remove the contrast-enhancing component seen on imaging. Some groups, however, have noted that fluorescent tissue boundaries often extend past the contrast-enhancing component seen on neuronavigation.[14] Thus, the extent of fluorescent tissue resection is becoming another important benchmark to measure tumor removal.[15]

There are numerous reports that demonstrate high rates of extensive resection can be achieved with 5-ALA FGS in cases of recurrent malignant gliomas. Hickmann et al examined outcomes in 58 patients undergoing reoperation with 5-ALA for recurrent gliomas. Mean EOR based on MRI was 91.1% and ranged from 17.5 to 100%. More than 98% of tumor volume resection was achieved in the majority (57.1%) of surgeries. Complete resection of all fluorescent tissue was achieved in 64.1% of all surgeries and was associated with a significantly greater contrast-enhancing EOR, demonstrating 5-ALA's role in promoting identification of enhancing tumor.[15] Within a subgroup of 33 recurrent high-grade gliomas, Della Puppa et al reported a GTR (>98% resection) rate of 94%.[14] Other smaller studies have also demonstrated high rates of complete tumor resection. Tykocki et al examined outcomes in 5-ALA-guided surgery in both primary and recurrent malignant glioma. Of the three patients with recurrent tumors, all demonstrated fluorescence and underwent GTR.[16] Archavlis et al reported that GTR and STR could be achieved in 59 and 41%, respectively, of 17 patients undergoing 5-ALA-guided re-resection of a malignant glioma. However, 47% of these tumors involved at least one eloquent region, limiting the ability to achieve a GTR.[17]

Other groups have examined 5-ALA's ability to improve upon other tumor-identifying methods. Quick-Weller et al examined EOR when 5-ALA guidance was used in conjunction with intraoperative MRI and demonstrated complete resection in all seven patients within the cohort.[18] Coburger et al also compared EOR of GBM for patients undergoing intraoperative MRI with or without 5-ALA guidance. In contrast to the report by Quick-Weller et al, these authors found for the six patients with recurrent tumor that EOR was similar whether or not 5-ALA was used.[19] However, such results have to be cautiously interpreted given the limited number of patients.

## 4.4 Impact on Progression Free Survival, Overall Survival, and Morbidity

There is evidence that 5-ALA FGS improves both PFS and OS when used for newly diagnosed high-grade malignant gliomas.[11] However, very few studies have been able to examine the impact of surgery using 5-ALA on PFS and OS in the context of recurrent disease. In Hickmann et al, the 58 patients undergoing reoperation with 5-ALA FGS for recurrent gliomas had longer OS compared to 65 patients undergoing repeat surgery without 5-ALA (when patients with long-term survival > 5 years were excluded from the control arm). However, no significant impact on PFS was observed.[15] Archavlis et al compared outcomes in 17 patients undergoing 5-ALA FGS and dense-dose temozolomide, and interstitial irradiation to historical controls treated with dense-dose temozolomide alone. Although it is difficult to isolate which particular therapies may have been responsible for the benefit, the authors reported an improved PFS of 3.5 months and survival after the experimental treatment by 3 months in the multimodal treatment group.[17] Aside from these few reports, there is only the indirect relationship demonstrating that surgery utilizing 5-ALA increases EOR and greater EOR leads to improved PFS and OS in patients with recurrent gliomas.

One concern with 5-ALA FGS is that if greater EOR is achieved, this may lead to higher rates of neurological deficits postoperatively if appropriate monitoring and mapping techniques are not used. In Ringel et al, re-resection (not involving 5-ALA-guided surgery) was associated with an 8% rate of new permanent neurological deficits, slightly higher than the 5% rate observed for the initial surgery.[6] However, Stummer et al did not see an impact of the use of 5-ALA on postoperative total stroke-scale scores between the experimental and control arm, suggesting that while 5-ALA FGS can improve EOR, the increased EOR does not increase neurological impairment.[11] A follow-up study suggested that within 48 hours, the rate of deterioration as measured by the National Institutes of Health Stroke Scale (NIH-SS) was more frequent in a cohort of patients operated on using 5-ALA FGS compared to controls. However, by 3 months, this difference was not significant.[20] In the study by Hickmann et al, there was no reported increase in new focal neurologic deficit based on whether fluorescence was observed intraoperatively or not. There was also no significant correlation between greater EOR and new focal deficits.[15] Overall, it appears that increased EOR using 5-ALA may lead to worsening of neurological deficits in the short-term but that the rate of deficits are comparable to conventional surgery over time.

## 4.5 Recurrent Tumor Fluorescence and Histological Correlation

One concern with the use of 5-ALA fluorescence is that its utility may be impacted by recurrent tumor characteristics, adjuvant therapies, and the timing of these therapies. Tissue changes such as gliosis, necrosis, and vascular hyalinization are frequently seen after adjuvant radiotherapy and chemotherapy[21,22,23,24,25,26,27,28] and their effect on both tumor and normal tissue as well as the impact on the blood–brain barrier (BBB) could potentially change the sensitivity and specificity of 5-ALA.

One point of interest is the percentage of recurrent tumors that are 5-ALA positive. Hickmann et al reported positive fluorescence in 84.1% of reoperations. The vast majority of these patients (87.3%) had undergone adjuvant therapy before recurrence, with 49.2% receiving radiotherapy in conjunction with some type of chemotherapy. Fluorescent tumors were more

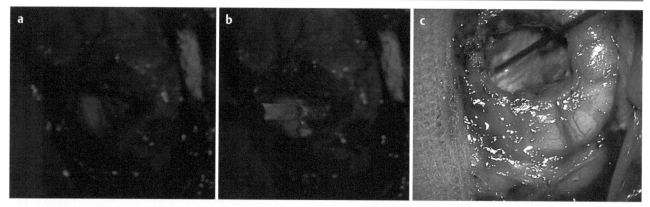

**Fig. 4.1** Intraoperative images of the use of a wavelength-specific lighted suction device to aid in 5-aminolevulinic acid (5-ALA) fluorescence-guided surgery. **(a)** Initially, no fluorescence tissue is observed deep within a resection cavity. **(b)** After providing more focused wavelength-specific excitation light within the resection cavity, areas of fluorescent tissue become more visible, demonstrating the critical need for adequate light exposure. **(c)** As seen under white light, identification of this pathological tissue would be difficult without the aid of 5-ALA.

frequently contrast enhancing on MRI, WHO grade IV, and isocitrate dehydrogenase (IDH) mutated. All tumors with positive MRI contrast enhancement but negative intraoperative fluorescence demonstrated oligodendroglial differentiation, and all but one MRI nonenhancing, nonfluorescent tumors were oligodendroglial tumors.[15] Nabavi et al found that all 36 patients in their cohort displayed some degree of 5-ALA fluorescence. Of these, 97% had received standard radiotherapy and 67% had received some type of chemotherapy.[29] In Kamp et al, only 1 of 13 patients was 5-ALA negative. Interestingly, all patients had received radiotherapy except for the one 5-ALA negative patient.[30] Utsuki et al reported that six of seven recurrent GBMs and five of six recurrent anaplastic astrocytomas were fluorescent.[31] Collectively, these studies demonstrate that the vast majority of recurrent gliomas are 5-ALA positive.

Other reports have investigated the correlation between 5-ALA fluorescence and the histological presence or absence of tumor cells. Nabavi et al examined 36 patients with recurrent glioma who underwent 5-ALA FGS. For biopsied areas that appeared nonpathologic under white light but fluoresced, the positive predictive value (PPV) was 93% for the presence of tumor. For tissue that appeared pathologic under white light and fluoresced, the PPV was even greater at 99.5%. However, within normal-appearing tissue under white light, there was a difference in PPV based on the fluorescence intensity with areas of strong and weak fluorescence having a PPV for tumor of 96.9 and 90.3%, respectively.[29] Lau et al examined the correlation of intensity of 5-ALA fluorescence with the degree of tumor cellularity. A total of 211 biopsies from 59 patients were included in the study, 110 of which were from patients with recurrent high-grade glioma. For tissue with a maximum 5-ALA fluorescence intensity (intensity score of 3) within the recurrent group, the PPV for presence of tumor was 93.8%, which is similar to newly resected GBM and grade III gliomas. For nonfluorescent tissue, the negative predictive value for absence of tumor was 31.0%.[13] Therefore, while strong tissue fluorescence is a good predictor for the presence of tumor, the absence of fluorescence is not necessarily a good marker for the absence of tumor. The authors also reported that for the recurrent glioma group, a fluorescence intensity grading scale and tumor cellularity grading scale did correlate with a Spearman correlation coefficient of 0.62.[13]

Given this, it is important to consider factors that influence fluorescence intensity. Emitted tissue fluorescence in 5-ALA-guided surgery is greatly dependent upon exposure of protoporphyrin IX to a light source (e.g., microscope light). Barriers to light penetration may include the depth of the surgical field, presence of overhanging tissue, shadows created by instruments, magnification and focus settings of the microscope, and even patient positioning. This is especially relevant in the setting of recurrent tumor when resection may take place within a preexisting deep cavity. If exposure to light is diminished, patches of tumor cells may not fluoresce intensely and, thus, be discredited as normal brain tissue. Devices that provide more focused wavelength-specific excitation light to a target area may lead to improved visualization of tumor fluorescence, even in lesions within prior resection cavities (▶ Fig. 4.1). Video 4.1 depicts this technique.

It is also important to consider what factors impact false-positive fluorescence at the time of reoperation. Kamp et al retrospectively examined 313 patients who underwent resection for suspected contrast-enhancing tumor recurrence and assessed 5-ALA fluorescence in the resected tissue samples sent for pathology. Thirteen out of 313 patients demonstrated only reactive changes without active recurrent tumor tissue, and of these 13, the majority demonstrated some degree of 5-ALA fluorescence. Seven displayed solid, five displayed vague, and one displayed no 5-ALA fluorescence intraoperatively.[30] In the study by Nabavi et al, reactive or regressive tissue demonstrated a false-positive rate of only 3.5%. Of note, the authors reported that neither necrotic areas nor scar tissue displayed any fluorescence.[29] The cohorts between these two studies were slightly different as about half the patients in the Kamp et al study had undergone a reoperation and an intensified adjuvant salvage therapy. Utsuki et al reported on positive fluorescent signal without histological evidence of tumor in 5 of 11 patients with recurrent malignant glioma (false-positive rate of 45.4%) and was thought to be related to leaky BBB as these false-positive areas were found in areas of peritumoral edema and inflammatory cell/reactive astrocyte infiltration.[31]

# 4.6 Conclusion

In summary, 5-ALA fluorescence guidance is a safe technique that positively impacts EOR of recurrent high-grade gliomas without causing worse neurological deficits. Although some small nonrandomized cohorts of patients demonstrate possible improvement in PFS and OS, further studies are needed to provide clear evidence of this in the context of recurrent disease. Fortunately, the majority of recurrent tumors appear to be 5-ALA positive, but how various adjuvant treatments and inherent tumor characteristics impact the degree of fluorescence positivity is still incompletely understood.

# References

[1] Barker FG, II, Prados MD, Chang SM, et al. Radiation response and survival time in patients with glioblastoma multiforme. J Neurosurg. 1996; 84(3): 442–448

[2] Albert FK, Forsting M, Sartor K, Adams HP, Kunze S. Early postoperative magnetic resonance imaging after resection of malignant glioma: objective evaluation of residual tumor and its influence on regrowth and prognosis. Neurosurgery. 1994; 34(1):45–60, discussion 60–61

[3] Vecht CJ, Avezaat CJ, van Putten WL, Eijkenboom WM, Stefanko SZ. The influence of the extent of surgery on the neurological function and survival in malignant glioma. A retrospective analysis in 243 patients. J Neurol Neurosurg Psychiatry. 1990; 53(6):466–471

[4] Simpson JR, Horton J, Scott C, et al. Influence of location and extent of surgical resection on survival of patients with glioblastoma multiforme: results of three consecutive Radiation Therapy Oncology Group (RTOG) clinical trials. Int J Radiat Oncol Biol Phys. 1993; 26(2):239–244

[5] Sanai N, Polley M-Y, McDermott MW, Parsa AT, Berger MS. An extent of resection threshold for newly diagnosed glioblastomas. J Neurosurg. 2011; 115(1):3–8

[6] Ringel F, Pape H, Sabel M, et al. SN1 study group. Clinical benefit from resection of recurrent glioblastomas: results of a multicenter study including 503 patients with recurrent glioblastomas undergoing surgical resection. Neuro-oncol. 2016; 18(1):96–104

[7] Suchorska B, Weller M, Tabatabai G, et al. Complete resection of contrast-enhancing tumor volume is associated with improved survival in recurrent glioblastoma-results from the DIRECTOR trial. Neuro-oncol. 2016; 18(4):549–556

[8] Perrini P, Gambacciani C, Weiss A, et al. Survival outcomes following repeat surgery for recurrent glioblastoma: a single-center retrospective analysis. J Neurooncol. 2017; 131(3):585–591

[9] Orringer D, Lau D, Khatri S, et al. Extent of resection in patients with glioblastoma: limiting factors, perception of resectability, and effect on survival. J Neurosurg. 2012; 117(5):851–859

[10] Willems PW, Taphoorn MJ, Burger H, Berkelbach van der Sprenkel JW, Tulleken CA. Effectiveness of neuronavigation in resecting solitary intracerebral contrast-enhancing tumors: a randomized controlled trial. J Neurosurg. 2006; 104(3):360–368

[11] Stummer W, Pichlmeier U, Meinel T, Wiestler OD, Zanella F, Reulen HJ, ALA-Glioma Study Group. Fluorescence-guided surgery with 5-aminolevulinic acid for resection of malignant glioma: a randomised controlled multicentre phase III trial. Lancet Oncol. 2006; 7(5):392–401

[12] Stupp R, Mason WP, van den Bent MJ, et al. European Organisation for Research and Treatment of Cancer Brain Tumor and Radiotherapy Groups, National Cancer Institute of Canada Clinical Trials Group. Radiotherapy plus concomitant and adjuvant temozolomide for glioblastoma. N Engl J Med. 2005; 352(10):987–996

[13] Lau D, Hervey-Jumper SL, Chang S, et al. A prospective phase II clinical trial of 5-aminolevulinic acid to assess the correlation of intraoperative fluorescence intensity and degree of histologic cellularity during resection of high-grade gliomas. J Neurosurg. 2016; 124(5):1300–1309

[14] Della Puppa A, Ciccarino P, Lombardi G, Rolma G, Cecchin D, Rossetto M. 5-Aminolevulinic acid fluorescence in high grade glioma surgery: surgical outcome, intraoperative findings, and fluorescence patterns. BioMed Res Int. 2014; 2014:232561

[15] Hickmann AK, Nadji-Ohl M, Hopf NJ. Feasibility of fluorescence-guided resection of recurrent gliomas using five-aminolevulinic acid: retrospective analysis of surgical and neurological outcome in 58 patients. J Neurooncol. 2015; 122(1):151–160

[16] Tykocki T, Michalik R, Bonicki W, Nauman P. Fluorescence-guided resection of primary and recurrent malignant gliomas with 5-aminolevulinic acid. Preliminary results. Neurol Neurochir Pol. 2012; 46(1):47–51

[17] Archavlis E, Tselis N, Birn G, Ulrich P, Zamboglou N. Salvage therapy for recurrent glioblastoma multiforme: a multimodal approach combining fluorescence-guided resurgery, interstitial irradiation, and chemotherapy. Neurol Res. 2014; 36(12):1047–1055

[18] Quick-Weller J, Lescher S, Forster M-T, Konczalla J, Seifert V, Senft C. Combination of 5-ALA and iMRI in re-resection of recurrent glioblastoma. Br J Neurosurg. 2016; 30(3):313–317

[19] Coburger J, Hagel V, Wirtz CR, König R. Surgery for glioblastoma: impact of the combined use of 5-aminolevulinic acid and intraoperative MRI on extent of resection and survival. PLoS One. 2015; 10(6):e0131872

[20] Stummer W, Tonn J-CC, Mehdorn HM, et al. ALA-Glioma Study Group. Counterbalancing risks and gains from extended resections in malignant glioma surgery: a supplemental analysis from the randomized 5-aminolevulinic acid glioma resection study. Clinical article. J Neurosurg. 2011; 114(3):613–623

[21] Brandes AA, Tosoni A, Spagnolli F, et al. Disease progression or pseudoprogression after concomitant radiochemotherapy treatment: pitfalls in neurooncology. Neuro-oncol. 2008; 10(3):361–367

[22] Chamberlain MC, Glantz MJ, Chalmers L, Van Horn A, Sloan AE. Early necrosis following concurrent Temodar and radiotherapy in patients with glioblastoma. J Neurooncol. 2007; 82(1):81–83

[23] Chaskis C, Neyns B, Michotte A, De Ridder M, Everaert H. Pseudoprogression after radiotherapy with concurrent temozolomide for high-grade glioma: clinical observations and working recommendations. Surg Neurol. 2009; 72 (4):423–428

[24] de Wit MCY, de Bruin HG, Eijkenboom W, Sillevis Smitt PAE, van den Bent MJ. Immediate post-radiotherapy changes in malignant glioma can mimic tumor progression. Neurology. 2004; 63(3):535–537

[25] Giglio P, Gilbert MR. Cerebral radiation necrosis. Neurologist. 2003; 9(4):180–188

[26] Gunjur A, Lau E, Taouk Y, Ryan G. Early post-treatment pseudo-progression amongst glioblastoma multiforme patients treated with radiotherapy and temozolomide: a retrospective analysis. J Med Imaging Radiat Oncol. 2011; 55(6):603–610

[27] Kumar AJ, Leeds NE, Fuller GN, et al. Malignant gliomas: MR imaging spectrum of radiation therapy- and chemotherapy-induced necrosis of the brain after treatment. Radiology. 2000; 217(2):377–384

[28] Taal W, Brandsma D, de Bruin HG, et al. Incidence of early pseudoprogression in a cohort of malignant glioma patients treated with chemoirradiation with temozolomide. Cancer. 2008; 113(2):405–410

[29] Nabavi A, Thurm H, Zountsas B, et al. 5-ALA Recurrent Glioma Study Group. Five-aminolevulinic acid for fluorescence-guided resection of recurrent malignant gliomas: a phase II study. Neurosurgery. 2009; 65(6):1070–1076, discussion 1076–1077

[30] Kamp MA, Felsberg J, Sadat H, et al. 5-ALA-induced fluorescence behavior of reactive tissue changes following glioblastoma treatment with radiation and chemotherapy. Acta Neurochir (Wien). 2015; 157(2):207–213, discussion 213–214

[31] Utsuki S, Oka H, Sato S, et al. Histological examination of false positive tissue resection using 5-aminolevulinic acid-induced fluorescence guidance. Neurol Med Chir (Tokyo). 2007; 47(5):210–213, discussion 213–214

# 5 5-Aminolevulinic Acid in Low-Grade Gliomas

*Georg Widhalm, Mitchel S. Berger, and Johannes Wölfer*

**Abstract**

5-aminolevulinic acid (5-ALA)-induced tumor fluorescence represents a powerful tool to optimize the resection of high-grade gliomas (HGG). Use of 5-ALA for the fluorescence-guided surgery (FGS) of low-grade glioma (LGG) tumors in patients is actively being studied. Currently, 5-ALA-induced fluorescence helps identify anaplastic tumor areas in diffuse infiltrating gliomas without MRI contrast enhancement that would have gone unnoticed otherwise, potentially subjecting patients to insufficient therapies. Further, specific imaging and metabolic parameters that enhance the propensity of suspected low-grade tumors to show significant and surgically useful fluorescence have been identified. However, the task of intraoperatively identifying the margins of a diffuse, straight LGG cannot yet be reliably addressed by the technique in its current setup, even though the differences of 5-ALA metabolism between LGG and HGG seem to be only quantitative rather than qualitative. Introducing methods such as fluorescence spectroscopy or confocal microscopy might considerably expand the field of FGS in order to optimize intraoperative visualization and thus maximize resection of LGG.

*Keywords:* 5-ALA, low-grade gliomas, anaplastic focus, sampling error, fluorescence spectroscopy, confocal microscopy

## 5.1 Introduction

Selective intraoperative visualization of malignant gliomas has become feasible with the introduction of 5-aminolevulinic acid (5-ALA)-induced fluorescence into the neurosurgical field in the last years. Fluorescence-guided resection using 5-ALA has been established as standard for surgery of high-grade gliomas (HGG) at many neurosurgical centers worldwide. Low-grade gliomas (LGG) were generally thought to be inaccessible to this technique, but recent data do provide support in estimating its usefulness in a subgroup of these tumors that do not show the classical hallmarks of malignant gliomas. This chapter will try to span the distance between the evidence for the use of 5-ALA in LGGs with the current visualization techniques and the possibly extended range of indications with future developments.

## 5.2 Low-Grade Gliomas

### 5.2.1 Background

Diffusely infiltrating gliomas (DIGs) represent the most common primary brain tumors in adults.[1] Based on specific histopathological criteria defined by the World Health Organization (WHO), the usually slow-growing LGG (WHO grade II) are distinguished from the aggressive HGG (WHO grades III and IV).[1] Annually, 2,700 to 4,600 cases of LGG are diagnosed in the United States, and such tumors frequently present in the second to fourth decade.[2,3] The first clinical symptom of LGG is the occurrence of new epileptic seizures in up to 80% of cases.[2]

Further frequent symptoms include changes of mental status, clinical signs of increased intracranial pressure, and focal neurological deficits.[4]

### 5.2.2 Preoperative Imaging

MRI represents the imaging technique of choice to further investigate suspected LGG.[5] To detect a potential disruption of the blood–brain barrier (BBB), additional administration of contrast medium during the MR investigation is of major importance.[5] Contrary to HGG, significant contrast enhancement (CE) on MRI is usually absent in LGG.[6] To further characterize suspected LGG, advanced MRI methods such as MR spectroscopy (MRS), perfusion MRI, diffusion-weighted images (DWI), and diffusion tensor imaging (DTI) were established in the last decade.[5,7] Additionally, positron emission tomography (PET) using amino acid tracers such as [18]F-fluoroethyl-L-tyrosine (FET) and [11]C-methionine (MET) is a powerful technique to characterize suspected LGG.[8,9,10]

### 5.2.3 Treatment

Generally, the primary treatment in patients with suspected LGG is surgical resection whenever possible. The formerly often advocated "watch and wait" strategy has been replaced by an early and aggressive surgical treatment approach. This has been supported by a Norwegian retrospective study comparing early surgery to observation after biopsy of suspected LGG tumors.[11] Early surgical management was associated with better overall survival.[11] Nowadays, there is clear evidence that more extensive resections of LGG result in improved patient outcomes.[12,13,14] Additionally, maximal resection of LGG tumors prolongs the time span to malignant transformation.[15] Consequently, the current aim of surgery in suspected LGG is maximum safe tumor removal with preservation of neurological function. The Response Assessment in Neuro-Oncology (RANO) criteria define a complete resection of LGG as total removal of the abnormality on preoperative MRI T2-weighted/fluid-attenuated inversion recovery (FLAIR) sequences.[6,16] To avoid new postoperative neurological deficits and to achieve maximal safe resection, brain mapping and intraoperative stimulation have nowadays become indispensable techniques in LGG surgery.[17] Additionally, intraoperative navigation with DTI data provides a powerful tool to localize and avoid injury to relevant white matter tracts in LGG surgery.[7] Ultrasound may be used as an easily available adjunct, even though echodensity of LGG is variable and often incongruent to T2 and/or FLAIR by MRI.[18]

After surgical resection, a postoperative "watch and wait" strategy with regular imaging follow-up, but without initial adjuvant treatment, is frequently conducted in LGG patients.[19] However, new molecular markers such as isocitrate dehydrogenase 1 (IDH1)/IDH2 mutation and 1p19q co-deletion status are important prognostic factors that also impact treatment decisions with such tumors.[1,20]

### 5.2.4 Shortcomings of LGG Surgery and Current Solutions

Suspected LGG pose a special challenge for the neurosurgeon both in the preoperative planning phase and during resection itself. Typically, surgery of gliomas with nonsignificant CE on MRI is associated with specific drawbacks. First of all, incomplete resection of LGG is reported in the literature in 54 to 88% of cases resulting in worse patient prognosis.[12,15,21,22] One of the major causes for incomplete resection is insufficient visualization of the margin of LGG during resection since these tumors demonstrate only slight differences in macroscopic appearance and texture consistency compared to normal brain. Moreover, histopathological undergrading of gliomas due to the so-called sampling error is not uncommon.[8,23] Gliomas often show histopathological heterogeneity, and thus circumscribed intratumoral areas of malignant transformation, so-called anaplastic foci, may arise in initial pure LGG.[23] Missing such an anaplastic focus can lead to histopathological undergrading and inadequate postoperative patient management.

To improve LGG resection, the use of neuronavigation, navigation-guided tissue sampling from a PET or MRI/MRS "hotspot" to avoid undergrading, and intraoperative MRI have been proposed.[10,24,25,26] However, navigation systems tend to lose their initial accuracy during the course of resection due to brain shift, while intraoperative MRI is time-consuming and expensive, and therefore not widely available. Consequently, different surgical tools are required to overcome the current limitations of LGG surgery.

## 5.3 5-Aminolevulinic Acid in Low-Grade Glioma

Intraoperative visualization of malignant brain tumor tissue using 5-ALA-induced fluorescence is a well-validated tool to optimize resection. 5-ALA fluorescence-guided surgery (FGS) is relatively inexpensive, widely available, and remains unaffected by intraoperative brain shift. Although this method has been primarily applied in HGG with significant CE on MRI,[27,28] there has been growing interest to analyze the value of 5-ALA-induced fluorescence in suspected LGG with nonsignificant CE as well.

### 5.3.1 Background

Initially, the breakdown of the BBB was felt to be a prerequisite of visible 5-ALA-induced fluorescence in brain tumors, and thus only HGG with significant CE were thought to be amenable to this technique.[28] Currently, additional factors such as the metabolism of 5-ALA to protoporphyrin IX (PpIX) in the heme biosynthesis pathway are known to play a crucial role for the presence of 5-ALA-induced fluorescence.[29] According to current knowledge, the principles of PpIX accumulation in HGG cells seem to apply to LGG as well. Most of them pertain to increased uptake, production, and/or decreased utilization of PpIX during heme biosynthesis.[30,31,32,33] The initial 5-ALA uptake into tumor cells is only partially understood, but altogether the differences between LGG and HGG seem to be based more on quantitative than on qualitative properties. In this sense, one of the key factors of 5-ALA metabolization in glioma cells seems to be the expression of the enzyme ferrochelatase.[34] This enzyme degrades fluorescing PpIX into nonfluorescing heme by the incorporation of iron (Fe).[34] Recently, a downregulation of ferrochelatase mRNA expression was found in glioblastomas as compared to low-grade astrocytomas.[34] This explains why a better fluorescence effect can be expected in HGG rather than LGG.

### 5.3.2 Initial Observations

In the first observations of two studies including 10 LGG patients, no visible 5-ALA tumor fluorescence could be found in any of these cases.[35,36] Similarly, Stummer et al were not able to detect visible 5-ALA-induced fluorescence in a patient suffering from a secondary HGG in the nonenhancing LGG portion.[28] Interestingly, however, the authors found focal fluorescence in the contrast-enhancing intratumoral area with malignant transformation.[28] In 2007, Ishihara et al performed an ex vivo analysis of glioma specimens of different WHO grades derived from fluorescence resections using 5-ALA.[37] In this analysis, no visible fluorescence was detected in any of the specimens of the two analyzed WHO grade II gliomas.[37] In contrast, specimens with fluorescence visible as well as absent were observed in the two analyzed WHO grade III gliomas.[37]

### 5.3.3 Clinical Studies

Based on these initial observations, the first clinical study to better characterize 5-ALA tumor fluorescence in suspected LGG was performed by Widhalm et al in 2010.[38] Altogether, 17 patients with suspected DIGs, but without significant CE on preoperative MRI, were included.[38] 5-ALA-induced fluorescence was observed in a subgroup of these patients.[38] A circumscribed intratumoral area of fluorescence was found in eight of nine gliomas classified as WHO grade III after histopathologic analysis.[38] In contrast, no visible fluorescence was detected in any intratumoral region of all eight histologically confirmed WHO grade II gliomas.[38] A subsequent study from this group included 59 patients with suspected LGG.[39] They found that 23 of 26 WHO grade III gliomas demonstrated focal intratumoral fluorescence, whereas 29 of 33 WHO grade II gliomas did not reveal any visible fluorescence at all after 5-ALA administration.[39] In this study, high sensitivity (89%), specificity (88%), and positive (85%) and negative (91%) predictive values of visible fluorescence for high-grade histology were found.[39] In 2011, Ewelt et al reported similar findings in an independent patient cohort.[40] In their study, the authors found visible fluorescence in 12 of 17 WHO grade III and IV gliomas, but no visible fluorescence in 12 of 13 WHO grade II gliomas.[40] In the largest series to date (2017), Jaber et al found visible fluorescence in 59 of 76 WHO grade III gliomas.[41] In contrast, visible fluorescence was absent in 69 of 82 WHO grade II gliomas.[41] In summary, it can be stated that the vast majority of WHO grade II gliomas do not show visible fluorescence, whereas most WHO grade III/IV gliomas demonstrate visible (focal) 5-ALA-induced fluorescence.

## 5.3.4 Imaging Parameters

### Amount of Contrast Enhancement on Preoperative MRI

The breakdown of the BBB and thus the presence of visible CE on MRI seems to be one important indicator of visible 5-ALA-induced fluorescence.[28] In this sense, a recent study found a positive correlation of 5-ALA-induced fluorescence with the amount of CE on preoperative MRI in radiologically suspected LGG.[39] In this study, visible fluorescence was observed especially in gliomas with patchy/faint CE (53%) and focal CE (88%), whereas such visible fluorescence was frequently absent in gliomas with no CE (87%).[39] Similarly, in a further study, visible 5-ALA-induced fluorescence was found in 78% of gliomas with CE on MRI, but only in 16% of gliomas with no CE.[41]

### Metabolic Activity According to PET

The metabolic activity assessed by PET seems to serve as a further powerful indicator of visible 5-ALA-induced fluorescence in suspected LGG. A significantly higher PET uptake of either MET or FET was found in gliomas with visible (focal) fluorescence as compared to nonfluorescing gliomas.[38,39,40] Recently, an FET-PET uptake ratio of more than 1.9 was identified as a strong predictor for visible fluorescence in gliomas.[41] Interestingly, regions of focal fluorescence in suspected LGG topographically correlated with the intratumoral area of maximum MET-PET tracer uptake as well.[38,39]

## 5.3.5 Histopathology and Molecular Markers

### Histopathology

In radiologically suspected LGG, a correlation between visible 5-ALA-induced fluorescence and specific histopathological findings has been found. The proliferation rate assessed by the MIB-1 labeling index (LI) was found to be significantly higher in fluorescing gliomas than in nonfluorescing gliomas.[38,39,41] Moreover, the proliferation rate was found to be significantly higher in tumor regions with visible fluorescence compared to nonfluorescing areas within the same glioma[38] (▶ Fig. 5.1). Additionally, visible 5-ALA-induced fluorescence correlated with a MIB-1 LI over 10% in suspected LGG.[38] However, in a recent publication, it was shown that visible 5-ALA-induced fluorescence correlates not only with the proliferation rate in gliomas with nonsignificant CE, but also with specific histopathological criteria of anaplasia defined by the WHO.[1,39] According to the data of this study, cell density, nuclear pleomorphism, and mitotic rate were found to be significantly higher in

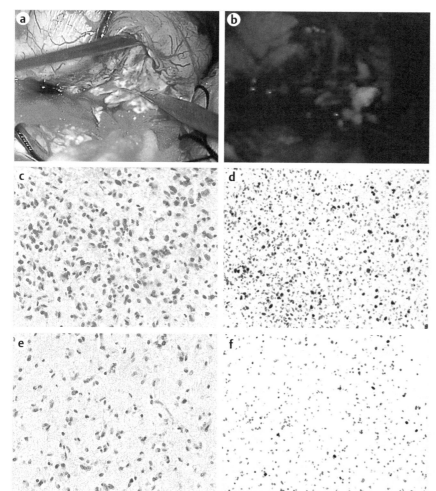

Fig. 5.1 Illustrative case of 5-aminolevulinic acid (5-ALA) fluorescence application during resection of a suspected low-grade glioma. (a) During surgery after preoperative administration of 5-ALA, the tumor tissue does not show clear signs of malignancy under white-light microscopy, (b) but with the violet–blue excitation light a focal area of unequivocal fluorescence can be detected. (c) According to histopathological analysis, this fluorescing area corresponds to anaplastic glioma tissue (anaplastic focus) with (d) a high proliferation rate. (e) In contrast, the nonfluorescing area corresponds only to low-grade glioma tissue with (f) a low proliferation rate. (Reproduced from Widhalm[42] with permission.)

intratumoral regions with focal fluorescence as compared to nonfluorescing areas.[39] These clinical studies highlight the ability of visible 5-ALA-induced fluorescence to intraoperatively identify focal intratumoral areas of malignant transformation without being affected by brain shift (Video 5.1).

### Molecular Markers

In recent years, correlations between visible 5-ALA-induced tumor fluorescence and a series of increasingly accepted and clinically relevant molecular markers have been sought. However, a recent study could not find a correlation of visible fluorescence with either the methyl guanine methyltransferase (MGMT) promoter methylation status or the detection of a 1p/19q co-deletion in gliomas.[41] Regarding the IDH mutational status, conflicting data are present in the current literature. While Kim et al[43] described enhanced 5-ALA-induced tumor fluorescence in malignant gliomas with IDH1 mutations in 2015, three other recent publications uniformly found that visible fluorescence was more common in IDH wild type/negative gliomas.[44,45,46]

### Optimized Patient Management

Visible 5-ALA-induced fluorescence provides the surgeon with an effective technique to intraoperatively identify anaplastic foci in gliomas with nonsignificant CE independent from brain shift. Thus, this method reduces the risk of histopathological undergrading of gliomas and the so-called sampling error. This also reflects in the observation that a high portion of suspected LGG does end up being histopathologically classified as HGG, if the 5-ALA fluorescence technique is applied for tissue sampling (*authors' personal experience*). This optimized intraoperative tissue sampling procedure in suspected LGG results in a more precise histopathological diagnosis and thus enables the allocation of glioma patients to standard of care postoperative treatment.

## 5.4 Indications for 5-ALA in Suspected LGG with Current Visualization Techniques

In routine clinical practice, radiologically suspected LGG with nonsignificant CE on preoperative MRI are not uncommon. According to a recent study, gliomas with the following characteristics are especially good candidates for preoperative administration of 5-ALA[41]:

- The existence of any, even patchy or faint, CE in MRI T1 contrast-enhanced images.
- In case of missing CE, [18]FET-PET images with uptake ratios (standardized uptake value [SUV]) greater than 1.9 (▶ Fig. 5.2).

Additionally, tumor size, CE, and patient age are significant predictors. Almost any tumor (i.e., > 96%) with patchy or faint CE, with a volume greater than 7 cm$^3$, in a patient older than 44 years will demonstrate fluorescence, while five of six tumors without CE will not.[41] If, above all, a negative FET-PET is available, the probability of finding intraoperative fluorescence drops to zero.[41] However, since PET negative cases can be observed even in HGG,[10] and PET imaging is not available at many centers, one might advocate administering 5-ALA in every case of a suspected LGG to rule out the existence of an intratumoral anaplastic region with malignant transformation.

## 5.5 Future Directions

Despite the described clinical benefits of 5-ALA in suspected LGG, specific limitations of this technique must be addressed. First, the current assessment of intraoperative fluorescence is subjective and thus observer dependent.[29] In this sense, vague fluorescence might not be recognized by selected neurosurgeons. Moreover, 5-ALA is not currently able to help visualize

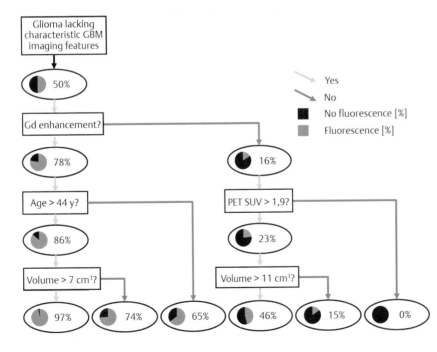

**Fig. 5.2** Gliomas lacking glioblastoma features on preoperative imaging, and 5-aminolevulinic acid (5-ALA) induced fluorescence. In this estimation, gliomas lacking characteristic glioblastoma features without typical ring-like contrast enhancement on preoperative MRI (no, weak/patchy, or strong homogeneous contrast enhancement) were evaluated. The estimation starts at equipoise concerning the prediction of the intraoperative 5-ALA fluorescence signal (i.e., fluorescence probability is rated 50% by the surgeon). Under this assumption, blood–brain barrier disruption (MRI T1 + gadolinium [Gd]) is the strongest predictor, followed by patient age or positive PET finding, and tumor volume[18] (for details see text). The probability of detecting a usable fluorescence signal intraoperatively may thus be estimated depending on the constellation of findings and available modalities. GBM, glioblastoma; PET, positron emission tomography; SUV, standardized uptake value. (Adapted from Wölfer and Stummer[47] with permission.)

tumor fluorescence in the majority of LGG.[29,37,38,39,40,41] Finally, a small subgroup of anaplastic foci cannot be visualized by the 5-ALA technique, hence remaining undetected.[39]

Recently, there has been a development of techniques, which may enhance 5-ALA fluorescence detection even in LGG cases without openly visible fluorescence signal with standard fluorescence modified operative microscopes. Apart from enhancing microscope optics, camera sensitivity, or light sources, two fluorescence detection techniques seem to be promising.

## 5.5.1 Quantitative Spectroscopic Fluorescence Measurements

Apart from creating more objective quantitative data (i.e., tissue concentrations of PpIX), observation sensitivity can be increased with the help of spectroscopic techniques (▶ Fig. 5.3). Recently, small and handheld devices have become available for this purpose.[48,49,50,51] Spectroscopic fluorescence measurements in LGG patients after the application of 5-ALA have demonstrated diagnostically useable PpIX accumulation in almost half of the tissue specimens that would have gone unnoticed by the surgeon's visual perception alone.[51] Sensitivity of fluorescence detection was increased around 100-fold compared to state-of-the-art visible fluorescence technologies in the first

cases of LGG, with LGG tissue still showing PpIX concentrations 5 to 50 times higher than in the normal brain.[51]

Based on the promising data in this pilot study, we are currently recruiting patients at the University of California, San Francisco (UCSF; Mitchel Berger, Georg Widhalm) in a cooperation study with the Dartmouth-Hitchcock Medical Center (David Roberts) to analyze the clinical value of such handheld spectroscopic probes to visualize LGG tissue as well as intratumoral heterogeneity in a large patient cohort.

## 5.5.2 Confocal Microscopy

Rasterizing a tissue surface with a focused light or laser beam and retrieving the returned light through an aperture simultaneously adapted to each illuminated voxel is the basic idea of confocal microscopy (for a sketch of the principle, see ▶ Fig. 5.4). The technique allows for increased three-dimensional resolution down to subcellular levels by two mechanisms. Structures not within the desired optic plane are less brightly illuminated, and scattered light from outside this same optic plane is rejected by the adapted pinhole aperture within the light path toward the detecting unit (usually a charge-coupled device camera or a photomultiplier). In the case of LGG surgery, this means the possibility of capturing PpIX fluorescence from the mitochondria of scattered glioma cells that are

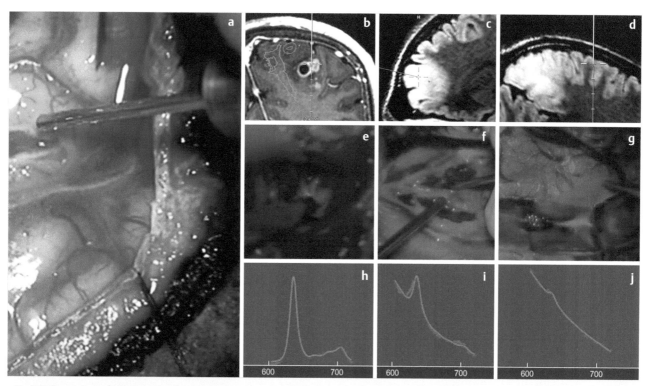

**Fig. 5.3** Comparison of intraoperative fluorescence spectroscopy in a high-grade glioma, low-grade glioma, and normal cortex. **(a)** During surgery, a small spectroscopic probe is applied that is capable of measuring the 5-aminolevulinic acid (5-ALA) induced absolute protoporphyrin IX (PpIX) tissue concentration. **(b)** In the contrast-enhancing tumor of a high-grade glioma verified by neuronavigation, **(e)** an intense fluorescence signal (*5-ALA grade 3*) is detected and **(h)** a very high PpIX concentration is measured with the probe. **(c)** In the tumor on FLAIR (fluid-attenuated inversion recovery) images confirmed by neuronavigation of a nonenhancing low-grade glioma, **(f)** no visible fluorescence (*5-ALA grade 0*) can be identified with the conventional violet–blue excitation light, **(i)** but still a considerably elevated PpIX concentration can be measured with the probe that is, however, markedly lower than in the high-grade glioma. **(d)** In the region of normal cortex, **(g)** no visible fluorescence (*5-ALA grade 0*) is present and **(j)** the measured PpIX concentration is very low. (Data derived from a cooperation study of the University of California, San Francisco [UCSF] with the Dartmouth-Hitchcock Medical Center.)

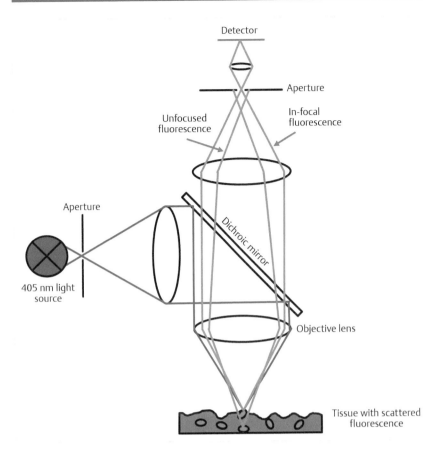

Detector

Aperture

In-focal
fluorescence

Unfocused
fluorescence

Dichroic mirror

Aperture

405 nm light
source

Objective lens

Tissue with scattered
fluorescence

**Fig. 5.4** Principle of confocal microscopy for potential improved visualization of low-grade gliomas. Confocal microscopy allows for increased three-dimensional resolution down to subcellular levels. Resolution is improved by illuminating a surface with a focused light beam and simultaneously registering the returning light signal through an aperture tuned to the desired optic plane. Illuminating and returning light can be separated by a dichroic mirror if their wavelengths are different (as is the shown case with 5-aminolevulinic acid [5-ALA] fluorescence). Rasterizing is either effected by moving the sample under the fixed illuminating beam or, more commonly, by inserting a tilting mirror between the beam divider and the objective lens. Alternative setups (e.g., **V**-shaped without the need of a beam divider) have been described.[52]

not identifiable by conventional wide field microscopy. Though first applied more than 10 years ago, this method still awaits its transformation into a portable, easy-to-use and affordable setup.[52,53] Using this technique, intraoperative and histological findings were found to correlate well when trying to identify the margin of macroscopically nonfluorescing LGG.[22] The rather small field of view (mostly reported to be around 500 × 500 μm) and the need for separate visualization, however, make the method difficult to incorporate into a normal resection workflow. Even some highly integrated variant of intraoperative confocal microscopy might, however, just document the fact that glioma margins are ill defined, so that other, for example, functional considerations would still have to take the lead in tailoring a resection. Altogether, technical implementation and the clinical value of the principle remain to be established.

## 5.6 Conclusion

While being firmly established in the resection of HGG, the neurosurgical focus on 5-ALA-induced fluorescence has recently been expanded to LGG. According to the current literature, 5-ALA-induced fluorescence is a reliable intraoperative marker for detection of anaplastic foci independent of brain shift during surgery of suspected LGG. Tissue sampling from such intratumoral areas of focal fluorescence enables a more precise histopathological diagnosis and thus allocation of patients to the proper adjuvant postoperative treatment. Consequently, we advocate administering 5-ALA to suspected LGG

patients to rule out the existence of intratumoral regions with malignant transformation.

In contrast, the vast majority of LGG cannot be visualized by the current operative microscope fluorescence techniques since the achievable concentrations and fluorescence intensities are usually much lower than in HGG. However, at least two promising technologies are being explored in LGG with fluorescence spectroscopy and confocal microscopy to potentially overcome these current limitations.

## References

[1] Louis DN, Ohgaki H, Wiestler OD, Cavenee WK. WHO Classification of Tumours of the Central Nervous System. 4th ed. New York, NY: WHO Press; 2016

[2] Forst DA, Nahed BV, Loeffler JS, Batchelor TT. Low-grade gliomas. Oncologist. 2014; 19(4):403–413

[3] Schiff D, Brown PD, Giannini C. Outcome in adult low-grade glioma: the impact of prognostic factors and treatment. Neurology. 2007; 69(13):1366–1373

[4] Grier JT, Batchelor T. Low-grade gliomas in adults. Oncologist. 2006; 11(6): 681–693

[5] Cha S. Neuroimaging in neuro-oncology. Neurotherapeutics. 2009; 6(3):465–477

[6] van den Bent MJ, Wefel JS, Schiff D, et al. Response assessment in neuro-oncology (a report of the RANO group): assessment of outcome in trials of diffuse low-grade gliomas. Lancet Oncol. 2011; 12(6):583–593

[7] Nimsky C, Ganslandt O, Fahlbusch R. Implementation of fiber tract navigation. Neurosurgery. 2006; 58(4) s uppl 2:ONS-292–ONS-303, discussion ONS-303–ONS-304

[8] Kunz M, Thon N, Eigenbrod S, et al. Hot spots in dynamic (18)FET-PET delineate malignant tumor parts within suspected WHO grade II gliomas. Neuro-oncol. 2011; 13(3):307–316

[9] Smits A, Baumert BG. The clinical value of PET with amino acid tracers for gliomas WHO grade II. Int J Mol Imaging. 2011; 2011:372509

[10] Widhalm G, Krssak M, Minchev G, et al. Value of 1H-magnetic resonance spectroscopy chemical shift imaging for detection of anaplastic foci in diffusely infiltrating gliomas with non-significant contrast-enhancement. J Neurol Neurosurg Psychiatry. 2011; 82(5):512–520

[11] Jakola AS, Myrmel KS, Kloster R, et al. Comparison of a strategy favoring early surgical resection vs a strategy favoring watchful waiting in low-grade gliomas. JAMA. 2012; 308(18):1881–1888

[12] Smith JS, Chang EF, Lamborn KR, et al. Role of extent of resection in the long-term outcome of low-grade hemispheric gliomas. J Clin Oncol. 2008; 26(8):1338–1345

[13] Hervey-Jumper SL, Berger MS. Role of surgical resection in low- and high-grade gliomas. Curr Treat Options Neurol. 2014; 16(4):284

[14] Sanai N, Berger MS. Glioma extent of resection and its impact on patient outcome. Neurosurgery. 2008; 62(4):753–764, discussion 264–266

[15] Sanai N, Polley MY, Berger MS. Insular glioma resection: assessment of patient morbidity, survival, and tumor progression. J Neurosurg. 2010; 112(1):1–9

[16] Vogelbaum MA, Jost S, Aghi MK, et al. Application of novel response/progression measures for surgically delivered therapies for gliomas: response assessment in Neuro-Oncology (RANO) Working Group. Neurosurgery. 2012; 70(1):234–243, discussion 243–244

[17] De Witt Hamer PC, Robles SG, Zwinderman AH, Duffau H, Berger MS. Impact of intraoperative stimulation brain mapping on glioma surgery outcome: a meta-analysis. J Clin Oncol. 2012; 30(20):2559–2565

[18] Petridis AK, Anokhin M, Vavruska J, Mahvash M, Scholz M. The value of intraoperative sonography in low grade glioma surgery. Clin Neurol Neurosurg. 2015; 131(7):64–68

[19] Stupp R, Janzer RC, Hegi ME, Villemure J-G, Mirimanoff RO. Prognostic factors for low-grade gliomas. Semin Oncol. 2003; 30(6) s uppl 19:23–28

[20] Eckel-Passow JE, Lachance DH, Molinaro AM, et al. Glioma groups based on 1p/19q, IDH, and TERT promoter mutations in tumors. N Engl J Med. 2015; 372(26):2499–2508

[21] Capelle L, Fontaine D, Mandonnet E, et al. French Réseau d'Étude des Gliomes. Spontaneous and therapeutic prognostic factors in adult hemispheric World Health Organization Grade II gliomas: a series of 1097 cases: clinical article. J Neurosurg. 2013; 118(6):1157–1168

[22] Sanai N, Snyder LA, Honea NJ, et al. Intraoperative confocal microscopy in the visualization of 5-aminolevulinic acid fluorescence in low-grade gliomas. J Neurosurg. 2011; 115(4):740–748

[23] Paulus W, Peiffer J. Intratumoral histologic heterogeneity of gliomas. A quantitative study. Cancer. 1989; 64(2):442–447

[24] Black PM, Alexander E, III, Martin C, et al. Craniotomy for tumor treatment in an intraoperative magnetic resonance imaging unit. Neurosurgery. 1999; 45(3):423–431, discussion 431–433

[25] Mert A, Kiesel B, Wöhrer A, et al. Introduction of a standardized multimodality image protocol for navigation-guided surgery of suspected low-grade gliomas. Neurosurg Focus. 2015; 38(1):E4

[26] Roberts DW, Strohbehn JW, Hatch JF, Murray W, Kettenberger H. A frameless stereotaxic integration of computerized tomographic imaging and the operating microscope. J Neurosurg. 1986; 65(4):545–549

[27] Stummer W, Novotny A, Stepp H, Goetz C, Bise K, Reulen HJ. Fluorescence-guided resection of glioblastoma multiforme by using 5-aminolevulinic acid-induced porphyrins: a prospective study in 52 consecutive patients. J Neurosurg. 2000; 93(6):1003–1013

[28] Stummer W, Stocker S, Wagner S, et al. Intraoperative detection of malignant gliomas by 5-aminolevulinic acid-induced porphyrin fluorescence. Neurosurgery. 1998; 42(3):518–525, discussion 525–526

[29] Hadjipanayis CG, Widhalm G, Stummer W. What is the surgical benefit of utilizing 5-aminolevulinic acid for fluorescence-guided surgery of malignant gliomas? Neurosurgery. 2015; 77(5):663–673

[30] Colditz MJ, Jeffree RL. Aminolevulinic acid (ALA)-protoporphyrin IX fluorescence guided tumour resection. Part 1: clinical, radiological and pathological studies. J Clin Neurosci. 2012; 19(11):1471–1474

[31] Colditz MJ, Leyen Kv, Jeffree RL. Aminolevulinic acid (ALA)-protoporphyrin IX fluorescence guided tumour resection. Part 2: theoretical, biochemical and practical aspects. J Clin Neurosci. 2012; 19(12):1611–1616

[32] Peng Q, Warloe T, Berg K, et al. 5-Aminolevulinic acid-based photodynamic therapy. Clinical research and future challenges. Cancer. 1997; 79(12):2282–2308

[33] Van Hillegersberg R, Van den Berg JW, Kort WJ, Terpstra OT, Wilson JH. Selective accumulation of endogenously produced porphyrins in a liver metastasis model in rats. Gastroenterology. 1992; 103(2):647–651

[34] Teng L, Nakada M, Zhao SG, et al. Silencing of ferrochelatase enhances 5-aminolevulinic acid-based fluorescence and photodynamic therapy efficacy. Br J Cancer. 2011; 104(5):798–807

[35] Hefti M, von Campe G, Moschopulos M, Siegner A, Looser H, Landolt H. 5-aminolevulinic acid induced protoporphyrin IX fluorescence in high-grade glioma surgery: a one-year experience at a single institution. Swiss Med Wkly. 2008; 138(11)(–)(12):180–185

[36] Utsuki S, Oka H, Sato S, et al. Possibility of using laser spectroscopy for the intraoperative detection of nonfluorescing brain tumors and the boundaries of brain tumor infiltrates. Technical note. J Neurosurg. 2006; 104(4):618–620

[37] Ishihara R, Katayama Y, Watanabe T, Yoshino A, Fukushima T, Sakatani K. Quantitative spectroscopic analysis of 5-aminolevulinic acid-induced protoporphyrin IX fluorescence intensity in diffusely infiltrating astrocytomas. Neurol Med Chir (Tokyo). 2007; 47(2):53–57, discussion 57

[38] Widhalm G, Wolfsberger S, Minchev G, et al. 5-Aminolevulinic acid is a promising marker for detection of anaplastic foci in diffusely infiltrating gliomas with nonsignificant contrast enhancement. Cancer. 2010; 116(6):1545–1552

[39] Widhalm G, Kiesel B, Woehrer A, et al. 5-Aminolevulinic acid induced fluorescence is a powerful intraoperative marker for precise histopathological grading of gliomas with non-significant contrast-enhancement. PLoS One. 2013; 8(10):e76988

[40] Ewelt C, Floeth FW, Felsberg J, et al. Finding the anaplastic focus in diffuse gliomas: the value of Gd-DTPA enhanced MRI, FET-PET, and intraoperative, ALA-derived tissue fluorescence. Clin Neurol Neurosurg. 2011; 113(7):541–547

[41] Jaber M, Wölfer J, Ewelt C, et al. The value of 5-aminolevulinic acid in low-grade gliomas and high-grade gliomas lacking glioblastoma imaging features: an analysis based on fluorescence, magnetic resonance imaging, 18F-fluoroethyl tyrosine positron emission tomography, and tumor molecular factors. Neurosurgery. 2016; 78(3):401–411, discussion 411

[42] Widhalm G. Intra-operative visualization of brain tumors with 5-aminolevulinic acid-induced fluorescence. Clin Neuropathol. 2014; 33(4):260–278

[43] Kim JE, Cho HR, Xu WJ, et al. Mechanism for enhanced 5-aminolevulinic acid fluorescence in isocitrate dehydrogenase 1 mutant malignant gliomas. Oncotarget. 2015; 6(24):20266–20277

[44] Hickmann A-K, Nadji-Ohl M, Hopf NJ. Feasibility of fluorescence-guided resection of recurrent gliomas using five-aminolevulinic acid: retrospective analysis of surgical and neurological outcome in 58 patients. J Neurooncol. 2015; 122(1):151–160

[45] Nakae S, Murayama K, Sasaki H, et al. Prediction of genetic subgroups in adult supra tentorial gliomas by pre- and intraoperative parameters. J Neurooncol. 2017; 131(2):403–412

[46] Saito K, Hirai T, Takeshima H, et al. Genetic factors affecting intraoperative 5-aminolevulinic acid-induced fluorescence of diffuse gliomas. Radiol Oncol. 2017; 51(2):142–150

[47] Wölfer J, Stummer W. Fluoreszenz-gestützte Gliomresektion. In: Simon M, ed. Gliomchirurgie. Berlin: Springer; 2017

[48] Haj-Hosseini N, Richter J, Andersson-Engels S, Wårdell K. Optical touch pointer for fluorescence guided glioblastoma resection using 5-aminolevulinic acid. Lasers Surg Med. 2010; 42(1):9–14

[49] Kairdolf BA, Bouras A, Kaluzova M, et al. Intraoperative spectroscopy with ultrahigh sensitivity for image-guided surgery of malignant brain tumors. Anal Chem. 2016; 88(1):858–867

[50] Kim A, Khurana M, Moriyama Y, Wilson BC. Quantification of in vivo fluorescence decoupled from the effects of tissue optical properties using fiber-optic spectroscopy measurements. J Biomed Opt. 2010; 15(6):067006

[51] Valdés PA, Jacobs V, Harris BT, et al. Quantitative fluorescence using 5-aminolevulinic acid-induced protoporphyrin IX biomarker as a surgical adjunct in low-grade glioma surgery. J Neurosurg. 2015; 123(3):771–780

[52] Meza D, Wang D, Wang Y, Borwege S, Sanai N, Liu JTC. Comparing high-resolution microscopy techniques for potential intraoperative use in guiding low-grade glioma resections. Lasers Surg Med. 2015; 47(4):289–295

[53] Olivo M, Wilson BC. Mapping ALA-induced PPIX fluorescence in normal brain and brain tumour using confocal fluorescence microscopy. Int J Oncol. 2004; 25(1):37–45

# 6 Intraoperative Fluorescence Guidance in Meningiomas

*Pablo A. Valdes Quevedo, Alexandra J. Golby, and David W. Roberts*

## Abstract

Fluorescence guidance has become a useful adjunct for neurosurgeons. The main fluorescent markers in clinical use for meningiomas include 5-aminolevulinic acid-induced protoporphyrin IX, indocyanine green, and fluorescein sodium. These markers have been used with microscope- and spectroscopy-based technologies for tumor surgery and delineation of intracranial vasculature. This chapter reviews the main clinical applications of fluorescence guidance in meningiomas.

*Keywords:* fluorescence-guided surgery, 5-aminolevulinic acid, protoporphyrin IX, indocyanine green, meningiomas, optical spectroscopy

## 6.1 Introduction

Fluorescence guidance has become a burgeoning field of research and increasingly adopted surgical adjunct for clinical applications in neurosurgery.[1,2] Multiple technologies including microscope systems and single probe spectroscopic or microscopic-based tools have been developed for clinical implementation. These technologies have been coupled to various fluorescent agents including 5-aminolevulinic-acid-induced protoporphyrin IX (ALA-PpIX), fluorescein, and indocyanine green (IGC). Cranial and spinal applications of fluorescence guidance in neurosurgery include use in brain tumors such as gliomas, metastases, and meningiomas.[1,3,4,5,6] Here, we present an overview of the neurosurgical literature using fluorescence guidance in meningiomas.

## 6.2 5-Aminolevulinic-Acid-Induced Protoporphyrin IX

The most widely used fluorescent agent for neurosurgical resection of intracranial tumors is ALA-PpIX.[1,2] Briefly, ALA is administered orally prior to surgery, which leads to uptake of ALA with subsequent production and selective accumulation of PpIX in tumor cells. PpIX is the active fluorescent compound with two major excitation peaks at 405 and 633 nm and two major emission peaks at 635 and 710 nm.[3,5] The largest experience with ALA-PpIX was a phase III randomized controlled trial in glioblastoma, which demonstrated almost doubling of complete resection rates and improved progression-free survival in patients, which has led to its widespread use in Europe.[4]

The clinical experience and literature on the use of 5-ALA in meningioma resection are more limited, and as such the clinical role of ALA-PpIX is not yet as firmly grounded as it is for high-grade gliomas. For example, a recent review noted the following distribution of publication numbers per tumor type: pediatric brain tumors 5, spinal tumors 7, meningioma 10, low-grade glioma 14, metastases 15, and high-grade glioma 51.[6] The largest reported series on meningiomas is that of Millesi et al.[7] The authors analyzed 204 meningiomas undergoing ALA-PpIX

fluorescence-guided surgery and highlighted various key observations of relevance to meningioma, which have been further elaborated and confirmed in the literature. This study reported Simpson grade resection I to IV in 45, 22, 17, and 16% of tumors, respectively; positive fluorescence was seen in 91% (185/204) of cases with no correlation between location, histology, and fluorescence appearance; a mostly homogeneous pattern of fluorescence (75%, 113/150 analyzed cases)[8]; 89 cases with dural tails on MRI demonstrating no visible fluorescence, of which 5/16 analyzed histopathologically contained tumor cells; 7 cases of satellite lesions detected with PpIX fluorescence, which would have otherwise gone undetected; tumor-infiltrated bone flaps with positive fluorescence in 100% of cases (13/13); and fluorescence in adjacent cortex in 25% (20/80) of cases with a significant difference in cases with a disrupted arachnoid (41 vs. 11%, $p = 0.002$) but no correlation with WHO grade. (Of note, the authors did not provide histopathologic confirmation regarding the degree or status of tumor infiltration in the evaluated arachnoid or cortex.)

One of the first reports using ALA-PpIX was that of Coluccia et al[9] on a cohort of 33 patients with intracranial meningiomas (32, WHO grades I–II) and (1, WHO grade III), which noted that 94% (31/34) of patients demonstrated visible levels of fluorescence with no correlation to histology, MIB index, mitotic index, or preoperative brain edema. These results are similar to the first report on ALA-PpIX in meningiomas by Kajimoto et al[10] who reported on 24 patients, with 83% (20/24) demonstrating visible fluorescence with no correlation between histology and fluorescence. Cornelius et al[11] studied 31 meningiomas across WHO grades I to III (19, 8, and 4, respectively), in which 94% were positive for fluorescence; in their study, they did report a correlation between subjective intensity and WHO grade ($\rho = 0.557$; $p = 0.001$). Coluccia et al, similar to others,[10,12] did note the presence of positive fluorescent tumor infiltrating skull in one case, highlighting the ability of ALA-PpIX to delineate *infiltrated margins beyond the tumor bulk and into skull.* Kajimoto et al[10] also note histologic confirmation not only of skull invasion, but also invasion of hypertrophied dura with a sensitivity of 100% (5/5) and specificity of 83% (5/6).

Della Puppa et al[13] reported the use of ALA-PpIX in 12 patients with bone-invading meningiomas, noting a sensitivity of 89% and specificity of 100% for detecting bone invasion with positive predictive value (PPV) = 100%, negative predictive value (NPV) = 83%, overall accuracy = 93%, and no residual bone invasion on postoperative MRI. This study further highlighted relationships between bone invasion, hyperostosis, and fluorescence. All fluorescent samples had bone invasion (100%, 57/57) and 30% (7/23) of nonfluorescent samples had bone invasion and hyperostosis, and none of the nonhyperostotic samples had fluorescence, that is, all false-negatives were found in hyperostotic bone (7/23). This study demonstrates a strong association between bone invasion and fluorescence as well as a weaker association between hyperostosis and fluorescence.

Whitson et al[14] used confocal microscopy and histology to investigate tumor infiltration and the dural margins. They note a high specificity in which uninvolved dura demonstrated no fluorescence. They also note a decreased sensitivity in which microscopic amounts of tumor cells contained no significant fluorescence; for example, less than 1 mm of tumor tail showed no fluorescence. Bekelis et al[15] applied a quantitative probe in a case of a skull base meningioma showing significantly improved sensitivity in detecting significant levels of PpIX despite no visible fluorescence. Cornelius et al[16] used PpIX fluorescence as an adjunct to MRI- and PET-guided resection to help identify a skull base meningioma with bony and dural infiltration.

Wilbers et al[17] presented a case report of an atypical WHO grade II meningioma where distinct fluorescence was noted not just in gross tumor, but also in adjacent dura, arachnoid, and cortex with histologic confirmation, suggesting that arachnoid may be a source of tumor recurrence despite macroscopic gross total resection of tumor and adjacent dura; that is, despite achieving Simpson grade I resection. In a similar report of an atypical meningioma, Scheichel et al[18] observed histopathologically confirmed visible fluorescence in the periosteal layer, inner temporalis muscle fascia, temporalis muscle, and bone in addition to the solid tumor, highlighting the limitation of standard white light resection to identify these infiltrating tumor remnants.

Most studies with ALA-PpIX are in cranial meningiomas, while studies on spinal applications have been much more limited. Eicker et al[19] looked at 26 patients with intradural spinal tumors, which included 8 meningiomas (WHO grade I) using ALA-PpIX. Seven of the eight meningiomas demonstrated

bright pink fluorescence with a PPV of 100%. The authors noted that fluorescence was of particular utility in recurrent cases with adherent, scarred tissue to help dissect tumor from spinal cord. Muroi et al[20] report on the utility of ALA-PpIX in one case of a spinal meningioma where on macroscopic, white light inspection at the end of resection, the authors judged they had achieved a Simpson grade II resection, but on final inspection with fluorescence identified a small tumor remnant that was subsequently resected without dural removal.

The aforementioned studies have used a modified surgical microscope with ultraviolet excitation light and collection emission filters greater than 450 nm to visualize the emitted red–pink fluorescence through the surgical oculars and onto a color camera.[5,7,9,12,13,17] As such, assessments of fluorescence in meningioma surgery have been qualitative in nature, noting a "strong" or "weak" fluorescence without measuring the actual quantitative levels of PpIX (▶ Fig. 6.1). That is, such qualitative assessments do not take into account the nonlinear, attenuating effects of tissue optical properties; that is, absorption and scattering on the excitation light and emitted fluorescence.[21] These attenuating effects can lead to inaccurate assessments of the tissue fluorescence, such as intraoperative qualitative assessment of "no visible fluorescence" in areas where there might actually be significant levels of fluorescent PpIX biomarker.[2,22,23]

Recent advances at the interface between neurosurgery and optical engineering have developed new optical probes that

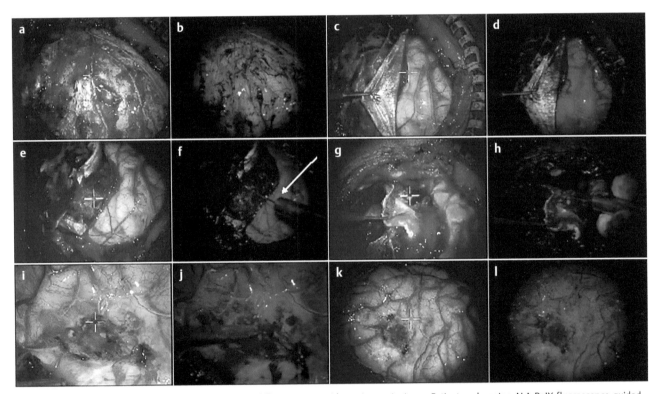

**Fig. 6.1** Aminolevulinic acid protoporphyrin IX (ALA-PpIX) fluorescence guidance in meningioma. Patient undergoing ALA-PpIX fluorescence-guided resection for a meningioma under standard white light and violet–blue light illumination mode for fluorescence imaging **(a,b)** prior to dural opening without any visible fluorescence; **(c,d)** immediately after dural opening with visualization of the underlying convexity meningioma not visualized through the overlying dura; **(e,f)** further exposure of the tumor bulk with use of an intraoperative quantitative probe (*white arrow*); **(g,h)** exposure of the tumor bulk noting differences in PpIX fluorescence at the tumor and no visible fluorescence in nearby dura; **(i,j)** near the end of the resection after removal of the tumor bulk with a small remnant of residual fluorescent tissue; and **(k,l)** at the end of the resection with no residual tumor noted under both standard white light and confirmatory fluorescence mode.

enable intraoperative and in vivo quantitative assessments of PpIX.[2,8,15,22,23,24,25,26] Valdes et al[8] reported on 15 meningiomas using ALA-PpIX, noting that meningiomas demonstrated high, homogenous fluorescence, and no correlation between visible fluorescence characteristics and MR contrast enhancement. The authors performed quantitative assessments on 10 of 15 patients for a total of 49 interrogated sites, noting the diagnostic significance of quantitative ALA-PpIX: diagnostically high PpIX levels were measured in 69% of histologically confirmed tumor tissues that *did not demonstrate visible fluorescence.* Tumor had a statistically significant higher mean concentration of PpIX ($c_{PpIX}$) of $1.694 \pm 0.440$ µg/mL compared to normal dura (i.e., control) with an average $c_{PpIX}$ of $0.006 \pm 0.003$ µg/mL ($p = 0.002$). Furthermore, 39% (13/33) of confirmed tumor specimens did not display visible fluorescence (that is, false-negative), but 69% (9/13) of these nonvisibly fluorescent tumor specimens contained PpIX levels greater than 0.010 µg/mL. Receiver operating characteristic (ROC) analysis demonstrated a statistically significant improvement in diagnostic performance for quantitative fluorescence compared to qualitative fluorescence ($p = 0.007$). Using a quantitative approach, the authors were able to balance the need for improved sensitivity (i.e., lower cutoff threshold value, $c_{PpIX} = 0.001$, accuracy of 90%, PPV of 91%, specificity of 81%, NPV of 87%, and sensitivity of 94%) at the cost of decreased specificity and vice versa, improved specificity (i.e., higher cutoff threshold value, $c_{PpIX} = 0.0114$; accuracy of 84%, PPV of 100%, specificity of 100%, NPV of 67%, and sensitivity of 76%) at the cost of decreased sensitivity.

These studies highlight the utility of PpIX as a surgical adjunct for meningioma resection. Qualitative assessments of PpIX provide the surgeon an additional tool to help identify not just tumor bulk, but also perhaps of more value, infiltrating margins including dural margins, satellite lesions, and infiltrated bone. This tool can help maximize resection while helping to minimize resection of noninfiltrated bone and/or dura. Furthermore, quantitative measurements provide a more sensitive tool for qualitative assessments to further improve sensitivity, and hopefully, decrease overall recurrence rates.

## 6.3 Indocyanine Green

Unlike PpIX, ICG is excited (e.g., main peak at 800 nm) and emits (e.g., main peak at 830–840 nm)[2] in the near infrared spectrum of light and works primarily as an agent to identify vascularity. In the case of tumor resection, this helps identify tumor via the enhanced permeability retention effect.[5,27] Lee et al used ICG in 18 patients with WHO grade I and II meningiomas, of which 14 demonstrated significantly higher fluorescence compared to adjacent brain. In this study, the authors relied on the enhanced permeability and retention (EPR) effect to visualize tumors with ICG, by giving the patient a large dose (~10 times greater) than the typical angiographic dose. The authors reported a PPV of 71%, NPV of 87%, specificity of 39%, sensitivity of 96%, and overall ROC area under the curve (AUC) of 0.68, which, compared to standard white light imaging, improved overall sensitivity but decreased overall specificity (39% down from 100%).

ICG has also been used in the resection of meningiomas as a vascular imaging tool specifically applied to imaging the tumor–sinus relationships.[28] In d'Avella et al, the authors note the utility of angiographic doses of ICG for identifying and preserving the venous collaterals during radical resection of parasagittal meningiomas with total superior sagittal sinus occlusion.[29] The authors note the utility of ICG to confirm intraoperatively total sinus occlusion, and identification of cortical and collateral veins distinct from tumor draining vessels. Ueba et al[30] reported on 10 cases in which they used "transdural ICG imaging" to localize cortical arteries, veins and venous sinus during resection of meningiomas, and found this tool of particular utility in visualizing the dural attachment and the venous sinus to optimize safe dural opening. Han et al[31] used ICG to visualize the pial vascular supply of the optic nerve before and after resection of a compressing tuberculum meningioma, noting improving blood flow, and concluding that ICG enabled more accurate assessment of the pial vascular supply, which could serve as a prognostic indicator of improvement in visual function in these patients.

A major advantage and difference of ICG imaging in these studies compared to ALA-PpIX is the ability to excite tissue fluorophores and collect fluorescence emissions of longer wavelengths, which can lead to detection of deeper seated lesions to a depth of approximately 1 cm compared to the more superficial tissue detection offered by 405-nm excitation light with ALA-PpIX guidance (i.e., < 0.2 mm).

## 6.4 Fluorescein

Fluorescein is analogous to ICG in terms of its physiologic mechanism as a vascular agent and its ability to accumulate in tumors via the enhanced permeability effect.[2] Similar to PpIX, fluorescein's fluorescent properties are in the visible range of the spectrum, with a main excitation peak at 494 nm and a main emission peak at 521 nm[3]. The work by da Silva et al[32,33] used standard white light microscopy without dedicated filters after sodium fluorescein administration to identify the yellow "pigmentation" provided by fluorescein accumulation, which was evident 10 minutes following administration and persisted for hours, and included tumor, cerebrospinal fluid, and dura, but not cranial nerves. Sanai et al[34] used an intraoperative confocal system to visualize microscopic tissue in multiple pathologies including eight meningiomas down to micrometer resolutions with a dedicated 488-nm excitation light and emission filter in the range of 505 to 585 nm. Their confocal tool enabled intraoperative in vivo highlighting of classic histopathologic findings including meningothelial meningiomas with whorls and psammoma bodies, and fibrous meningioma cells with spindle-shaped morphology. In a follow-up study of 24 meningiomas,[35] the authors reported a confocal-to-histology concordance of 90%, and similar to work on PpIX with meningiomas, they also reported dural invasion detected by confocal imaging.

## 6.5 Conclusion

The neurosurgical armamentarium is growing in the number of tools utilized to help guide resection of brain tumors, thus helping maximize the extent of tumor resection and minimize the risk of surgical complications. Fluorescence guidance is a valuable adjunct that is gaining traction for resection of meningiomas, helping identify tumor bulk, invading tumor at both the dural and skull margins, and otherwise missed satellite lesions. The reported diagnostic accuracies for meningiomas using basic qualitative assessment of the fluorescence, specifically with ALA-PpIX guidance, are encouraging as a tumor biomarker. Additional agents such as ICG can further help enable the surgeon in identifying adjacent arterial and venous structures to help the surgeon maximize the safety of the procedure while pushing the limits of the ability to resect tumor.

Current fluorescence-guided resection of meningiomas has various limitations that need to be addressed. First, we are starting to better understand the full diagnostic value of PpIX, fluorescein, and ICG for meningiomas, but the experience is quite limited when compared to gliomas. Future work should focus on providing a better understanding of the extent and accuracy to which these biomarkers can be used to guide resection and provide validated PPV, NPV, specificity, sensitivity, and classification accuracy for meningiomas. The issue of qualitative versus quantitative fluorescence is a technological problem with fluorescence guidance in general. As noted earlier, efforts are underway to standardize assessments of fluorescence with the development of quantitative technologies. Future developments will aim to develop quantitative fluorescence technologies that enable surgeons across the world to make more accurate and objective assessments of the tissue fluorescence, thus improving overall diagnostic accuracies. Another limitation of current implementations is the issue of depth detection. Clinical systems for ALA or fluorescence are designed to detect surface fluorescence, whereas ICG systems can detect deeper fluorescence, yet no clinical system provides an estimate of depth or fluorescence quantification at depth. Future developments will seek to exploit near-infrared (NIR) compounds like ICG or the far-red spectrum of PpIX to detect fluorescence at depth.

The applications of fluorescence in meningiomas are just starting to be investigated, and with the advent of new imaging technologies (e.g., fluorescence-enabled microscopes, spectroscopy probes, quantitative imaging systems) and multiple fluorophores (e.g., ALA-PpIX, ICG, fluorescein), the benefits and limits of fluorescence in meningiomas are yet to be fully understood and exploited. The neurosurgeon is tasked with the exciting opportunity to both develop and implement these new, emerging fluorescence technologies to help maximize tumor resection and improve safety, thus helping improve overall patient quality of life and overall survival.

# References

[1] Hadjipanayis CG, Widhalm G, Stummer W. What is the surgical benefit of utilizing 5-aminolevulinic acid for fluorescence-guided surgery of malignant gliomas? Neurosurgery. 2015; 77(5):663–673

[2] Valdés PA, Roberts DW, Lu FK, Golby A. Optical technologies for intraoperative neurosurgical guidance. Neurosurg Focus. 2016; 40(3):E8

[3] Pogue BW, Gibbs-Strauss S, Valdés PA, Samkoe K, Roberts DW, Paulsen KD. Review of neurosurgical fluorescence imaging methodologies. IEEE J Sel Top Quantum Electron. 2010; 16(3):493–505

[4] Stummer W, Pichlmeier U, Meinel T, Wiestler OD, Zanella F, Reulen HJ, ALA-Glioma Study Group. Fluorescence-guided surgery with 5-aminolevulinic acid for resection of malignant glioma: a randomised controlled multicentre phase III trial. Lancet Oncol. 2006; 7(5):392–401

[5] Valdes PA, Jacobs VL, Paulsen KD, Roberts DW, Leblond F. In vivo fluorescence detection in surgery: a review of principles, methods, and applications. Curr Med Imaging Rev. 2011

[6] Kamp MA, Krause Molle Z, Munoz-Bendix C, et al. Various shades of red: a systematic analysis of qualitative estimation of ALA-derived fluorescence in neurosurgery. Neurosurg Rev. 2016

[7] Millesi M, Kiesel B, Mischkulnig M, et al. Analysis of the surgical benefits of 5-ALA-induced fluorescence in intracranial meningiomas: experience in 204 meningiomas. J Neurosurg. 2016; 125(6):1408–1419

[8] Valdes PA, Bekelis K, Harris BT, et al. 5-Aminolevulinic acid-induced protoporphyrin IX fluorescence in meningioma: qualitative and quantitative measurements in vivo. Neurosurgery. 2014; 10 suppl 1:74–82, discussion 82–83

[9] Coluccia D, Fandino J, Fujioka M, Cordovi S, Muroi C, Landolt H. Intraoperative 5-aminolevulinic-acid-induced fluorescence in meningiomas. Acta Neurochir (Wien). 2010; 152(10):1711–1719

[10] Kajimoto Y, Kuroiwa T, Miyatake S, et al. Use of 5-aminolevulinic acid in fluorescence-guided resection of meningioma with high risk of recurrence. Case report. J Neurosurg. 2007; 106(6):1070–1074

[11] Cornelius JF, Slotty PJ, Kamp MA, Schneiderhan TM, Steiger HJ, El-Khatib M. Impact of 5-aminolevulinic acid fluorescence-guided surgery on the extent of resection of meningiomas–with special regard to high-grade tumors. Photodiagn Photodyn Ther. 2014; 11(4):481–490

[12] Morofuji Y, Matsuo T, Hayashi Y, Suyama K, Nagata I. Usefulness of intraoperative photodynamic diagnosis using 5-aminolevulinic acid for meningiomas with cranial invasion: technical case report. Neurosurgery. 2008; 62(3) suppl 1:102–103, discussion 103–104

[13] Della Puppa A, Rustemi O, Gioffrè G, et al. Predictive value of intraoperative 5-aminolevulinic acid-induced fluorescence for detecting bone invasion in meningioma surgery. J Neurosurg. 2014; 120(4):840–845

[14] Whitson WJ, Valdes PA, Harris BT, Paulsen KD, Roberts DW. Confocal microscopy for the histological fluorescence pattern of a recurrent atypical meningioma: case report. Neurosurgery. 2011; 68(6):E1768–E1772, discussion E1772–E1773

[15] Bekelis K, Valdés PA, Erkmen K, et al. Quantitative and qualitative 5-aminolevulinic acid-induced protoporphyrin IX fluorescence in skull base meningiomas. Neurosurg Focus. 2011; 30(5):E8

[16] Cornelius JF, Slotty PJ, Stoffels G, Galldiks N, Langen KJ, Steiger HJ. 5-Aminolevulinic acid and (18)F-FET-PET as metabolic imaging tools for surgery of a recurrent skull base meningioma. J Neurol Surg B Skull Base. 2013; 74(4):211–216

[17] Wilbers E, Hargus G, Wölfer J, Stummer W. Usefulness of 5-ALA (Gliolan®)-derived PPX fluorescence for demonstrating the extent of infiltration in atypical meningiomas. Acta Neurochir (Wien). 2014; 156(10):1853–1854

[18] Scheichel F, Ungersboeck K, Kitzwoegerer M, Marhold F. Fluorescence-guided resection of extracranial soft tissue tumour infiltration in atypical meningioma. Acta Neurochir (Wien). 2017; 159(6):1027–1031

[19] Eicker SO, Floeth FW, Kamp M, Steiger HJ, Hänggi D. The impact of fluorescence guidance on spinal intradural tumour surgery. Eur Spine J. 2013; 22(6):1394–1401

[20] Muroi C, Fandino J, Coluccia D, Berkmann S, Fathi AR, Landolt H. 5-Aminolevulinic acid fluorescence-guided surgery for spinal meningioma. World Neurosurg. 2013; 80(1–2):223.e1–223.e3

[21] Bradley RS, Thorniley MS. A review of attenuation correction techniques for tissue fluorescence. J R Soc Interface. 2006; 3(6):1–13

[22] Valdés PA, Leblond F, Kim A, et al. Quantitative fluorescence in intracranial tumor: implications for ALA-induced PpIX as an intraoperative biomarker. J Neurosurg. 2011; 115(1):11–17

[23] Valdés PA, Leblond F, Jacobs VL, Wilson BC, Paulsen KD, Roberts DW. Quantitative, spectrally-resolved intraoperative fluorescence imaging. Sci Rep. 2012; 2:798

[24] Valdés PA, Jacobs V, Harris BT, et al. Quantitative fluorescence using 5-aminolevulinic acid-induced protoporphyrin IX biomarker as a surgical adjunct in low-grade glioma surgery. J Neurosurg. 2015; 123(3):771–780

[25] Valdés PA, Kim A, Brantsch M, et al. δ-aminolevulinic acid-induced protoporphyrin IX concentration correlates with histopathologic markers of malignancy in human gliomas: the need for quantitative fluorescence-guided resection to identify regions of increasing malignancy. Neuro-oncol. 2011; 13 (8):846–856

[26] Valdes PA, Angelo JP, Choi HS, Gioux S. qF-SSOP: real-time optical property corrected fluorescence imaging. Biomed Opt Express. 2017; 8(8):3597–3605

[27] Lee JY, Pierce JT, Thawani JP, et al. Near-infrared fluorescent image-guided surgery for intracranial meningioma. J Neurosurg. 2018; 128:380–390

[28] Ferroli P, Acerbi F, Albanese E, et al. Application of intraoperative indocyanine green angiography for CNS tumors: results on the first 100 cases. Acta Neurochir Suppl (Wien). 2011; 109:251–257

[29] d'Avella E, Volpin F, Manara R, Scienza R, Della Puppa A. Indocyanine green videoangiography (ICGV)-guided surgery of parasagittal meningiomas occluding the superior sagittal sinus (SSS). Acta Neurochir (Wien). 2013; 155 (3):415–420

[30] Ueba T, Okawa M, Abe H, et al. Identification of venous sinus, tumor location, and pial supply during meningioma surgery by transdural indocyanine green videography. J Neurosurg. 2013; 118(3):632–636

[31] Han SJ, Magill ST, Tarapore PE, Horton JC, McDermott MW. Direct visualization of improved optic nerve pial vascular supply following tuberculum meningioma resection: case report. J Neurosurg. 2016; 125(3): 565–569

[32] da Silva CE, da Silva VD, da Silva JL. Sodium fluorescein in skull base meningiomas: a technical note. Clin Neurol Neurosurg. 2014; 120:32–35

[33] da Silva CE, da Silva VD, da Silva JL. Skull base meningiomas and cranial nerves contrast using sodium fluorescein: a new application of an old tool. J Neurol Surg B Skull Base. 2014; 75(4):255–260

[34] Sanai N, Eschbacher J, Hattendorf G, et al. Intraoperative confocal microscopy for brain tumors: a feasibility analysis in humans. Neurosurgery. 2011; 68(2) suppl operative:282–290, discussion 290

[35] Eschbacher J, Martirosyan NL, Nakaji P, et al. In vivo intraoperative confocal microscopy for real-time histopathological imaging of brain tumors. J Neurosurg. 2012; 116(4):854–860

# 7 5-Aminolevulinic Acid and Brain Metastases

*Marcel A. Kamp, Marion Rapp, Jan Frederick Cornelius, Hans-Jakob Steiger, and Michael Sabel*

## Abstract

Cerebral metastases are one of the most common intracerebral neoplasms. It was questioned if the 5-aminolevulinic acid (5-ALA) technique is feasible to visualize cerebral metastases and metastatic infiltration, subsequently improves the degree of surgical resection, and lowers the high local recurrence rates. However, only about half of cerebral metastases reveal 5-ALA-derived tumor fluorescence. A very limited number of retrospective studies have suggested that the 5-ALA technique does not allow a reliable visualization of residual parts or the infiltration zone after metastasis resection. Predictors for 5-ALA-induced fluorescence of cerebral metastases have not yet been identified. However, the dichotomized 5-ALA fluorescence behavior might be an indicator for a more aggressive behavior of cerebral metastases.

*Keywords:* cerebral metastases, cerebral metastasis, 5-ALA, fluorescence-guided resection, recurrence, protoporphyrin IX

## 7.1 Introduction

Cerebral metastases are neoplasms that originate from malignant tumors outside the central nervous system (CNS), spread secondarily to the brain, and are not connected with the primary tumor. About 50% of cerebral metastases originate from non–small cell lung cancer (NSCLC) or small cell lung cancer (SCLC), about 20% from breast cancer, and 5 to 20% from melanoma.[1,2] Metastases are the most common cerebral neoplasms with an estimated incidence of about 200,000 patients in the United States each year.[3,4] Approximately 20 to 40% of cancer patients develop cerebral metastases, about 20% dural metastases, and 8% leptomeningeal metastases.[5] However, the incidence of occult cerebral metastases might even be higher based on autopsy studies.[6] Modern targeted cancer therapies further alter the incidence and behavior of cerebral metastases. For example, the introduction of human epidermal growth factor receptor 2 (HER2) targeted therapies in HER2-positive breast cancer patients led to a clinically observed increase in the incidence of cerebral metastases over historical estimates.[7] Similarly, the CNS is the first site of tumor progression in 46% of patients with an anaplastic lymphoma kinase (ALK) rearranged NSCLC treated with crizotinib.[8] On the other hand, subtyping of different tumor entities, development of new chemotherapies, and induction of targeted therapies have dramatically improved systemic control and patient outcomes. As the outcome of cancer patients is improving and cerebral metastases are observed more frequently, the adequate therapy of cerebral metastases is an increasing challenge in modern neuro-oncology. Achieving long-lasting local tumor control with low morbidity and mortality and providing patients with favorable quality of life (QOL) should be major goals in the treatment of cerebral metastases.

## 7.2 Evidence for the Surgical Resection of Cerebral Metastases

Treatment options for cerebral metastases include surgery, single-fraction stereotactic radiosurgery (SRS), radiation therapy, and chemotherapy. Different factors, such as the patient's clinical and neurological condition, number and location of the metastases, and—if applicable—the histopathological diagnosis of the primary tumor, influence the choice of the favored therapy. Therefore, treatment of cerebral metastases is multimodal and interdisciplinary.

Surgical resection of cerebral metastases is still a key modality in the treatment of oligometastatic patients. Its impact has been evaluated in a series of prospective, randomized, and controlled studies comparing resection of single cerebral metastases combined with a whole-brain radiation therapy (WBRT) in comparison to WBRT alone: The key study by Patchell et al and a later Dutch study provided evidence for a significant benefit of a combined treatment as compared to WBRT alone, resulting in an improved progression-free, functionally independent progression-free, and improved overall survival of patients.[9,10,11,12] Even after induction of other therapy modalities such as SRS, surgery for single cerebral metastases is one of the major therapeutic approaches and included in the common recommendations and international guidelines (level I evidence).[13,14,15,16,17] In practice, surgery should be considered for large tumors with a diameter of more than 2 to 3 cm, for surgically accessible metastases, and for symptomatic patients who are otherwise healthy.

## 7.3 Standard Surgical Technique and Associated Problems

The aim of surgery is to completely remove the cerebral metastasis as safely as possible and to achieve long-lasting tumor control.[18] The surgical standard procedure is a microsurgical, white-light-assisted, circumferential resection from the surrounding brain tissue assuming that the cerebral metastasis is well circumscribed. A gliotic pseudocapsule might facilitate complete en bloc resection of cerebral metastases. In contrast to a piecemeal resection, en bloc resections were considered to lower the risk of neurological complications, local recurrence, and leptomeningeal dissemination.[19,20] Frequently, modern neurosurgical techniques are integrated during metastasis resection. A neuronavigation system may help plan the craniotomy, while the intraoperative use of ultrasound may help with the surgical approach for localizing the cerebral metastases. Surgical associated neurological deficits might be prevented by preoperative functional imaging (e.g., by functional MRI or transcortical magnet stimulation) or intraoperative neurophysiologic mapping (e.g., by intraoperative neurophysiological monitoring and awake surgery) to determine location of eloquent cortical tissue and white fiber connections.

The standard technique of metastasis resection results in up to 30% incomplete surgical resections and, without any additional adjuvant therapy, up to 60% local tumor progression.[21,22,23,24] The local recurrence rate after surgery alone was 46% after 1 year in a prospective, randomized American multicenter study and after 2 years 53 and 59% in a retrospective Korean and the prospective, randomized EORTC 22952–26001 trail, respectively.[22,23,24] One explanation for the high local recurrence rate is an irregular tumor–brain interface or an infiltrative growth pattern of cerebral metastases.[25] Another explanation for the high local recurrence rate might be unintended residual tumor tissue after assumed gross total resection.[21] In fact, residual tumor tissue was observed in up to 20% after intended complete surgical resection of cerebral metastases.[21,26] A supramarginal resection with extension of the surgical resection after complete gross total resection to a depth of additional 5 mm might address infiltrative tumor tissue or residual parts and might subsequently result in a lower local recurrence rate.[27,28]

## 7.4 A Rationale for 5-ALA-Derived Fluorescence Detection of Cerebral Metastases

5-aminolevulinic acid (5-ALA) fluorescence-guided surgery (FGS) of high-grade glioma maximizes the extent of surgical resection and improves progression-free survival.[29] 5-ALA-derived fluorescence is also observed in culture with several malignancies outside the CNS such as lung adenocarcinoma, pleural carcinoma, breast carcinoma, colon carcinoma, and malignant melanoma cells.[30,31,32,33,34,35] Apart from these experimental results, various diagnostic and therapeutic approaches utilize 5-ALA-derived fluorescence including multiple prospective, randomized, and controlled studies that have provided evidence for the use of 5-ALA (and hexylaminolevulinate) for detection of bladder cancer.[36,37,38,39,40,41,42,43] This technique was shown to increase detection of bladder malignancies and to lower their recurrence rates.[44] Additional phase I or II studies evaluating the value of 5-ALA-derived fluorescence for intraoperative diagnosis or resection were conducted in patients suffering from breast, gastrointestinal, renal, prostate, or ovarian cancer.[45] An interesting phase I study showed 95% sensitivity and 94% specificity in 5-ALA fluorescence-based detection of residual tumor tissue during laparoscopic partial nephrectomies.[45,46]

We therefore questioned whether 5-ALA FGS will visualize cerebral metastases and metastatic infiltration, subsequently improving the degree of surgical resection and lowering local recurrence rates.

## 7.5 5-ALA Fluorescence of Metastatic Brain Tumors

Utsuki et al first described 5-ALA-induced fluorescence in 9 of 11 cerebral metastases (81.8%).[47] Since that first study, 12 additional studies reported 5-ALA fluorescence of cerebral metastases, of which 6 studies had ≥ 10 patients. For these six studies with more than nine patients, the proportion of 5-ALA-positive metastases ranged from 30 to 81.8%.[47,48,49,50,51,52] In all, they included 233 patients with a total of 120 5-ALA fluorescent metastases (51.5%). Therefore, more than half of cerebral metastases exhibit either faint or strong 5-ALA-induced fluorescence (▶ Fig. 7.1).

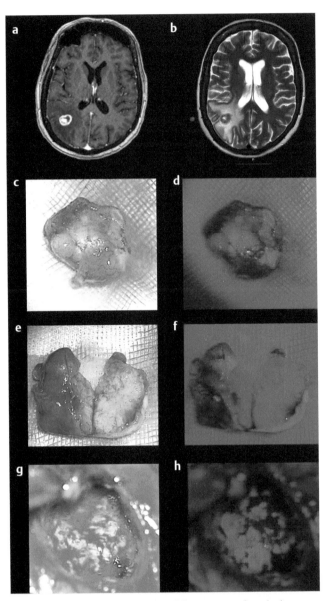

Fig. 7.1 5-Aminolevulinic acid (5-ALA) fluorescence of cerebral metastases: an example. The figure shows the 5-ALA-derived fluorescence of cerebral metastases of a clear-cell renal cancer. The 58-year-old female patients suffered from a renal cancer (classified as grade IV according to the UICC classification) with pulmonal and cerebral metastases. A right parietal metastasis was resected (preoperative MRI scans: **a**, contrast-enhanced T1 sequence; **b**, T2 sequence). Interestingly, the capsule of the metastases but not the core partially showed 5-ALA-derived fluorescence (**c–f**). The 5-ALA fluorescent tumor bed showed a 5-ALA-induced fluorescent but biopsies taken for histopathological analysis revealed no tumor infiltration (**g,h**). (Images **a** and **b** are provided courtesy of Institute for Diagnostic and Interventional Radiology, Medical Faculty, Heinrich-Heine-University, Düsseldorf.)

## 7.6 Does 5-ALA-Induced Fluorescence of Cerebral Metastases Improve the Degree of Surgical Resection?

Unintended residual tumor tissue after assumed complete surgical resection of cerebral metastases is considered to be one explanation for their high local recurrence rate.[21] Does 5-ALA enable visualization of the infiltration zone and residual tumor tissue in 5-ALA fluorescent metastases? This question cannot definitely be answered. In one retrospective study, the resection cavity was assessed for residual fluorescence after macroscopic complete metastases resection in 42 of 52 patients. Residual 5-ALA-induced fluorescence was observed in 24 patients (57.2%).[48] In 18 patients, biopsies were taken from fluorescent tissue, but tumor tissue was demonstrated in only 6/18 patients (33%).[48] A later study analyzed the correlation between 5-ALA fluorescence of cerebral metastases and the extent of the surgical resection as assessed by an early postoperative MRI. Dichotomized 5-ALA fluorescence had no statistical influence on the degree of surgical resection.[49] Furthermore, 5-ALA-induced fluorescence of the metastases did not necessarily correlate with the 5-ALA-derived fluorescence of the resection cavity. Utsuki et al observed diffuse 5-ALA-induced fluorescence of the tumor-free edematous zone surrounding cerebral metastases.[47] Metastases with little 5-ALA-induced fluorescence might even exhibit strong 5-ALA-induced fluorescence of their resection cavity.[48] Unspecific 5-ALA-induced fluorescence might be evoked by diffuse leakage of protoporphyrin IX (PpIX) into areas of edema. However, the precise mechanism is unclear.

Recently, tumor detection by 5-ALA-derived fluorescence was compared to intraoperative MRI. The sensitivity and specificity for detecting 5-ALA fluorescent solid metastases was equal for 5-ALA and for intraoperative MRI in a recent retrospective analysis with eight included patients.[51] The 5-ALA technique showed a slightly higher specificity in detection of the infiltration zone as compared to an intraoperative MRI. However, the difference was not statistically significant.[51]

In conclusion, recent studies do not suggest that 5-ALA allows reliable visualization of residual tumor after metastatic surgical resection. Furthermore, a strongly fluorescent resection cavity does not necessarily contain residual tumor tissue. However, the evidence is poor and further studies are required.

## 7.7 Predictors for 5-ALA-Induced Fluorescence of Cerebral Metastases

If about half of all cerebral metastases reveal faint 5-ALA-induced fluorescence, are there any predictors for 5-ALA-induced fluorescence of cerebral metastases? To date, none of the studies have found a statistically significant correlation between 5-ALA-induced fluorescence and either the histopathological subtype of a metastasis or its primary site.[48,49,50]

## 7.8 5-ALA-Induced Fluorescence as a Marker to Assess the Risk of Local Recurrence

Recently, a significant correlation between 5-ALA-induced fluorescence of cerebral metastases and the local in-brain progression rate was observed. Patients with 5-ALA fluorescent metastases had a significantly lower risk of a local recurrence as compared to patients with nonfluorescent metastases.[49] However, this study included a heterogeneous population with patients suffering from different primary tumors, different tumor stages, and different adjuvant therapy concepts. If only the 64 patients receiving standardized adjuvant WBRT after resection of the cerebral metastases were considered, there was a trend toward a relation of 5-ALA fluorescence and local recurrence rate, but the results no longer reached significance.[49] The dichotomized 5-ALA fluorescence pattern might be an indicator for a more aggressive behavior of cerebral metastases. Previously, the tumor infiltration pattern of cultured lung tumor cell lines was considered to influence 5-ALA fluorescence intensities.[30] However, less is known about a potential correlation between tumor aggressiveness and 5-ALA-induced fluorescence behavior.

Expression of certain molecular markers correlates with the 5-ALA-induced fluorescence of brain tumors and has an influence on tumor migration and invasion. Aquaporin-4 is overexpressed in 5-ALA fluorescent metastases in comparison to normal tissue[53] and may play an important role in tumor cell migration and invasion. In breast cancer cell lines, small interfering RNA (siRNA) knockdown of aquaporin-4 results in an inhibition of cell proliferation, migration, and invasion.[54] Aquaporin-4 expression is considered to play a role in cancer cell metastatic spread in lung adenocarcinomas.[55] A previous study analyzed aquaporin-4 transcription in 576 different normal lung and NSCLC samples. A higher aquaporin-4 expression was observed in a subset of lung adenocarcinomas and higher transcript and protein levels of aquaporin-4 were associated with a more favorable prognosis.[56]

Another crucial molecule that impacts the 5-ALA-induced fluorescence behavior of cerebral tumors is the enzyme ferrochelatase. In mitochondria, 5-ALA is converted to PpIX, which is strongly fluorescent after blue-light excitation. In a further step, the ferrochelatase incorporates iron (Fe) ions into PpIX to form heme. Downregulation of the ferrochelatase in malignant tumor cells leads to an accumulation of PpIX and subsequently to 5-ALA-induced fluorescence of the tumor tissue. Ferrochelatase downregulation results in a strong 5-ALA-induced fluorescence of gastric and colorectal cancer cell lines.[57] Ferrochelatase might further have a direct influence on the outcome of tumor patients as recently observed for desmoid tumors. Overexpression of ferrochelatase was found in more aggressive forms of desmoid tumors and was associated with a poor clinical outcome.[58]

## 7.9 Conclusion

Only about half of cerebral metastases reveal 5-ALA-derived tumor fluorescence. A very limited number of retrospective studies have suggested that the 5-ALA technique does not allow a reliable visualization of residual parts or the infiltration zone after metastasis resection. Predictors for 5-ALA-induced fluorescence of cerebral metastases have yet not been identified. However, the dichotomized 5-ALA fluorescence behavior might be an indicator for a more aggressive behavior of cerebral metastases.

# References

[1] Borgelt B, Gelber R, Kramer S, et al. The palliation of brain metastases: final results of the first two studies by the Radiation Therapy Oncology Group. Int J Radiat Oncol Biol Phys. 1980; 6(1):1–9

[2] Kocher M, Wittig A, Piroth MD, et al. Stereotactic radiosurgery for treatment of brain metastases. A report of the DEGRO Working Group on Stereotactic Radiotherapy. Strahlenther Onkol. 2014; 190(6):521–532

[3] Gavrilovic IT, Posner JB. Brain metastases: epidemiology and pathophysiology. J Neurooncol. 2005; 75(1):5–14

[4] Patchell RA. The management of brain metastases. Cancer Treat Rev. 2003; 29 (6):533–540

[5] DeAngelis LM. Brain tumors. N Engl J Med. 2001; 344(2):114–123

[6] Shojania KG, Burton EC, McDonald KM, Goldman L. Changes in rates of autopsy-detected diagnostic errors over time: a systematic review. JAMA. 2003; 289(21):2849–2856

[7] Lin NU, Winer EP. Brain metastases: the HER2 paradigm. Clin Cancer Res. 2007; 13(6):1648–1655

[8] Takeda M, Okamoto I, Nakagawa K. Clinical impact of continued crizotinib administration after isolated central nervous system progression in patients with lung cancer positive for ALK rearrangement. J Thorac Oncol. 2013; 8(5):654–657

[9] Patchell RA, Tibbs PA, Walsh JW, et al. A randomized trial of surgery in the treatment of single metastases to the brain. N Engl J Med. 1990; 322(8):494–500

[10] Vecht CJ, Haaxma-Reiche H, Noordijk EM, et al. Treatment of single brain metastasis: radiotherapy alone or combined with neurosurgery? Ann Neurol. 1993; 33(6):583–590

[11] Noordijk EM, Vecht CJ, Haaxma-Reiche H, et al. The choice of treatment of single brain metastasis should be based on extracranial tumor activity and age. Int J Radiat Oncol Biol Phys. 1994; 29(4):711–717

[12] Mintz AH, Kestle J, Rathbone MP, et al. A randomized trial to assess the efficacy of surgery in addition to radiotherapy in patients with a single cerebral metastasis. Cancer. 1996; 78(7):1470–1476

[13] Tsao MN, Rades D, Wirth A, et al. International practice survey on the management of brain metastases: Third International Consensus Workshop on Palliative Radiotherapy and Symptom Control. Clin Oncol (R Coll Radiol). 2012; 24(6):e81–e92

[14] Kalkanis SN, Kondziolka D, Gaspar LE, et al. The role of surgical resection in the management of newly diagnosed brain metastases: a systematic review and evidence-based clinical practice guideline. J Neurooncol. 2010; 96(1):33–43

[15] Soffietti R, Ducati A, Rudà R. Brain metastases. Handb Clin Neurol. 2012; 105:747–755

[16] Soffietti R, Trevisan E, Rudà R. Targeted therapy in brain metastasis. Curr Opin Oncol. 2012; 24(6):679–686

[17] Goeckenjan G, Sitter H, Thomas M, et al. German Respiratory Society, German Cancer Society. Prevention, diagnosis, therapy, and follow-up of lung cancer: interdisciplinary guideline of the German Respiratory Society and the German Cancer Society. Pneumologie. 2011; 65(1):39–59

[18] Al-Shamy G, Sawaya R. Management of brain metastases: the indispensable role of surgery. J Neurooncol. 2009; 92(3):275–282

[19] Suki D, Abouassi H, Patel AJ, Sawaya R, Weinberg JS, Groves MD. Comparative risk of leptomeningeal disease after resection or stereotactic radiosurgery for solid tumor metastasis to the posterior fossa. J Neurosurg. 2008; 108(2):248–257

[20] Patel AJ, Suki D, Hatiboglu MA, et al. Factors influencing the risk of local recurrence after resection of a single brain metastasis. J Neurosurg. 2010; 113 (2):181–189

[21] Kamp MA, Rapp M, Bühner J, et al. Early postoperative magnet resonance tomography after resection of cerebral metastases. Acta Neurochir (Wien). 2015; 157(9):1573–1580

[22] Patchell RA, Tibbs PA, Regine WF, et al. Postoperative radiotherapy in the treatment of single metastases to the brain: a randomized trial. JAMA. 1998; 280(17):1485–1489

[23] Yoo H, Kim YZ, Nam BH, et al. Reduced local recurrence of a single brain metastasis through microscopic total resection. J Neurosurg. 2009; 110(4):730–736

[24] Kocher M, Soffietti R, Abacioglu U, et al. Adjuvant whole-brain radiotherapy versus observation after radiosurgery or surgical resection of one to three cerebral metastases: results of the EORTC 22952–26001 study. J Clin Oncol. 2011; 29(2):134–141

[25] Kamp MA, Slotty PJ, Cornelius JF, Steiger HJ, Rapp M, Sabel M. The impact of cerebral metastases growth pattern on neurosurgical treatment. Neurosurg Rev. 2016

[26] Benveniste RJ, Ferraro N, Tsimpas A. Yield and utility of routine postoperative imaging after resection of brain metastases. J Neurooncol. 2014; 118(2):363–367

[27] Kamp MA, Rapp M, Slotty PJ, et al. Incidence of local in-brain progression after supramarginal resection of cerebral metastases. Acta Neurochir (Wien). 2015; 157(6):905–910, discussion 910–911

[28] Kamp MA, Dibué M, Niemann L, et al. Proof of principle: supramarginal resection of cerebral metastases in eloquent brain areas. Acta Neurochir (Wien). 2012; 154(11):1981–1986

[29] Stummer W, Pichlmeier U, Meinel T, Wiestler OD, Zanella F, Reulen HJ, ALA-Glioma Study Group. Fluorescence-guided surgery with 5-aminolevulinic acid for resection of malignant glioma: a randomised controlled multicentre phase III trial. Lancet Oncol. 2006; 7(5):392–401

[30] Gamarra F, Lingk P, Marmarova A, et al. 5-aminolevulinic acid-induced fluorescence in bronchial tumours: dependency on the patterns of tumour invasion. J Photochem Photobiol B. 2004; 73(1–2):35–42

[31] Huber RM, Gamarra F, Hautmann H, et al. 5-Aminolaevulinic acid (ALA) for the fluorescence detection of bronchial tumors. Diagn Ther Endosc. 1999; 5 (2):113–118

[32] Tsai T, Ji HT, Chiang PC, Chou RH, Chang WS, Chen CT. ALA-PDT results in phenotypic changes and decreased cellular invasion in surviving cancer cells. Lasers Surg Med. 2009; 41(4):305–315

[33] Ali AH, Takizawa H, Kondo K, et al. 5-Aminolevulinic acid-induced fluorescence diagnosis of pleural malignant tumor. Lung Cancer. 2011; 74(1):48–54

[34] Moan J, Bech O, Gaullier JM, et al. Protoporphyrin IX accumulation in cells treated with 5-aminolevulinic acid: dependence on cell density, cell size and cell cycle. Int J Cancer. 1998; 75(1):134–139

[35] Campbell DL, Gudgin-Dickson EF, Forkert PG, Pottier RH, Kennedy JC. Detection of early stages of carcinogenesis in adenomas of murine lung by 5-aminolevulinic acid-induced protoporphyrin IX fluorescence. Photochem Photobiol. 1996; 64(4):676–682

[36] Riedl CR, Daniltchenko D, Koenig F, Simak R, Loening SA, Pflueger H. Fluorescence endoscopy with 5-aminolevulinic acid reduces early recurrence rate in superficial bladder cancer. J Urol. 2001; 165(4):1121–1123

[37] Filbeck T, Pichlmeier U, Knuechel R, Wieland WF, Roessler W. Do patients profit from 5-aminolevulinic acid-induced fluorescence diagnosis in transurethral resection of bladder carcinoma? Urology. 2002; 60(6):1025–1028

[38] Filbeck T, Pichlmeier U, Knuechel R, Wieland WF, Roessler W. Clinically relevant improvement of recurrence-free survival with 5-aminolevulinic acid induced fluorescence diagnosis in patients with superficial bladder tumors. J Urol. 2002; 168(1):67–71

[39] Kriegmair M, Zaak D, Rothenberger KH, et al. Transurethral resection for bladder cancer using 5-aminolevulinic acid induced fluorescence endoscopy versus white light endoscopy. J Urol. 2002; 168(2):475–478

[40] Zaak D, Hungerhuber E, Schneede P, et al. Role of 5-aminolevulinic acid in the detection of urothelial premalignant lesions. Cancer. 2002; 95(6):1234–1238

[41] Babjuk M, Soukup V, Petrík R, Jirsa M, Dvorácek J. 5-aminolaevulinic acid-induced fluorescence cystoscopy during transurethral resection reduces the risk of recurrence in stage Ta/T1 bladder cancer. BJU Int. 2005; 96(6):798–802

[42] Schumacher MC, Holmäng S, Davidsson T, Friedrich B, Pedersen J, Wiklund NP. Transurethral resection of non-muscle-invasive bladder transitional cell cancers with or without 5-aminolevulinic Acid under visible and fluorescent light: results of a prospective, randomised, multicentre study. Eur Urol. 2010; 57(2):293–299

[43] Stenzl A, Penkoff H, Dajc-Sommerer E, et al. Detection and clinical outcome of urinary bladder cancer with 5-aminolevulinic acid-induced fluorescence

cystoscopy : A multicenter randomized, double-blind, placebo-controlled trial. Cancer. 2011; 117(5):938–947

[44] Lee JY, Cho KS, Kang DH, et al. A network meta-analysis of therapeutic outcomes after new image technology-assisted transurethral resection for non-muscle invasive bladder cancer: 5-aminolaevulinic acid fluorescence vs hexyla-minolevulinate fluorescence vs narrow band imaging. BMC Cancer. 2015; 15:566

[45] Nokes B, Apel M, Jones C, Brown G, Lang JE. Aminolevulinic acid (ALA): photodynamic detection and potential therapeutic applications. J Surg Res. 2013; 181(2):262–271

[46] Hoda MR, Popken G. Surgical outcomes of fluorescence-guided laparoscopic partial nephrectomy using 5-aminolevulinic acid-induced protoporphyrin IX. J Surg Res. 2009; 154(2):220–225

[47] Utsuki S, Miyoshi N, Oka H, et al. Fluorescence-guided resection of metastatic brain tumors using a 5-aminolevulinic acid-induced protoporphyrin IX: pathological study. Brain Tumor Pathol. 2007; 24(2):53–55

[48] Kamp MA, Grosser P, Felsberg J, et al. 5-aminolevulinic acid (5-ALA)-induced fluorescence in intracerebral metastases: a retrospective study. Acta Neurochir (Wien). 2012; 154(2):223–228, discussion 228

[49] Kamp MA, Fischer I, Bühner J, et al. 5-ALA fluorescence of cerebral metastases and its impact for the local-in-brain progression. Oncotarget. 2016; 7(41): 66776–66789

[50] Marbacher S, Klinger E, Schwyzer L, et al. Use of fluorescence to guide resection or biopsy of primary brain tumors and brain metastases. Neurosurg Focus. 2014; 36(2):E10

[51] Coburger J, Engelke J, Scheuerle A, et al. Tumor detection with 5-aminolevulinic acid fluorescence and Gd-DTPA-enhanced intraoperative MRI at the border of contrast-enhancing lesions: a prospective study based on histopathological assessment. Neurosurg Focus. 2014; 36(2):E3

[52] Takahashi K, Ikeda N, Nonoguchi N, et al. Enhanced expression of coproporphyrinogen oxidase in malignant brain tumors: CPOX expression and 5-ALA-induced fluorescence. Neuro-oncol. 2011; 13(11):1234–1243

[53] Suero Molina EJ, Ardon H, Schroeteler J, et al. Aquaporin-4 in glioma and metastatic tissues harboring 5-aminolevulinic acid-induced porphyrin fluorescence. Clin Neurol Neurosurg. 2013; 115(10):2075–2081

[54] Li YB, Sun SR, Han XH. Down-regulation of AQP4 inhibits proliferation, migration and invasion of human breast cancer cells. Folia Biol (Praha). 2016; 62(3):131–137

[55] Xie Y, Wen X, Jiang Z, Fu HQ, Han H, Dai L. Aquaporin 1 and aquaporin 4 are involved in invasion of lung cancer cells. Clin Lab. 2012; 58(1–2):75–80

[56] Warth A, Muley T, Meister M, et al. Loss of aquaporin-4 expression and putative function in non-small cell lung cancer. BMC Cancer. 2011; 11:161

[57] Kemmner W, Wan K, Rüttinger S, et al. Silencing of human ferrochelatase causes abundant protoporphyrin-IX accumulation in colon cancer. FASEB J. 2008; 22(2):500–509

[58] Salas S, Brulard C, Terrier P, et al. Gene expression profiling of desmoid tumors by cDNA microarrays and correlation with progression-free survival. Clin Cancer Res. 2015; 21(18):4194–4200

# 8 5-Aminolevulinic Acid and Indocyanine Green: Fluorescence-Guided Resection of Spinal Cord Intramedullary Tumors

*Toshiki Endo, Tomoo Inoue, and Teiji Tominaga*

**Abstract**

During surgery for intramedullary spinal cord tumors, it is important to detect the boundaries between the lesion and the normal spinal cord. Better visualization of the border will increase the likelihood for the maximum degree of resection without damaging the surrounding spinal cord. For this purpose, we describe here the utility of 5-aminolevulinic acid (5-ALA) and indocyanine green (ICG) videoangiography during intramedullary spinal cord tumor surgery. In astrocytic and ependymal tumors, 5-ALA induces red fluorescence in tumors, which helps surgeons delineate lesions from the surrounding spinal cord, especially with ependymomas. ICG videoangiography is useful for removing hypervascular tumors including hemangioblastomas. By locating feeders as well as drainers, ICG helps surgeons better understand the angioarchitectures around the tumors and perform reliable surgical resections. In cavernous angioma surgery, ICG videoangiography highlights lesions as an avascular area. Both 5-ALA and ICG are useful surgical adjuncts during intramedullary spinal cord tumor surgery. With appropriate use of fluorescence-guided surgery in spinal cord surgery, neurosurgeons are more likely to achieve both maximum tumor removal and preservation of spinal cord functions.

*Keywords:* 5-aminolevulinic acid, endoscope, indocyanine green, intramedullary tumor, spinal cord tumors, neuromonitoring

## 8.1 Introduction

In spinal cord tumor surgery, the goal is to achieve both maximum tumor resection and functional preservation. In this chapter, we describe the utility of fluorescence-guided resection in spinal cord intramedullary tumor surgery. Specifically, we describe the application of 5-aminolevulinic acid (5-ALA) during spinal cord ependymoma and astrocytoma surgery. We also present clinical cases (hemangioblastoma and cavernous angioma) in which indocyanine green (ICG) videoangiography was utilized.

## 8.2 Protocols

### 8.2.1 5-Aminolevulinic Acid

Patients were orally administered 5-ALA (20 mg/kg bodyweight; Cosmo Bio Co., Ltd, Tokyo, Japan) 2 hours before the induction of anesthesia. For intraoperative detection of 5-ALA fluorescence, an operative microscope (Carl Zeiss Co., Oberkochen, Germany), which can switch from conventional white light to violet–blue excitation light, was used. To avoid potential skin phototoxicity, all patients were protected from light sources for 24 hours after 5-ALA administration.

### 8.2.2 Indocyanine Green

For intraoperative ICG videoangiography, 0.3 mg/kg of ICG (Santen, Tokyo, Japan), diluted with 3.0 mL of saline, followed by 10 mL of saline were injected intravenously. A Pentero operating microscope (Carl Zeiss Co.) was used to excite and visualize ICG.

## 8.3 5-Aminolevulinic Acid in Ependymoma Surgery

### 8.3.1 Overview

Spinal cord ependymoma is the most common intramedullary tumor and accounts for 35 to 40% of such tumors.[1] Once gross total resection is achieved, intramedullary ependymoma is potentially curable with an excellent prognosis and a low recurrence rate.[2,3] The most important tip for gross total resection of intramedullary ependymoma is to find the cleavage plane between the tumor and the normal spinal cord parenchyma.[4] This is often difficult at the rostral and caudal ends of the tumor cavity or in the anterior medial fissure.[5] The former portion is connected to the cavity and central canal, and the plane is often unclear. Small branches from the anterior spinal artery frequently feed the tumors. Care must be taken to preserve the anterior commissure and the anterior spinal vasculature since gliosis on the ventral side of the tumor can be severe due to repeated hemorrhage. In the following section, we describe each step of the surgical procedure for 5-ALA fluorescence-guided resection of ependymoma.

### 8.3.2 Surgical Procedure

To separate the posterior median sulcus and approach the tumor, patients were usually positioned prone. At our facility, we routinely monitor motor evoked potentials (MEPs) and somatosensory evoked potentials (SSEPs) in all spinal cord tumor operations. SSEPs were elicited from the posterior tibial and ulnar nerves (pulse duration 0.20 ms, frequency 4.7 Hz, and intensity 10–30 mA). Transcranial stimulation was applied for MEPs under the following conditions: biphasic 5 train stimuli; pulse duration = 0.5 ms; pulse interval = 2 ms; and intensity = 150–200 mA (MS-120B, Nihon Koden, Tokyo, Japan). Evoked muscles included the biceps, hypothenar, tibialis anterior, and gastrocnemius. The surgical procedure began after the neuromonitoring team completed their setup and confirmed responses.

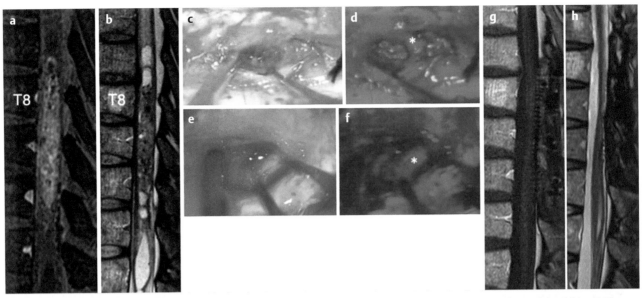

**Fig. 8.1** 5-aminolevulinic acid (5-ALA) fluorescence-guided resection in ependymoma. Preoperative contrast-enhanced T1-weighted **(a)** and T2-weighted **(b)** sagittal MRI revealing a heterogeneously enhanced intramedullary T8–T10 tumor with cyst formation extending to T7. **(c–f)** Intraoperative images. Note that the images obtained using white light (left column) are coupled with images using 5-ALA fluorescence (right). **(c,d)** After dissection of the posterior medial sulcus, the tumor, which had a vivid red fluorescence (*asterisk*), was encountered. **(e,f)** At the ventrocaudal edge of the tumor, yellow tissue was left untouched based on negative 5-ALA fluorescence (*asterisk*). Postoperative contrast-enhanced T1-weighted **(g)** and T2-weighted **(h)** sagittal MRI confirmed no recurrence of the tumor 5 years after the operation.

### 8.3.3 Representative Cases

Following dissection of the posterior median sulcus, we encountered gray tumors in the midline (▶ Fig. 8.1c). As shown in ▶ Fig. 8.1, strong fluorescence was apparent in the tumor (▶ Fig. 8.1d). As we reported previously, spinal cord ependymoma tumors frequently reveal strong 5-ALA-induced fluorescence.[5] In our case series, seven of nine cases showed strong fluorescence, which was dependent on MIB-1 labeling indexes.

In one case, we were unable to dissect a yellow tissue of the tumor at the ventrocaudal end (▶ Fig. 8.1e). Observation using violet–blue excitation light showed no 5-ALA fluorescence (▶ Fig. 8.1f). Therefore, we did not think it was necessary to proceed with further radical dissection of the ventral spinal cord, and we closed the case.

Preoperatively, his postoperative neurological recovery was remarkable. The last follow-up was 5 years after the surgery. The patient was free from tumor recurrence, and could walk and run without assistance.

In another case (▶ Fig. 8.2; Video 8.1), 5-ALA-induced protoporphyrin IX (PpIX) fluorescence was observed at the caudal border of the tumor (▶ Fig. 8.2e). We thus resected this portion and encountered yellowish tissue (▶ Fig. 8.2g). We did not remove the yellowish tissue since it exhibited no fluorescence (▶ Fig. 8.2h). Importantly, postoperative histological evaluations confirmed the findings of PpIX fluorescence. Tumor cells were evident where 5-ALA fluorescence was positive at the tumor border (▶ Fig. 8.2f). Following fluorescence-guided resection, this patient experienced postoperative neurological recovery and a long-term recurrence-free period.

### 8.3.4 Summary

As the representative cases indicate, tumor fluorescence derived from 5-ALA enabled neurosurgeons to identify the tumor during resection and to better identify the resection border. 5-ALA fluorescence-guided surgery (FGS) was easy and did not require the interruption of surgery.[5] Moreover, this technique was useful for differentiating tumors from nontumor tissues, thus facilitating complete resections of intramedullary ependymomas without permanent neurological deterioration.

## 8.4 5-Aminolevulinic Acid in Astrocytoma Surgery

### 8.4.1 Overview

In general, the prognosis of spinal cord high-grade astrocytoma remains poor. According to previous reports, estimated median survival ranges from 10 to 72 months and 9 to 13.1 months in anaplastic astrocytoma and glioblastoma, respectively.[6,7,8] Among various prognostic factors, the extent of surgical resection might improve patient outcomes. For instance, McGirt et al reported the beneficial effects of radical resection in increasing overall survival in high-grade astrocytoma cases.[7] However, pursuing radical tumor resection can sometimes be harmful, since a clear cleavage plane between the tumor and the normal spinal cord does not exist in most cases of spinal cord astrocytoma.[9]

In treating spinal cord astrocytoma, we believe that treatment protocols should rely on histological grades. Therefore,

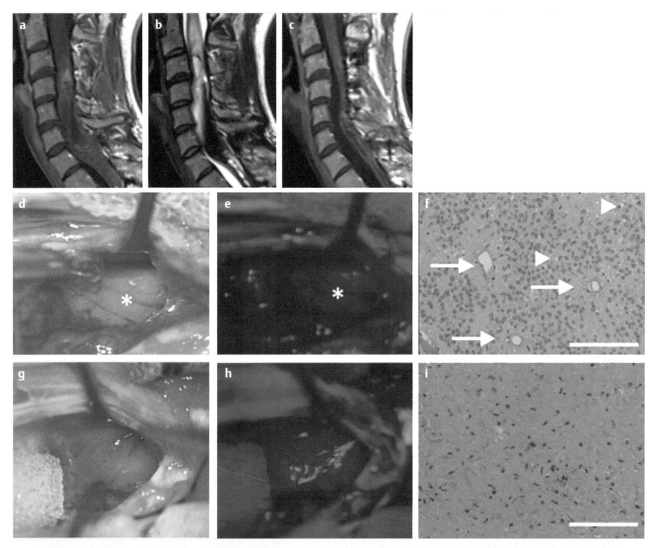

**Fig. 8.2** 5-aminolevulinic acid (5-ALA) fluorescence-guided resection in ependymoma. Preoperative contrast-enhanced T1-weighted **(a)** and T2-weighted **(b)** sagittal MRI revealing a heterogeneously enhanced intramedullary tumor at the C4 level with an intratumoral cyst. **(c)** Postoperative T1-weighted sagittal MRI confirmed complete tumor resection with no signs of recurrence. **(d,e)** At the caudal end of the tumor, a residual tumor was visualized with 5-ALA fluorescence (*asterisk*). **(f)** Characteristic perivascular pseudorosettes (*arrows*) and ependymal rosettes (*arrowheads*) were observed in the tissue with 5-ALA positive fluorescence. Hematoxylin and eosin stain. Scale bars = 200 mm. **(g,h)** With 5-ALA fluorescence guidance, complete tumor resection was accomplished. **(i)** Postoperative histological analysis confirmed the absence of tumor in areas with 5-ALA negative fluorescence. Scale bars = 200 mm. (Reproduced with permission from Inoue et al.[5])

when the preoperative diagnosis included astrocytoma, open biopsy or partial resections were indicated to determine the pathological diagnosis. Based on the diagnosis and histological grade, decisions were made for further surgical intervention and/or postoperative adjuvant chemotherapy and radiotherapy. In the following section, we describe our findings with 5-ALA FGS in spinal cord astrocytoma surgery.

## 8.4.2 Representative Case

Herein, we present the case of a 67-year-old man who had a 1-year history of progressive difficulty with walking and hypesthesia in the lower extremities. T2-weighted MRI demonstrated a hyperintense area in the conus medullaris (▶ Fig. 8.3). Contrast-enhanced MRI showed heterogeneous enhancement. To obtain a pathological diagnosis, open biopsy through a right

T12 hemilaminectomy was performed. During the procedure, it was noted that 5-ALA-induced fluorescence was strongly positive in sections of the tumor where the surgical specimens were collected (▶ Fig. 8.3d). Based on the fluorescence, the biopsy was completed and a histological diagnosis of anaplastic astrocytoma was established.

After the patient received local spinal irradiation with a total dose of 50 Gy at our radiology department, the patient was referred to us again due to rapid regrowth of the tumor (▶ Fig. 8.4a). Although the patient was ambulating with a cane, he experienced worsening of lower extremity muscle strength and difficulties in urinary voiding. In a second operation, after 5-ALA administration, vague and diffuse positive fluorescence was visualized inside the tumor (▶ Fig. 8.4c). It was difficult to determine tumor and spinal cord boundaries under standard white-light observation. Therefore, we removed the tumor

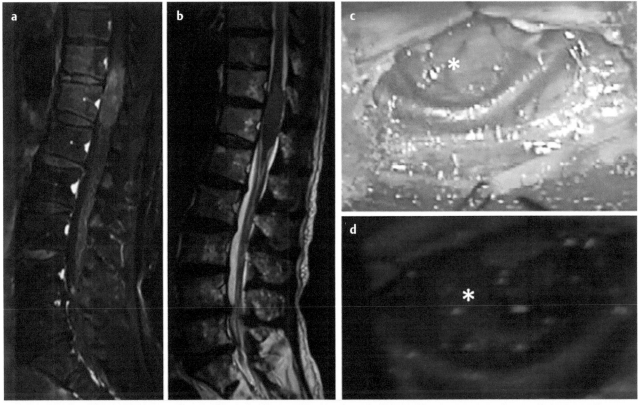

**Fig. 8.3** 5-aminolevulinic acid fluorescence-guided resection in spinal cord astrocytoma. Preoperative contrast-enhanced T1-weighted **(a)** sagittal MRI revealing a heterogeneously enhanced mass in the conus medullaris. T2-weighted MRI **(b)** indicating swelling and abnormal hyperintensity in the spinal cord. **(c,d)** Following T12 hemilaminectomy and dural incision, red fluorescence (*asterisk*) indicated the area suitable for histological analyses.

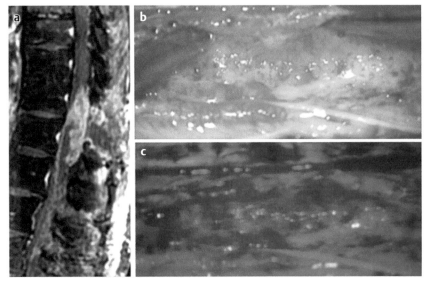

**Fig. 8.4** 5-aminolevulinic acid (5-ALA) fluorescence-guided resection in spinal cord astrocytoma. **(a)** Contrast-enhanced T1-weighted sagittal MRI revealing rapid growth of the enhanced mass in the conus medullaris. **(b)** Under microscopic inspection, it was difficult to find the margins between the tumor and spinal cord. **(c)** 5-ALA demonstrated diffuse and vague fluorescence.

under 5-ALA fluorescence guidance. However, this strategy still resulted in partial resection since amplitudes of the MEPs significantly decreased. After surgery, the patient's lower extremity symptoms worsened. The patient required wheelchair usage and self-intermittent catheterization for voiding. Later, the patient suffered intracranial dissemination and died 2 years after the first operation.

## 8.4.3 Summary

To date, experience with the administration of 5-ALA for spinal cord astrocytomas have been limited to a few case series.[10,11] Ewelt et al[11] reported a recurrent spinal glioma case in which positive 5-ALA fluorescence determined boundaries between the spinal cord and malignant gliomas when they perform

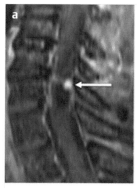
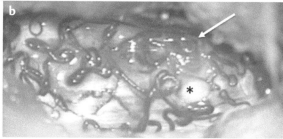
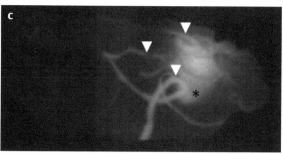

**Fig. 8.5** Indocyanine green (ICG) fluorescence-guided resection in hemangioblastoma. **(a)** Contrast-enhanced T1-weighted sagittal MRI revealing an enhanced mass (*arrow*) with a peritumoral cyst at the C6 level. **(b)** Following C6 hemilaminectomy, the tumor was visible dorsally on the spinal cord (*arrow*). The relationships between the tumor and surrounding vasculatures were not clear. Part of the tumor was embedded inside the spinal cord and was not visible (*asterisk*). **(c)** An image from ICG videoangiography. In the arterial phase, feeding arteries (*arrowheads*) were recognized. ICG fluorescence indicated that part of the tumor was embedded inside the spinal cord (*asterisk*).

palliative spinal corpectomy. Based on our original individual case and other cases reported in the literature, high-grade astrocytomas tend to be 5-ALA fluorescence positive. However, tumor and spinal cord boundaries were not as clearly defined as we experienced with the ependymoma cases. It may be true that a higher extent of surgical resection could improve overall survival. However, surgeons face a dilemma as such radical resections may cause patients to suffer new or worsening neurological deficits. Especially when the margins between tumors and normal tissue are unclear, surgical manipulation could lead to disruption of the adjacent microvasculature and edema of the surrounding tissue.[1,12] Even with recent advances in electrophysiological neuromonitoring, it is still difficult to perform radical surgical resection while preserving high-level functional outcomes in spinal cord astrocytoma.[13,14,15] A prospective study with a large number of cases is necessary to determine whether 5-ALA FGS can improve clinical outcomes in this clinical entity.

## 8.5 Indocyanine Green in Vascular Tumors (i.e., Hemangioblastoma and Cavernous Angioma)

### 8.5.1 Overview

Following the intravenous injection of ICG, intravascular fluorescence can be imaged with a surgical microscope.[16] ICG videoangiography was originally used to provide useful information in cerebrovascular[17] and spinal vascular surgeries.[18] Herein, we describe a case of hemangioblastoma and cavernous angioma, in which ICG videoangiography was useful in demonstrating tumor borders and angioarchitectures related to a tumor.

### 8.5.2 Representative Cases

#### Hemangioblastoma

A 57-year-old man was referred to us with a complaint of hypersensation in his right lower extremity. Preoperative MRI

indicated an enhanced solid mass lesion surrounded by an intraparenchymal cyst (▶ Fig. 8.5a). Following a right C6 hemilaminectomy, a part of the tumor was exposed (▶ Fig. 8.5b; Video 8.2). ICG videoangiography indicated the locations of the arterial feeders. With ICG fluorescence, the margins of the tumor that were partly embedded inside the spinal cord were clearly visible (▶ Fig. 8.5c). By understanding the angioarchitectures of this hypervascular tumor, we could safely achieve complete resection of the tumor. Postoperatively, the patient's symptoms improved remarkably.

#### Cavernous Angioma

A 43-year-old man presented with a sudden onset of weakness in the left upper and lower extremities. The patient also had decreased positional sense in the bilateral leg. MRI on admission demonstrated a heterogeneously enhanced mass lesion surrounded by intraparenchymal hemorrhage. Contrast-enhanced MRI also indicated the coexistence of a developmental venous anomaly located dorsally on the spinal cord (▶ Fig. 8.6a,b). Following C2 lower partial hemilaminotomy, C3 hemilaminectomy, and dural incision, an intramedullary cavernous angioma was recognized on the left dorsal spinal cord (▶ Fig. 8.6c). Through the arterial and venous phases, ICG videoangiography depicted the cavernous angiomas as avascular areas, while dorsal veins and normal spinal cord parenchymas were visualized. The lesions were safely removed while the posterior spinal veins were preserved. The pathological diagnosis was cavernous angioma. Postoperative MRI confirmed total resection and he did not experience new neurological symptoms. The patient could ambulate with a cane and remained stable for 4 years postoperatively in the last follow-up.

### 8.5.3 Summary

The utility of ICG in hypervascular tumors has been described and is well established.[19] ICG angiography can locate feeders and drainers and help surgeons perform safer surgical

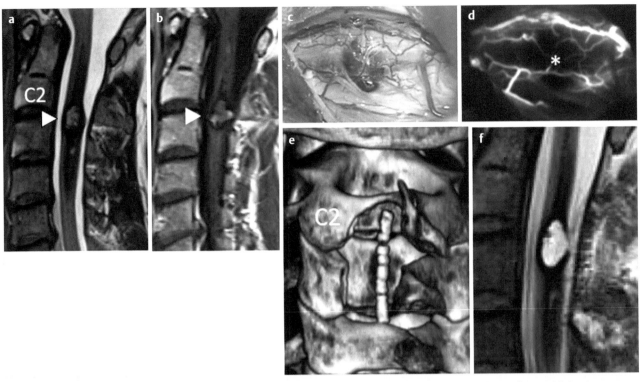

**Fig. 8.6** Indocyanine green (ICG) fluorescence-guided resection in intramedullary cavernous angioma. T2-weighted sagittal image **(a)** showing an area of mixed intensities in the spinal cord at C2/C3. Contrast-enhanced T1-weighted sagittal MRI **(b)** revealing a heterogeneously enhanced mass (*arrowheads* in **a** and **b**), compatible with the intramedullary cavernous angioma. **(c,d)** Intraoperative images on the left dorsal spinal cord. Under ICG fluorescence **(d)**, note an avascular area (*asterisk*) indicating intramedullary cavernous angioma. **(e)** Postoperative computed tomography scan (3D reconstruction image) showing the left dorsal opening of C2 and C3. **(f)** Postoperative T2-weighted sagittal MRI confirmed complete removal and no recurrence of the tumor 4 years after the operation.

resections. Furthermore, immediate postresection ICG videoangiography helped confirm the resection was complete.[20]

We also described the characteristics of ICG fluorescence in a unique case involving intramedullary cavernous angiomas.[21] Interestingly, following ICG injection, cavernous angiomas remained avascular, while the spinal cord parenchyma and spinal veins showed strong ICG fluorescence. This contrasting appearance indicated the location and possible outline of the lesions before the commencement of myelotomy.[21] By recognizing avascular areas in ICG videoangiography, surgeons can estimate the margins of intramedullary cavernous angiomas and the relationships between the lesion and the accompanying developmental venous anomaly.

Selective intra-arterial injection ICG fluorescence angiography further improved the temporary resolution and the flow dynamics related to spinal cord vascular lesions.[22] Recent technical advancements in ICG endoscopy are now applicable to spinal cord pathology.[23] FGS can demonstrate fine vasculatures related to spinal cord tumors and it definitely helps surgeons proceed with surgical removal in a safe and reliable manner.

## 8.6 Conclusion

5-ALA and ICG FGS are a feasible option for various spinal cord intramedullary tumors. Appropriate use of fluorescence in spinal cord surgery can increase the likelihood of achieving both maximal tumor removal and preservation of spinal cord functions.

## References

[1] McCormick PC, Torres R, Post KD, Stein BM. Intramedullary ependymoma of the spinal cord. J Neurosurg. 1990; 72(4):523–532

[2] Aghakhani N, David P, Parker F, Lacroix C, Benoudiba F, Tadie M. Intramedullary spinal ependymomas: analysis of a consecutive series of 82 adult cases with particular attention to patients with no preoperative neurological deficit. Neurosurgery. 2008; 62(6):1279–1285, discussion 1285–1286

[3] Chang UK, Choe WJ, Chung SK, Chung CK, Kim HJ. Surgical outcome and prognostic factors of spinal intramedullary ependymomas in adults. J Neurooncol. 2002; 57(2):133–139

[4] Kucia EJ, Bambakidis NC, Chang SW, Spetzler RF. Surgical technique and outcomes in the treatment of spinal cord ependymomas, part 1: intramedullary ependymomas. Neurosurgery. 2011; 68(1) suppl operative: 57–63, discussion 63

[5] Inoue T, Endo T, Nagamatsu K, Watanabe M, Tominaga T. 5-aminolevulinic acid fluorescence-guided resection of intramedullary ependymoma: report of 9 cases. Neurosurgery. 2013; 72(2) suppl operative:159–168, discussion 168

[6] Adams H, Avendaño J, Raza SM, Gokaslan ZL, Jallo GI, Quiñones-Hinojosa A. Prognostic factors and survival in primary malignant astrocytomas of the spinal cord: a population-based analysis from 1973 to 2007. Spine. 2012; 37 (12):E727–E735

[7] McGirt MJ, Goldstein IM, Chaichana KL, Tobias ME, Kothbauer KF, Jallo GI. Extent of surgical resection of malignant astrocytomas of the spinal cord: outcome analysis of 35 patients. Neurosurgery. 2008; 63(1):55–60, discussion 60–61

[8] Santi M, Mena H, Wong K, Koeller K, Olsen C, Rushing EJ. Spinal cord malignant astrocytomas. Clinicopathologic features in 36 cases. Cancer. 2003; 98(3):554–561

[9] Minehan KJ, Brown PD, Scheithauer BW, Krauss WE, Wright MP. Prognosis and treatment of spinal cord astrocytoma. Int J Radiat Oncol Biol Phys. 2009; 73(3):727–733

[10] Millesi M, Kiesel B, Woehrer A, et al. Analysis of 5-aminolevulinic acid-induced fluorescence in 55 different spinal tumors. Neurosurg Focus. 2014; 36(2):E11

[11] Ewelt C, Stummer W, Klink B, Felsberg J, Steiger HJ, Sabel M. Cordectomy as final treatment option for diffuse intramedullary malignant glioma using 5-ALA fluorescence-guided resection. Clin Neurol Neurosurg. 2010; 112(4):357–361

[12] Nagasawa DT, Smith ZA, Cremer N, Fong C, Lu DC, Yang I. Complications associated with the treatment for spinal ependymomas. Neurosurg Focus. 2011; 31(4):E13

[13] Kothbauer KF, Deletis V, Epstein FJ. Motor-evoked potential monitoring for intramedullary spinal cord tumor surgery: correlation of clinical and neurophysiological data in a series of 100 consecutive procedures. Neurosurg Focus. 1998; 4(5):e1

[14] Deletis V, Sala F. Intraoperative neurophysiological monitoring of the spinal cord during spinal cord and spine surgery: a review focus on the corticospinal tracts. Clin Neurophysiol. 2008; 119(2):248–264

[15] Matsuyama Y, Sakai Y, Katayama Y, et al. Surgical results of intramedullary spinal cord tumor with spinal cord monitoring to guide extent of resection. J Neurosurg Spine. 2009; 10(5):404–413

[16] Raabe A, Beck J, Gerlach R, Zimmermann M, Seifert V. Near-infrared indocyanine green video angiography: a new method for intraoperative assessment of vascular flow. Neurosurgery. 2003; 52(1):132–139, discussion 139

[17] Holling M, Brokinkel B, Ewelt C, Fischer BR, Stummer W. Dynamic ICG fluorescence provides better intraoperative understanding of arteriovenous fistulae. Neurosurgery. 2013; 73(1) suppl operative:93–98, discussion 99

[18] Endo T, Shimizu H, Sato K, et al. Cervical perimedullary arteriovenous shunts: a study of 22 consecutive cases with a focus on angioarchitecture and surgical approaches. Neurosurgery. 2014; 75(3):238–249, discussion 249

[19] Murakami T, Koyanagi I, Kaneko T, Iihoshi S, Houkin K. Intraoperative indocyanine green videoangiography for spinal vascular lesions: case report. Neurosurgery. 2011; 68(1) suppl operative:241–245, discussion 245

[20] Hwang SW, Malek AM, Schapiro R, Wu JK. Intraoperative use of indocyanine green fluorescence videography for resection of a spinal cord hemangioblastoma. Neurosurgery. 2010; 67(3) suppl operative:300–303, discussion 303

[21] Endo T, Aizawa-Kohama M, Nagamatsu K, Murakami K, Takahashi A, Tominaga T. Use of microscope-integrated near-infrared indocyanine green videoangiography in the surgical treatment of intramedullary cavernous malformations: report of 8 cases. J Neurosurg Spine. 2013; 18 (5):443–449

[22] Yamamoto S, Kim P, Kurokawa R, Itoki K, Kawamoto S. Selective intraarterial injection of ICG for fluorescence angiography as a guide to extirpate perimedullary arteriovenous fistulas. Acta Neurochir (Wien). 2012; 154(3): 457–463

[23] Ito A, Endo T, Inoue T, Endo H, Sato K, Tominaga T. Use of indocyanine green fluorescence endoscopy to treat concurrent perimedullary and dural arteriovenous fistulas in the cervical spine. World Neurosurg. 2017; 101:814. e1–814.e6

# 9 5-Aminolevulinic Acid Utility in Pediatric Brain Tumors, Other Adult Brain Tumors, and Photodynamic Therapy

*Nikita Lakomkin, Isabelle M. Germano, and Constantinos G. Hadjipanayis*

**Abstract**

The use of 5-aminolevulinic acid (5-ALA) as an agent for fluorescence-guided surgery (FGS) of high-grade gliomas (HGGs) has been associated with significantly improved extent of tumor resection and prolonged progression-free survival relative to conventional microsurgery. These findings have led to its approval by the European Medicines Agency and, more recently, the Food and Drug Administration (FDA). This compound is currently indicated for adult patients undergoing surgical intervention for suspected HGGs. However, various studies in the literature have proposed that other brain tumor etiologies may be amenable to 5-ALA-guided resection. Based on promising results in both laboratory studies and early clinical reports, 5-ALA may facilitate improved differentiation of neoplastic tissue during the resection of pediatric brain tumors. Additionally, the accumulation of fluorescence has been observed in a variety of other adult tumor types, including primary central nervous system lymphoma, hemangioblastomas, subependymomas, and germ cell tumors. 5-ALA-mediated tumor fluorescence has also been utilized in quantitative diagnostic techniques, such as through its incorporation of spectrometry, which may augment the ability to detect tumors that exhibit reduced fluorescence accumulation. Although the primary role of 5-ALA in the management of gliomas is the identification of neoplastic tissue, this compound can also be induced to directly and selectively destroy tumors via photodynamic therapy. Studies have begun to evaluate the feasibility, effectiveness, and safety of this treatment modality. In this chapter, the evidence regarding these emerging applications of 5-ALA will be discussed, as well as potential areas that merit further investigation.

*Keywords:* 5-ALA, lymphoma, hemangioblastoma, germ cell tumor, subependymomas, pituitary tumor, schwannoma, pediatric brain tumor, ependymoma, photodynamic therapy

## 9.1 Introduction

The utility of 5-aminolevulinic acid (5-ALA) in facilitating the intraoperative visualization of tumor tissue during the resection of high-grade gliomas (HGGs) is well established.[1,2,3,4,5,6] Intraoperative use of 5-ALA has been significantly associated with improved extent of tumor resection and prolonged progression-free survival for these patients.[7] This led to 5-ALA approval by the European Medicines Agency in 2007. In June 2017, 5-ALA was approved by the Food and Drug Administration (FDA) for the resection of suspected HGGs as an imaging agent to facilitate the real-time detection and visualization of malignant tissue during glioma surgery (https://www.fda.gov/downloads/AdvisoryCommittees/CommitteesMeetingMaterials/Drugs/MedicalImagingDrugsAdvisoryCommittee/UCM557136.pdf). Although its approval is limited to adult patients with suspected HGGs, recent studies have identified additional promising applications for 5-ALA. 5-ALA has been successfully employed in the resection of pediatric brain tumors, with very few reported adverse events.[8,9,10,11] In addition, substantial 5-ALA-induced tumor fluorescence has been observed in other adult tumor types besides HGGs, such as primary central nervous system (CNS) lymphomas, and was deemed to be a useful surgical adjunct for these patients.[12,13,14,15] 5-ALA has been used during surgery for hemangioblastoma, subependymoma, pituitary, and germ cell tumors in addition to meningioma, ependymoma, and brain metastatic tumors, which are discussed in other chapters. Treatment modalities employing 5-ALA for applications beyond tumor visualization have been proposed as well. Under specific conditions, this agent has been demonstrated to have direct cytotoxic effects on neoplasms, and in some cases result in improved survival.[16,17,18] This technique, known as photodynamic therapy (PDT), utilizes specific wavelengths of light to induce targeted damage of tumor tissue via mechanisms involving oxygen radical-mediated toxicity.[19,20,21] While these applications currently represent off-label uses for 5-ALA, preliminary findings may have important implications for the management of complex cranial tumor etiologies. In this chapter, we will review the following promising new areas to be assessed for the use of 5-ALA as adjuvant to resection of other adult tumors as well as brain tumors in the pediatric population. We will also discuss 5-ALA PDT for brain tumors.

## 9.2 Pediatric Tumors

Pediatric brain tumors present a number of unique challenges for surgical management. As in adult patients, complete resection is important in reducing the probability of recurrence and improving long-term outcomes.[22,23,24,25] Although 5-ALA has been demonstrated to be a valuable tool for the intraoperative tumor visualization in adults, literature describing the use of 5-ALA in pediatric tumors remains sparse. In the absence of large controlled trials, questions remain regarding therapeutic safety and efficacy in this patient population. The successful use of 5-ALA-enhanced visualization in the complete resection of a pediatric tumor was first reported by Ruge and Liu in 2009.[10] The authors described a 9-year-old patient presenting with a right temporal lobe pleomorphic xanthoastrocytoma, who underwent 5-ALA fluorescence-guided surgery (FGS). Intraoperative fluorescence was noted to have improved the visualization of the tumor bed and no serious side effects or complications were reported. These observations have since been corroborated by several additional case reports. Bernal García et al[26] reported the use of 5-ALA in the resection of a pediatric, left frontal meningeal sarcoma, while Eicker et al[27] described complete tumor resection in a 15-year-old patient with medulloblastoma (► Fig. 9.1). The postoperative course was uneventful for both patients. Despite these reports, larger case series have noted distinct variations in the level of fluorescence accumulation and consequent intraoperative utility among the

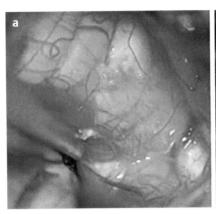
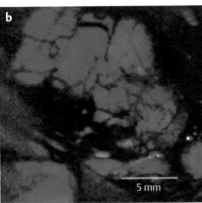

5 mm

**Fig. 9.1** (a) Intraoperative view of a pediatric medulloblastoma under white light. (b) Fluorescent tissue is visible under violet–blue light. (Reproduced with permission from Eicker et al.[27])

different tumor subtypes.[9,28] As in adult patients, HGGs appear to be most likely to fluoresce.

Due to the small numbers of patients included in these series and the substantial heterogeneity between cohorts, Stummer et al performed a survey study in order to compile data regarding the use of 5-ALA during the resection of pediatric brain tumors at centers across Europe.[11] Respondents were queried regarding tumor type, level of intraoperative fluorescence, 5-ALA administration practices, patient demographics, complications, and a variety of other relevant perioperative factors. Additionally, the respondents were asked to report the number of cases in which 5-ALA-induced fluorescence aided in the discrimination of high-grade tissue or informed intraoperative decision-making, which the authors used to gauge the "usefulness" of 5-ALA for these patients. Case information was collected for 78 patients, 28 of whom had fluorescence that was considered to be beneficial. Tumor fluorescence was observed most commonly in HGGs and ependymomas, representing 85 and 80% of tumors, respectively. However, 5-ALA appears to have been less effective for patients with gangliogliomas, medulloblastomas, and pilocytic astrocytomas, with evidence of tumor fluorescence to be as low as 15% for the pilocytic astrocytomas. The authors also addressed the relationship between tumor characteristics, such as location and recurrence, and the utility of 5-ALA. Although a greater percentage of patients with supratentorial tumors demonstrated useful fluorescence, this did not achieve statistical significance. The survey results also revealed distinct variations in 5-ALA administration practices between respondents where preoperative ingestion of the 5-ALA solution ranged from 2 to 6 hours. These early findings emphasize the importance of continued investigation to facilitate the development of evidence-based protocols for the use of this agent in pediatric patients.

Studies have also been carried out in vitro to describe the cellular response of pediatric brain tumors to 5-ALA. Schwake et al evaluated the 5-ALA uptake and fluorescence accumulation in the cell cultures of several pediatric tumor types.[29] Cultures encompassing gliomas, medulloblastomas, ependymomas, rhabdoid tumors, and primitive neuroectodermal tumor (PNET) were included in their analysis. All cell types had some level of 5-ALA-induced fluorescence, but the strength of emissions appeared to be dependent on tumor type. Glioblastoma (GBM) and ependymoma cell lines displayed strong signals, while the two medulloblastoma lines varied in their level of fluorescence. The other test cell cultures did not demonstrate a robust

response. These findings align with previously described observations in clinical cohorts.[9,11,28] The timing of maximal fluorescence following exposure to 5-ALA also revealed variability. Although most cells demonstrated peak fluorescence at 3 hours, one medulloblastoma culture displayed the strongest fluorescence signals 6 hours following 5-ALA exposure. While these findings may help optimize preoperative planning for patients with these tumor types, further investigations employing in vivo models are needed.

Although the intraoperative use of 5-ALA does not appear to introduce additional risks for adult patients with gliomas, safety profiles are not as well known in children where its use in resection is more rare.[30] To date, pediatric patients have not demonstrated adverse reactions following 5-ALA administration in most published reports.[8,9,10,27] However, one series assessing 16 pediatric brain tumor patients reported abnormal liver function tests (LFTs) related to 5-ALA use.[28] Among the overall cohort, postoperative alanine aminotransferase (ALT) and gamma-glutamyl transpeptidase (GGT) were significantly elevated compared to baseline, and were trending toward significance for aspartate aminotransferase (AST). While abnormal LFTs are known to be associated with 5-ALA administration in adults, they represent temporary changes and do not appear to have any detrimental effects on organ health.[30,31] Although these laboratory results were outside the normal ranges for several patients in this pediatric series, no liver dysfunction occurred. However, the authors found a significant correlation between decreased preoperative age and higher postoperative values, commenting on the importance of continued observation for this age group in future trials. Further studies are needed to explore potential differences in the metabolism of 5-ALA in pediatric patients as well as the relationship between age and adverse events.

## 9.3 Other Adult Tumors Types

### 9.3.1 Central Nervous System Lymphoma

Although the majority of the studies in the neurosurgical literature have examined the utility of 5-ALA in glioma resection, this compound has been employed for other adult brain tumor subtypes with favorable results. For instance, several reports

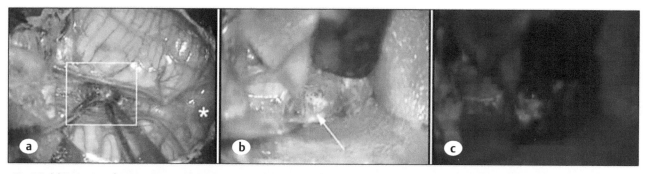

**Fig. 9.2** **(a)** Resection of a primary central nervous system lymphoma. **(b)** Closer view of the surgical site following exposure of the lesion. **(c)** Fluorescent emissions from the tumor under violet–blue light. (Reproduced with permission from Yamamoto et al.[33])

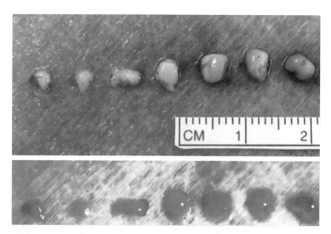

**Fig. 9.3** Biopsies of primary central nervous system lymphomas, which were visibly fluorescent in all but one case. (Reproduced with permission from Yamamoto et al.[36])

have highlighted the potential utility of 5-ALA-mediated fluorescence during surgical intervention for primary CNS lymphomas (▶ Fig. 9.2).[14,32,33] Primary CNS lymphomas are rare tumors that comprise 4% of CNS tumor diagnoses.[34] Since these lesions can be difficult to distinguish from other malignancies via imaging studies, a tissue biopsy is often required to make a definitive diagnosis and inform subsequent therapy.[35] The success of 5-ALA guidance in the resection of gliomas has led to several studies assessing this agent in the diagnosis of primary CNS lymphomas. The first published case detailing the intraoperative response of a primary CNS lymphoma to 5-ALA was published in 2014.[32] The patient was administered 5-ALA prior to open resection of a brain tumor located in the fourth ventricle. Although preoperative MRI features were suggestive of an HGG, postoperative histopathology demonstrated a large B-cell CNS lymphoma. Clear fluorescence of tumor tissue was visible during the surgery, indicating that further investigation into the role of 5-ALA for this tumor type was merited. To date, the largest case series describing the use of 5-ALA in primary CNS lymphoma was published by Yamamoto et al.[36] In this cohort, 41 patients underwent 5-ALA-guided biopsy that resulted in postoperative pathological confirmation of a primary CNS lymphoma. The authors recorded that tumors in 34 of these patients demonstrated positive fluorescence, resulting in a

true-positive rate of 82.9% (▶ Fig. 9.3). Although this rate is lower than the published values for HGGs, which have been reported to exceed 90%, it demonstrates that patients with lymphomas have the potential to benefit from fluorescence-guided visualization.[37] The authors of this study suggest that 5-ALA may increase the probability of obtaining a biopsy sample that is viable for pathological diagnosis of suspected lymphomas.

Despite the relatively high rate of 5-ALA-induced fluorescence, few studies have evaluated the role of 5-ALA during the resection of primary CNS lymphomas because resection is not generally recommended for these tumors.[38] Following the diagnosis of a primary CNS lymphoma, the standard of care consists of a course of chemotherapy, sometimes in conjunction with radiotherapy.[35] Unlike with gliomas, the debulking of primary CNS lymphomas does not appear to be associated with improved survival,[35,39,40] and the additional surgical risks introduced during partial or gross total resection are not typically considered justified due to the responsiveness of these lesions to adjuvant treatments such as methotrexate.[35,41]

## 9.3.2 Hemangioblastomas, Subependymomas, and Germ Cell Tumors

The benefits of 5-ALA guidance during resection have been reported for several other tumor types, including benign lesions and nonglial tumors. Several cases have been published describing the resection of hemangioblastomas under fluorescence guidance using 5-ALA.[42,43] Hemangioblastomas are benign masses that are primarily treated via resection. However, partial resection is associated with increased risk of recurrence, and tools that can potentially improve visualization with a greater consequent likelihood of complete resection may be beneficial in improving long-term outcomes.[44] Utsuki et al reported a case of strong 5-ALA-induced fluorescence in a cranial hemangioblastoma, showing that the visualization facilitated more complete resection.[43] One visual benefit of 5-ALA was reported by the authors to include visible fluorescence that allowed for identification of tumor in the associated peritumoral cyst. Because these cysts often do not contain tumor, surgeons may opt not to resect this portion of the lesion in order to mitigate the risk of damaging surrounding tissue. The authors proposed that 5-ALA can be employed to intraoperatively determine whether resection of the cyst wall is indicated based on the fluorescence emissions from this structure. Utsuki et al also published a larger case series of hemangioblastomas, in which all nine tumors fluoresced following 5-ALA administration.[42] In two cases, the cyst wall also had visible fluorescence, and was subsequently resected. Histopathological analysis revealed the presence of tumor in the cyst walls.

Other tumor types, including two cases of intense 5-ALA-mediated fluorescence accumulation in the resection of fourth ventricle subependymomas have been reported, with no residual lesion on postoperative MRI.[12] 5-ALA has also been used to facilitate the endoscopic biopsy of germ cell tumors.[15] The fluorescence signal was deemed to be useful in differentiating the tumor from the surrounding tissue due to the difficulty of visualizing the mass under normal illumination. These case reports demonstrate that fluorescence can be induced for diverse tumor types, and suggest that 5-ALA may be a valuable intraoperative tool for intervention beyond the resection of gliomas. However, it is difficult to draw definitive conclusions regarding the reliability of this technique. Larger cohorts are needed in order to determine the proportion of each tumor type that accumulates sufficient fluorescence in order to provide valuable intraoperative guidance, as well as to compute the rate of false-positive fluorescence signals. Additional studies are also needed to explore the utility of 5-ALA in providing significantly meaningful advantages regarding the extent of resection and patient outcomes in these surgical populations.

### 9.3.3 Pituitary and Schwannoma Tumors

Marbacher et al reported a series of 458 tumors that were resected or biopsied using 5-ALA visualization, including 12 pituitary adenomas and 7 schwannomas.[37] Of these, no schwannomas and only one adenoma resulted in clear fluorescence. By contrast, 99 of the 103 GBMs and 85 of the 110 meningiomas demonstrated significant fluorescence. These authors concluded that despite the benefits conferred by 5-ALA in HGG tumor visualization, this agent does not appear to be advantageous in the resection of adenomas or schwannomas. However, the presence of fluorescence in these tumors was documented based solely on observations by the surgeon, a known limitation of many 5-ALA studies.[20] Subjective evaluation of fluorescence levels can introduce inter-rater variability and potentially underrepresent the true rate of positive 5-ALA response for different tumor types.

### 9.3.4 Objective Determination of Fluorescence

In order to augment the differentiation of neoplasm from the surrounding parenchyma, methods facilitating the direct, quantitative measurement of fluorescence levels have also been proposed, including the addition of spectrometry.[45,46,47] Eljamel et al described their experiences incorporating an optical biopsy system during the resection of pituitary adenomas.[13] The authors used a probe constructed from a laser and fiberoptic cables that projected light at 440 nm onto the tissue and collected the resulting fluorescence emissions. The probe was connected to a spectrometer, which can be used to generate a fluorescence spectrum. The location and intensity of the peaks were subsequently used to determine the presence of fluorescent tumor tissue based on the known spectroscopic properties of PpIX. In their series of 30 consecutive pituitary adenoma patients, the sensitivity of the optical biopsy system was 95.5% and the specificity was 100%. These results highlight the potential for spectroscopy in facilitating detection of 5-ALA-induced fluorescence. Although it has been previously reported that spectroscopic analysis of fluorescence can result in reduced specificity, no false-positive diagnoses were recorded in this case series.[46] These findings are promising, particularly given the low rate of visually identified fluorescence for adenomas as reported by Marbacher et al.[37] A similar probe has also been used intraoperatively by Valdés et al during surgery for low grade gliomas.[48] However, rather than interpreting the fluorescence spectra, the authors used a mathematical model to estimate the actual concentration of PpIX in the sample. This model was designed to account for other fluorescence signals besides PpIX, as well as adjust for the effects on emissions as they pass through tissue prior to reaching the collection channel of the probe. The authors found that of the 20 tumor specimens without fluorescence apparent to the surgeon, 9 had detectable levels of PpIX accumulation via their approach. The sensitivity of the measurements employing the spectrometer was 58%, which compared favorably to the 21% sensitivity of direct observation by the surgeon. These studies demonstrate that incorporating quantitative diagnostic techniques has the potential to allow for broader application of 5-ALA-mediated intraoperative guidance in lower grade tumors that often exhibit reduced fluorescence accumulation.

## 9.4 Photodynamic Therapy

At present, the primary function of 5-ALA in neurosurgery is the intraoperative visualization of tumor tissue during biopsy or resection.[2] However, it has been reported that 5-ALA can, under specific conditions, have an antitumor effect directly on tumors by PDT.[18,49] The goal of PDT is to target the cancerous lesions with a nontoxic compound, followed by the trigger of its destructive properties to kill the tumor cells without harming the surrounding parenchyma.[50,51] A photosensitizer is administered to the patient and subsequently activated using a specific wavelength of light, which stimulates the release of reactive oxygen species (ROS; ▶ Fig. 9.4).[19] In the case of 5-ALA-based PDT, 5-ALA is metabolized to PpIX, which is then excited by a 635-nm laser.[52,53] This therapy results in the death of tumor cells via several mechanisms.[54] First, the ROS can cause damage to vital cell structures, including DNA, mitochondria, and the cell membrane, with subsequent activation of apoptosis-signaling pathways.[17,21] In addition, substantial necrosis coupled with damage to blood vessels has also been observed within tumors treated with PDT.[19] Some therapies have also been shown to stimulate leukocyte activation and recruitment, which drives the immune response against the neoplasms.[55] These techniques have been performed in the treatment of a variety of tumor types, including cervical, bladder, lung, skin, gastrointestinal, and head and neck cancers, using several classes of photosensitizers.[55,56] 5-ALA has already received FDA approval as a PDT agent, under the brand name Levulan, for topical use

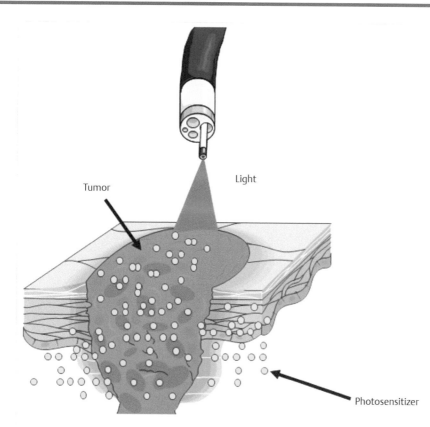

**Fig. 9.4** Illustration depicting the accumulation of the photosensitizing agent in tumor tissue, which is then induced to generate reactive oxygen species via laser excitation. (Reproduced with permission from Wachowska et al.[54])

Light

Tumor

Photosensitizer

during the treatment of actinic keratosis.[57] Beyond dermatological applications, 5-ALA PDT has also been considered for use in neuro-oncology due to the highly concentrated PpIX buildup in HGGs relative to normal tissue.[52]

Several laboratory studies have been performed to elucidate the mechanisms of 5-ALA's phototoxic effects as well as assess its potential viability for use in PDT for neuro-oncology.[17,58,59,60] Neumann et al investigated the cellular response to 5-ALA PDT in both rat and human pituitary adenoma cultures.[59] The authors found that 5-ALA alone did not induce cell destruction and that laser irradiation without prior 5-ALA administration similarly had no effect on proliferation. For cells exposed to both 5-ALA and 635-nm laser emissions, cell death was observed. The toxic effects of this PDT were reported to be modulated by 5-ALA dosage, with lower rates of surviving cells observed at higher 5-ALA concentrations. When this therapy was performed in different human adenoma cell cultures, which had been extracted from several subtypes of adenomas, the level of response varied. The dose of 5-ALA required for complete elimination of the cells was not uniform, indicating that tumor histology, even within a single tumor type, may be an important consideration in the clinical application of 5-ALA PDT. This technique has also been evaluated using in vivo rat glioma models.[60] Post-treatment analysis of extracted rat brains revealed that the destroyed tissue aligned with the size and location of the lesion noted on preoperative imaging studies. Minor damage of normal brain tissue was observed only for the highest tested laser intensity, and occurred with or without administration of 5-ALA prior to irradiation. Thus, 5-ALA-induced PpIX accumulation and toxicity appear to be isolated to

the tumor. Besides directly stimulating apoptotic pathways, it has also been proposed that 5-ALA PDT may inhibit other tumor properties. Etminan et al[17] studied the potential impact of 5-ALA PDT on the invasiveness of human gliomas, which were cultured in a three-dimensional matrix. It was found that cultures undergoing 5-ALA treatment and laser exposure demonstrated almost no migration, resulting in a statistically significant ($p < 0.001$) difference in invasion compared to untreated controls. Changes in cell shape and underlying structure of the cytoskeleton were also observed, which may have contributed to the modifications in the growth patterns of these cancer cells. Because the poor prognosis associated with GBM is attributed largely to the aggressive nature of this tumor type, the ability to not only destroy localized tumor cells, but also inhibit invasion has the potential to provide therapeutic benefit.

The application of 5-ALA PDT in clinical studies has yielded encouraging findings regarding its safety and efficacy in the treatment of brain tumor patients. One case of successful 5-ALA-mediated PDT was reported by Stummer et al.[18] The patient had undergone resection of a GBM, and presented with remote recurrence during the following year. This recurrence was deemed inoperable and subsequently treated with radiotherapy and temozolomide, but did not achieve a response. The patient subsequently opted for off-label treatment by 5-ALA-based PDT. The authors found that the mass was no longer visible on the MRI performed 24 hours following surgery, indicating a rapid and highly sensitive response. Temporary edema was observed on the MRI, but was not symptomatic and had returned to baseline by the subsequent follow-up imaging study. No complications occurred, and the patient's neurological status remained intact throughout this treatment course. The patient had follow-up for 56 months, throughout which he had no evidence of recurrence by imaging. The same research group published their experiences with an additional nine patients who also underwent 5-ALA PDT for recurrent GBM.[16] As in the first case, the tumor completely resolved on the postoperative images of six other patients, while partial reduction of the tumors occurred in the remaining three. Additionally, no adverse events secondary to PDT were reported. Overall, the median survival was reported to be 15 months. Although patients who underwent standard treatment were not included for comparison in this study, the authors described these results as promising given that the expected life span following diagnosis of recurrent GBM are typically 6 to 8 months. Further investigation would be necessary to demonstrate that 5-ALA PDT for HGGs is a promising adjuvant or alternative to conventional surgery and adjuvant external beam radiotherapy with concomitant and adjuvant chemotherapy.

The promise of 5-ALA-mediated PDT of brain tumors is further emphasized by its potential as a combined tool for both intraoperative visualization and postoperative cytotoxic therapy. Eljamel et al carried out a prospective trial to assess patient outcomes following 5-ALA FGS, followed by PDT in patients presenting with new GBM.[49] All 27 patients in this series underwent craniotomy and attempted maximal tumor resection, followed by a course of radiotherapy. The 13 patients who were randomly selected for the treatment group were preoperatively administered 5-ALA and Photofrin, another agent with known fluorescent and photosensitizing properties.[61] The tumor was visualized using laser illumination, and a spectroscopic probe was utilized to detect remaining fluorescent tissue and facilitate gross total resection of the tumor. Immediately following completion of the surgery, the patients then underwent PDT, which triggered the phototoxic properties of the 5-ALA and Photofrin in any residual tumors cells in the resection cavity. Over the next several days, the patients underwent four additional rounds of PDT and were given an additional dose of Photofrin prior to each therapy. At follow-up evaluation, the patients in the treatment group demonstrated excellent outcomes. The mean survival of this group was 52.8 weeks, compared to 24.6 weeks recorded in the control group. Patients who underwent PDT also had delayed tumor progression and a greater degree of improvement in functional status, as quantified by the Karnofsky performance status. These positive effects achieved statistical significance when compared to the patient group managed using standard resection and radiotherapy management. The mean hospital stay for both cohorts was 7 days. For the entire patient series, the only complications observed were three cases of deep vein thrombosis. Two of these events occurred in the treatment group, but were not considered to be related to the photodynamic drugs. However, patients in the treatment group experienced prolonged skin sensitivity, a known side effect of Photofrin and 5-ALA.[62] Skin sensitization is a well-known side effect of 5-ALA that can occur if a patient is exposed to bright lights within 24 to 48 hours after administration.[16,54] Based on these preliminary data, it appears that the use of photodynamic agents can have beneficial effects on patient outcomes without introducing substantial risk. Further study is necessary to quantify the impact of 5-ALA employed in the PDT of patients presenting with GBM.

## 9.5 Conclusion

5-ALA has promising indications as an adjuvant in the resection of CNS tumors other than HGGs, for which it is now approved in the United States. There is growing evidence that 5-ALA can be used in adult patients for certain benign and nonglial tumors. Similarly, preliminary evidence suggests that it could be beneficial for use in pediatric brain tumors where extent of resection is important for overall survival. Finally, 5-ALA seems to have a promising role as a therapeutic in PDT for HGGs. Clinical trials should be considered to bring further insights into these applications.

## References

[1] Coburger J, Engelke J, Scheuerle A, et al. Tumor detection with 5-aminolevulinic acid fluorescence and Gd-DTPA-enhanced intraoperative MRI at the border of contrast-enhancing lesions: a prospective study based on histopathological assessment. Neurosurg Focus. 2014; 36(2):E3

[2] Hadjipanayis CG, Widhalm G, Stummer W. What is the surgical benefit of utilizing 5-aminolevulinic acid for fluorescence-guided surgery of malignant gliomas? Neurosurgery. 2015; 77(5):663–673

[3] Panciani PP, Fontanella M, Schatlo B, et al. Fluorescence and image guided resection in high grade glioma. Clin Neurol Neurosurg. 2012; 114(1):37–41

[4] Stummer W, Novotny A, Stepp H, Goetz C, Bise K, Reulen HJ. Fluorescence-guided resection of glioblastoma multiforme by using 5-aminolevulinic acid-induced porphyrins: a prospective study in 52 consecutive patients. J Neurosurg. 2000; 93(6):1003–1013

[5] Tonn J-C, Stummer W. Fluorescence-guided resection of malignant gliomas using 5-aminolevulinic acid: practical use, risks, and pitfalls. Clin Neurosurg. 2008; 55:20–26

[6] Yamada S, Muragaki Y, Maruyama T, Komori T, Okada Y. Role of neurochemical navigation with 5-aminolevulinic acid during intraoperative MRI-guided resection of intracranial malignant gliomas. Clin Neurol Neurosurg. 2015; 130:134–139

[7] Stummer W, Pichlmeier U, Meinel T, Wiestler OD, Zanella F, Reulen HJ, ALA-Glioma Study Group. Fluorescence-guided surgery with 5-aminolevulinic acid for resection of malignant glioma: a randomised controlled multicentre phase III trial. Lancet Oncol. 2006; 7(5):392–401

[8] Barbagallo GMV, Certo F, Heiss K, Albanese V. 5-ALA fluorescence-assisted surgery in pediatric brain tumors: report of three cases and review of the literature. Br J Neurosurg. 2014; 28(6):750–754

[9] Preuß M, Renner C, Krupp W, et al. The use of 5-aminolevulinic acid fluorescence guidance in resection of pediatric brain tumors. Childs Nerv Syst. 2013; 29(8):1263–1267

[10] Ruge JR, Liu J. Use of 5-aminolevulinic acid for visualization and resection of a benign pediatric brain tumor. J Neurosurg Pediatr. 2009; 4(5):484–486

[11] Stummer W, Rodrigues F, Schucht P, et al. European ALA Pediatric Brain Tumor Study Group. Predicting the "usefulness" of 5-ALA-derived tumor fluorescence for fluorescence-guided resections in pediatric brain tumors: a European survey. Acta Neurochir (Wien). 2014; 156(12):2315–2324

[12] Bernal García LM, Cabezudo Artero JM, Marcelo Zamorano MB, Gilete Tejero I. Fluorescence-guided resection with 5-aminolevulinic acid of subependymomas of the fourth ventricle: report of 2 cases: technical case report. Neurosurgery. 2015; 11 suppl 2:E364–E371, discussion E371

[13] Eljamel MS, Leese G, Moseley H. Intraoperative optical identification of pituitary adenomas. J Neurooncol. 2009; 92(3):417–421

[14] Evers G, Kamp M, Warneke N, et al. 5-aminolaevulinic acid-induced fluorescence in primary central nervous system lymphoma. World Neurosurg. 2017; 98:375–380

[15] Takeda J, Nonaka M, Li Y, et al. 5-ALA fluorescence-guided endoscopic surgery for mixed germ cell tumors. J Neurooncol. 2017; 134(1):119–124

[16] Beck TJ, Kreth FW, Beyer W, et al. Interstitial photodynamic therapy of nonresectable malignant glioma recurrences using 5-aminolevulinic acid induced protoporphyrin IX. Lasers Surg Med. 2007; 39(5):386–393

[17] Etminan N, Peters C, Ficnar J, et al. Modulation of migratory activity and invasiveness of human glioma spheroids following 5-aminolevulinic acid-based photodynamic treatment. Laboratory investigation. J Neurosurg. 2011; 115(2):281–288

[18] Stummer W, Beck T, Beyer W, et al. Long-sustaining response in a patient with non-resectable, distant recurrence of glioblastoma multiforme treated by interstitial photodynamic therapy using 5-ALA: case report. J Neurooncol. 2008; 87(1):103–109

[19] Castano AP, Mroz P, Hamblin MR. Photodynamic therapy and anti-tumour immunity. Nat Rev Cancer. 2006; 6(7):535–545

[20] Ferraro N, Barbarite E, Albert TR, et al. The role of 5-aminolevulinic acid in brain tumor surgery: a systematic review. Neurosurg Rev. 2016; 39(4):545–555

[21] Onuki J, Chen Y, Teixeira PC, et al. Mitochondrial and nuclear DNA damage induced by 5-aminolevulinic acid. Arch Biochem Biophys. 2004; 432(2):178–187

[22] Brown TJ, Brennan MC, Li M, et al. Association of the extent of resection with survival in glioblastoma: a systematic review and meta-analysis. JAMA Oncol. 2016; 2(11):1460–1469

[23] Kramm CM, Wagner S, Van Gool S, et al. Improved survival after gross total resection of malignant gliomas in pediatric patients from the HIT-GBM studies. Anticancer Res. 2006; 26 5B:3773–3779

[24] McCrea HJ, Bander ED, Venn RA, et al. Sex, age, anatomic location, and extent of resection influence outcomes in children with high-grade glioma. Neurosurgery. 2015; 77(3):443–452, discussion 452–453

[25] Rutkowski S, von Hoff K, Emser A, et al. Survival and prognostic factors of early childhood medulloblastoma: an international meta-analysis. J Clin Oncol. 2010; 28(33):4961–4968

[26] Bernal García LM, Cabezudo Artero JM, Royano Sánchez M, Marcelo Zamorano MB, López Macías M. Fluorescence-guided resection with 5-aminolevulinic acid of meningeal sarcoma in a child. Childs Nerv Syst. 2015; 31(7):1177–1180

[27] Eicker S, Sarikaya-Seiwert S, Borkhardt A, et al. ALA-induced porphyrin accumulation in medulloblastoma and its use for fluorescence-guided surgery. Cent Eur Neurosurg. 2011; 72(2):101–103

[28] Beez T, Sarikaya-Seiwert S, Steiger H-J, Hänggi D. Fluorescence-guided surgery with 5-aminolevulinic acid for resection of brain tumors in children: a technical report. Acta Neurochir (Wien). 2014; 156(3):597–604

[29] Schwake M, Günes D, Köchling M, et al. Kinetics of porphyrin fluorescence accumulation in pediatric brain tumor cells incubated in 5-aminolevulinic acid. Acta Neurochir (Wien). 2014; 156(6):1077–1084

[30] Teixidor P, Arráez MÁ, Villalba G, et al. Safety and efficacy of 5-aminolevulinic acid for high grade glioma in usual clinical practice: a prospective cohort study. PLoS One. 2016; 11(2):e0149244

[31] Offersen CM, Skjoeth-Rasmussen J. Evaluation of the risk of liver damage from the use of 5-aminolevulinic acid for intra-operative identification and resection in patients with malignant gliomas. Acta Neurochir (Wien). 2017; 159(1):145–150

[32] Grossman R, Nossek E, Shimony N, Raz M, Ram Z. Intraoperative 5-aminolevulinic acid-induced fluorescence in primary central nervous system lymphoma. J Neurosurg. 2014; 120(1):67–69

[33] Yamamoto J, Kitagawa T, Akiba D, Nishizawa S. 5-aminolevulinic acid-induced fluorescence in cerebellar primary central nervous system lymphoma: a case report and literature review. Turk Neurosurg. 2015; 25(5):796–800

[34] Villano JL, Koshy M, Shaikh H, Dolecek TA, McCarthy BJ. Age, gender, and racial differences in incidence and survival in primary CNS lymphoma. Br J Cancer. 2011; 105(9):1414–1418

[35] Yun J, Iwamoto FM, Sonabend AM. Primary central nervous system lymphoma: a critical review of the role of surgery for resection. Arch Cancer Res. 2016; 4(2):71

[36] Yamamoto T, Ishikawa E, Miki S, et al. Photodynamic diagnosis using 5-aminolevulinic acid in 41 biopsies for primary central nervous system lymphoma. Photochem Photobiol. 2015; 91(6):1452–1457

[37] Marbacher S, Klinger E, Schwyzer L, et al. Use of fluorescence to guide resection or biopsy of primary brain tumors and brain metastases. Neurosurg Focus. 2014; 36(2):E10

[38] Batchelor T, Loeffler JS. Primary CNS lymphoma. J Clin Oncol. 2006; 24(8):1281–1288

[39] Bataille B, Delwail V, Menet E, et al. Primary intracerebral malignant lymphoma: report of 248 cases. J Neurosurg. 2000; 92(2):261–266

[40] Henry JM, Heffner RR, Jr, Dillard SH, Earle KM, Davis RL. Primary malignant lymphomas of the central nervous system. Cancer. 1974; 34(4):1293–1302

[41] Hoang-Xuan K, Bessell E, Bromberg J, et al. European Association for Neuro-Oncology Task Force on Primary CNS Lymphoma. Diagnosis and treatment of primary CNS lymphoma in immunocompetent patients: guidelines from the European Association for Neuro-Oncology. Lancet Oncol. 2015; 16(7):e322–e332

[42] Utsuki S, Oka H, Kijima C, Miyajima Y, Hagiwara H, Fujii K. Utility of intraoperative fluorescent diagnosis of residual hemangioblastoma using 5-aminolevulinic acid. Neurol India. 2011; 59(4):612–615

[43] Utsuki S, Oka H, Sato K, Shimizu S, Suzuki S, Fujii K. Fluorescence diagnosis of tumor cells in hemangioblastoma cysts with 5-aminolevulinic acid. J Neurosurg. 2010; 112(1):130–132

[44] Conway JE, Chou D, Clatterbuck RE, Brem H, Long DM, Rigamonti D. Hemangioblastomas of the central nervous system in von Hippel-Lindau syndrome and sporadic disease. Neurosurgery. 2001; 48(1):55–62, discussion 62–63

[45] Kim A, Khurana M, Moriyama Y, Wilson BC. Quantification of in vivo fluorescence decoupled from the effects of tissue optical properties using fiber-optic spectroscopy measurements. J Biomed Opt. 2010; 15(6):067006

[46] Stummer W, Tonn J-C, Goetz C, et al. 5-Aminolevulinic acid-derived tumor fluorescence: the diagnostic accuracy of visible fluorescence qualities as corroborated by spectrometry and histology and postoperative imaging. Neurosurgery. 2014; 74(3):310–319, discussion 319–320

[47] Valdés PA, Leblond F, Kim A, et al. Quantitative fluorescence in intracranial tumor: implications for ALA-induced PpIX as an intraoperative biomarker. J Neurosurg. 2011; 115(1):11–17

[48] Valdés PA, Jacobs V, Harris BT, et al. Quantitative fluorescence using 5-aminolevulinic acid-induced protoporphyrin IX biomarker as a surgical adjunct in low-grade glioma surgery. J Neurosurg. 2015; 123(3):771–780

[49] Eljamel MS, Goodman C, Moseley H. ALA and Photofrin fluorescence-guided resection and repetitive PDT in glioblastoma multiforme: a single centre phase III randomised controlled trial. Lasers Med Sci. 2008; 23(4):361–367

[50] Friesen SA, Hjortland GO, Madsen SJ, et al. 5-aminolevulinic acid-based photodynamic detection and therapy of brain tumors (review). Int J Oncol. 2002; 21(3):577–582

[51] Quirk BJ, Brandal G, Donlon S, et al. Photodynamic therapy (PDT) for malignant brain tumors–where do we stand? Photodiagn Photodyn Ther. 2015; 12(3):530–544

[52] Ewelt C, Nemes A, Senner V, et al. Fluorescence in neurosurgery: its diagnostic and therapeutic use. Review of the literature. J Photochem Photobiol B. 2015; 148:302–309

[53] Yang X, Palasuberniam P, Kraus D, Chen B. Aminolevulinic acid-based tumor detection and therapy: molecular mechanisms and strategies for enhancement. Int J Mol Sci. 2015; 16(10):25865–25880

[54] Wachowska M, Muchowicz A, Firczuk M, et al. Aminolevulinic acid (ALA) as a prodrug in photodynamic therapy of cancer. Molecules. 2011; 16:4140–4164

[55] Dolmans DEJGJ, Fukumura D, Jain RK. Photodynamic therapy for cancer. Nat Rev Cancer. 2003; 3(5):380–387

[56] Dougherty TJ, Gomer CJ, Henderson BW, et al. Photodynamic therapy. J Natl Cancer Inst. 1998; 90(12):889–905

[57] Jeffes EWB. Levulan: the first approved topical photosensitizer for the treatment of actinic keratosis. J Dermatolog Treat. 2002; 13 suppl 1:S19–S23

[58] Nemes A, Fortmann T, Poeschke S, et al. 5-ALA Fluorescence in native pituitary adenoma cell lines: resection control and basis for photodynamic therapy (PDT)? PLoS One. 2016; 11(9):e0161364

[59] Neumann LM, Beseoglu K, Slotty PJ, et al. Efficacy of 5-aminolevulinic acid based photodynamic therapy in pituitary adenomas-experimental study on rat and human cell cultures. Photodiagn Photodyn Ther. 2016; 14:77–83

[60] Olzowy B, Hundt CS, Stocker S, Bise K, Reulen HJ, Stummer W. Photoirradiation therapy of experimental malignant glioma with 5-aminolevulinic acid. J Neurosurg. 2002; 97(4):970–976

[61] Yang VXD, Muller PJ, Herman P, Wilson BC. A multispectral fluorescence imaging system: design and initial clinical tests in intra-operative Photofrin-photodynamic therapy of brain tumors. Lasers Surg Med. 2003; 32(3):224–232

[62] Agostinis P, Berg K, Cengel KA, et al. Photodynamic therapy of cancer: an update. CA Cancer J Clin. 2011; 61(4):250–281

# 10 Fluorescein-Guided Tumor Resection in Neurosurgical Oncology

*Joseph F. Georges and Peter Nakaji*

## Abstract

This chapter reviews fluorescein-guided resection of intracranial neoplasms such as gliomas, meningiomas, and metastases. Fluorescein's utility in the management of intracerebral abscesses and nonoperative lesions, such as central nervous system lymphoma, is also discussed. Fluorescein is the first fluorescent contrast agent to gain widespread clinical use, and its neurosurgical applications have undergone refinement alongside advancements in clinical fluorescence imaging technology. In the early 2010s, the first dedicated commercial surgical fluorescence microscope with fluorescein-specific excitation and emission filters was introduced. The introduction of dedicated fluorescence surgical microscopes led to renewed interest in optimizing protocols for fluorescein-guided tumor surgery. Recently, the neurosurgery field has moved toward administering lower doses of fluorescein for fluorescence-guided tumor resection. Data from studies of low-dose protocols indicate that fluorescein localizes well to intracranial lesions with disrupted blood–brain barriers in patterns similar to those of gadolinium contrast on magnetic resonance imaging (MRI). Current literature suggests that fluorescein contrast during tumor resection increases gross-total resection (GTR), with 100% GTR reported in one case series of fluorescein-guided glioblastoma resection. To date, no reports of significant deleterious effects have been reported with low-dose fluorescein for brain tumor visualization. This chapter focuses on studies that use a standardized administration protocol as reported after the introduction of commercial fluorescence surgical microscopes, with a review of the literature before this era. Although the utility of fluorescein for intraoperative visualization of intracranial tumors was first reported in the 1940s, the advantages of fluorescein guidance and techniques optimizing its administration and visualization continue to be discovered.

*Keywords:* extent of resection, fluorescein, fluorescence imaging, fluoroscopy, glioblastoma, intracranial neoplasm, intraoperative imaging, meningioma, metastasis, neurosurgical oncology, tumor resection

## 10.1 History

Fluorescein, discovered in 1871, was the first clinical fluorophore, and it has been broadly used in chemistry, biological sciences, and clinical medicine.[1] Clinically, other than in neurosurgery, fluorescein is routinely used in emergency departments to evaluate corneal abrasions with a Wood lamp. This technique exploits the robust fluorescence visualized when fluorescein is excited with the appropriate wavelength of light. Since the 1960s, fluorescein has been used in neurosurgery to detect cerebrospinal fluid leaks, and it is commonly used to detect dural compromise during transsphenoidal surgery.[2,3,4] In a landmark clinical study in 2006, Stummer et al[5] showed that fluorescence-guided tumor resection could improve brain tumor extent of resection (EOR). Since EOR is positively correlated with patient survival, neurosurgeons have aimed to discover additional fluorescent contrast agents to better visualize brain tumors and their margins intraoperatively.[6,7,8,9] In this chapter, we focus on the applications of fluorescein in neurosurgical oncology.

In 1947, Moore[10] made the first report of fluorescein localizing to brain tumors. In the initial studies prior to the advent of dedicated fluorescence surgical microscopes, ultraviolet light was used to excite the fluorophore, and fluorescence was visualized without dichroic filters in the light path.[10,11] This method (without the dichroic filters) highlighted fluorescein's high quantum yield and minimal photobleaching with excitation. These studies revealed that fluorescein localized to tumor regions and provided minimal fluorescence of normal brain.[10,11]

In the biological sciences, fluorescence imaging began to revolutionize data collection in the 1980s with the development of the first commercially available confocal microscope.[12] Advances in imaging technologies and the development of novel fluorophores created a new era of live-cell imaging, which allowed scientists to visualize cellular processes in real time. Development of clinical fluorescence imaging technology began to follow suit.

A surgical microscope capable of bright field and fluorescence imaging became available in 1998.[13] This technology was described in 1998 in the first report of a dedicated fluorescence microscope for fluorescein-guided brain tumor resection. Kuroiwa et al[13] used Zeiss OPMI MD and OPMI CS-NC operative microscopes (Carl Zeiss Meditec AG, Oberkochen, Germany) with appropriate excitation and emission filters to intraoperatively visualize tumors in patients with high-grade gliomas (HGGs). They reported that fluorescein localized well to areas where the blood–brain barrier was compromised, regions that also correlated with areas of gadolinium-based contrast on magnetic resonance imaging.

In 2003, Shinoda et al[11] compared the gross-total resection (GTR) rates of patients who underwent fluorescein-guided resection of glioblastoma (GBM) with the GTR rates of patients who underwent resection of GBM without fluorescein. In this study, fluorescein was administered in high doses after the dura was opened, and it was visualized under white light. The researchers reported that fluorescein localized to 100% of the GBMs in fluorescein-exposed patients and that it dramatically increased GTR rates (84.4% [27 of 32 patients with fluorescein] vs. 30.1% [22 of 73 patients without fluorescein]).

Before 2012, no study had evaluated the long-term clinical benefits of fluorescein-guided tumor resection. Results of a study correlating the effects of fluorescein-guided resection of brain tumors on progression-free survival (PFS) were published in 2012.[14] In this report, the outcomes of 10 glioma patients who underwent fluorescein-guided resection were compared with the outcomes of 12 similar controls. In the fluorescein group, mean PFS increased (mean > 7.2 vs. > 5.4 months).

In 2013, the Zeiss Pentero YE560 (YE560) became the first commercially available operative microscope with dedicated

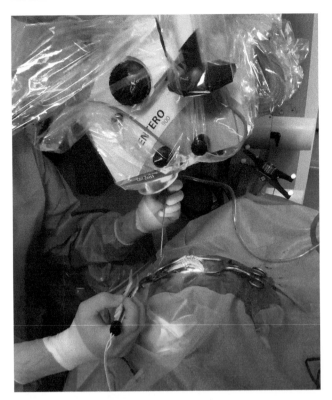

**Fig. 10.1** Fluorescence intraoperative surgical microscope. An intraoperative photograph shows the blue light from the Zeiss YE560 (Carl Zeiss Meditec AG) over a brain tumor exposure. (Reproduced with permission of Barrow Neurological Institute, Phoenix, Arizona.)

filter sets for fluorescein imaging. This microscope offers blue-light excitation and 540- to 690-nm emission filters for visualizing fluorescein (▶ Fig. 10.1). Peer-reviewed reports detailing this microscope's efficacy for intraoperative brain tumor imaging began to appear in 2013.[15,16] In 2015, Diaz et al[17] reported that YE560-guided resection of HGGs could yield 100% GTR. Since the introduction of dedicated filter sets for fluorescence imaging in surgical microscopes (now available from multiple manufacturers), most studies evaluating their usefulness have included similar dosing and imaging protocols for fluorescein. In this chapter, data are presented from studies that implement fluorescein-guided surgery that follows the clinical protocol commonly used with commercially available fluorescence surgical microscopes, such as the YE560 (▶ Table 10.1).[15,16,17,18,19,20,21,22]

## 10.2 High-Grade Gliomas

Multiple studies of fluorescein-guided brain tumor resection have focused on HGGs, reinforcing the fact that increased cytoreduction can improve survival of both newly diagnosed patients and patients with recurrent HGGs.[23,24] Since fluorescence guidance with 5-aminolevulinic acid (5-ALA) was reported to enhance glioma EOR, neurosurgeons have sought contrast agents with a similar utility that are approved for clinical use by the U.S. Food and Drug Administration. Fluorescein

was an obvious candidate; it had been used clinically for decades, was inexpensive, and provided bright fluorescence.[25] To date, the utility of fluorescein contrast in HGG surgery has been documented in at least 11 peer-reviewed publications.[26] These studies have investigated specificity, dosing, EOR, timing for use, and potential adverse effects.

Since the introduction of commercially available fluorescence surgical microscopes, four peer-reviewed studies have evaluated the sensitivity and specificity of fluorescein-guided glioma resection.[15,16,17,19] These reports show sensitivity and specificity of 90% and greater. For the surgeon, this means that fluorescence correlates reliably with high-grade tumors, and it appears to correspond well with enhancement on magnetic resonance images. In the current era (since 2013), GTR can be expected in up to 80% of glioma cases in which fluorescein guidance is used.[1]

## 10.3 Metastatic Disease

GTR of intracerebral metastases is an independent predictor of patient survival, PFS, and postsurgical neurological status.[27,28,29] Therefore, intraoperative techniques that increase the EOR, such as fluorescence-guided surgery, may improve patient survival and outcome. Several case series have evaluated the utility of fluorescein-guided resection of intracerebral metastases.[1,20,29] Initial studies did not use standardized fluorescein dosages or standardized imaging hardware. The lack of standardization precludes the accurate comparison of data from these studies. In this chapter, we focus on studies published since 2013, after the introduction of the YE560 and subsequent dose standardization. These studies have shown that fluorescein-guided microsurgery enhances EOR and GTR beyond the capabilities of traditional white-light microsurgery.[19,20] Current data show that fluorescein preferentially localizes to metastatic tissue within the brain compared to adjacent normal brain.[30] Furthermore, fluorescein appears to enable superior EOR of intracranial metastases compared to 5-ALA, although a direct comparison has never been performed.[20,31]

### 10.3.1 Usefulness and Extent of Resection

Researchers have subjectively assessed the usefulness of fluorescein-guided resection of intracerebral metastatic disease, and several authors have quantified the EOR by comparing intraoperative and postoperative magnetic resonance images. Use of intraoperative fluorescein contrast is considered helpful in identifying tumors and tumor margins in 95 to 97% of cases.[19,20] Furthermore, fluorescein-guided resection of intracerebral metastases can achieve 83 to 100% GTR. By comparison, traditional white-light microsurgery yields GTR of 54 to 76%.[32,33] Some users have noted that the fluorescence of fluorescein seems to extend slightly beyond the margin of the tumor, leading to the risk of supramaximal resection, although this possibility has not been rigorously studied. When operating at the periphery of metastatic lesions, surgeons should keep the possible extension of fluorescence in mind and should apply caution in eloquent regions of the brain until they are further interrogated.

**Table 10.1** Tumor resection with a commercial fluorescence surgical microscope (YE560) by lesion type

| Study | Cases | Lesion | Dose, mg/kg | Timing | Margins visualized | EOR | GTR | Findings |
|---|---|---|---|---|---|---|---|---|
| Acerbi et al[15] | 12 | GBM | 5–10 | After intubation | Inconclusive | 97.6% | 75% | Increases GTR |
| Diaz et al[17] | 12 | GBM | 3 | At induction of anesthesia | Yes | 100% | 100% | Increases GTR |
| Acerbi et al[18] | 20 | HGG | 5–10 | After intubation | Data quantified; sensitivity: 94%; specificity: 89.5% | 92.6% | 80% | FNA appears safe and increases rate of GTR |
| Hamamcıoğlu et al[19] | 30 | GBM, cerebral metastases, and lymphoma | 2–4 | After induction of anesthesia | Delineated in 97% | NA | Overall: 79% Glioma: 72.2% Metastases: 100% CNS lymphoma: 50% | Enhances GTR |
| Schebesch et al[16] | 31 | Glioma and metastases | 3–4 | After bone flap removed and immediately before durotomy | Glioma: margins visualized in 80.8% of cases Metastases: margins visualized in 100% of cases | NA | 80% | FNA helpful for tumor resection; margin visualization depends on histology and tumor pretreatment |
| Höhne et al[20] | 95 | Cerebral metastases | 2–5 | After induction of anesthesia | NA | Not quantified | 83% | Enhances EOR |
| Höhne et al[21] | 1 | Brain abscess | 5 | At induction of anesthesia: 30–45 min before surgery | Delineated capsule | NA | NA | Delineates abscess |
| Höhne et al[22] | 7 | Brain abscess | 5 | At induction of anesthesia: 30–45 min before surgery | Delineated capsule | NA | NA | Delineates abscess |

Abbreviations: CNS, central nervous system; EOR, extent of resection; FNA, fine-needle aspiration; GBM, glioblastoma; GTR, gross-total resection; HGG, high-grade glioma; NA, not available.

# 10.4 Intracranial Lesions: Meningiomas, Abscesses, and Lymphomas

Benefits of fluorescein-guided resection of meningiomas and other intracranial lesions are beginning to be reported in the neurosurgical literature. Currently, large case series have not reported the use of fluorescence guidance of the resection of these lesions with standardized protocols or the use of dedicated commercial fluorescence microscopes. We review case series and case reports published since 2010 that are specific to meningiomas, abscesses, and lymphomas.

## 10.4.1 Meningiomas

Fluorescein-guided resection of meningiomas has been reported for two types of lesions: convexity lesions and skull base lesions. In da Silva et al's[34] case series of five convexity meningiomas, fluorescein provided visualization of meningiomas and their dural tails, and it differentiated them from

surrounding tissue. Although the dura typically enhances with fluorescein, the dural tail specific to the meningioma could be differentiated from surrounding dura. In this case series, fluorescein was administered after tumor exposure. One gram (about 14 mg/kg for a 70-kg person) was injected and allowed to circulate for 10 minutes before imaging. White-light illumination was used, and imaging was conducted with a charge-coupled device camera. In this report of five cases, a Simpson grade I resection or better was achieved for four lesions, and a Simpson grade II was achieved for one lesion involving the sagittal sinus.

Preservation of cranial nerves and vasculature is a fundamental component of skull base surgery. Therefore, fluorescence guidance while resecting skull base tumors, such as meningiomas, has been investigated as a tool for differentiating tumor tissue from eloquent brain tissue. The first report of fluorescein-guided resection of skull base meningiomas was published by da Silva et al[35] in 2010, and the surgical literature is still limited to case reports and retrospective case series. These reports were conducted with bright field illumination after administration of 1-g fluorescein at the opening of the dura; they did not incorporate a specialized microscope, such as the YE560. These reports showed that fluorescein localized well to tumor regions and that cranial nerves were relatively devoid of fluorescence. Therefore, fluorescein contrast shows utility for differentiating tumor from eloquent skull base regions during tumor resection. However, more studies are needed.[36]

### 10.4.2 Abscesses

In 2016, Höhne et al[21] reported a case in which fluorescein was used to identify a brain abscess and suggested that the technique might aid resection. The following year, Höhne et al[22] reported a case series of seven patients who underwent fluorescein-guided evacuation of intracerebral abscesses. As of mid-2017, this study is the largest to investigate the utility of fluorescein guidance during evacuation of intracerebral abscesses. Patients in the study received 5 mg/kg fluorescein 30 to 45 minutes before surgery, and intraoperative fluorescence imaging was performed with the YE560. Five resections were completed with neuronavigation, and two resections were completed without intraoperative navigation. In all seven patients who had procedures, fluorescein provided bright contrast to the abscess capsule and assisted with complete intraoperative removal. No adverse events were associated with fluorescein administration.

### 10.4.3 Lymphomas

Primary central nervous system (CNS) lymphoma is typically treated with chemoradiotherapy. Therefore, reports of fluorescein-guided resection of this lesion are limited.[19,37] In two case series, the authors described the utility of fluorescein guidance in the resection of primary CNS lymphomas, describing seven such lymphomas in one series and two in the other. All cases were preoperatively diagnosed as HGGs. The patients were administered 2 to 10 mg/kg fluorescein immediately after induction of anesthesia, and intraoperative imaging was performed with the YE560. The reports showed that fluorescein sharply delineated lymphoma from normal brain. GTR was achieved in five cases, and subtotal resections were conducted in the additional cases because of intraoperative diagnosis of lymphoma or involvement of eloquent brain tissue.[15,19,37]

## 10.5 Dosing and Administration

Various concentrations of fluorescein have been studied for HGG resection. Doses have ranged from 2 to 10 mg/kg.[15,16,17,18,19] Despite the varying concentrations, authors have reported similar sensitivity, specificity, and EOR. Conventional wisdom suggests that the minimum dose to generate the desired effect is preferable.

In the current era of fluorescence-guided microsurgery of gliomas and intracerebral metastases, a dose of 3 to 5 mg/kg body weight has been used. Fluorescein is typically administered intravenously 2 to 3 hours before surgery to differentiate any tumor from normal brain (▶ Fig. 10.2; Video 10.1). This protocol has shown fluorescein contrast to localize similarly to gadolinium.[19,20] To date, no adverse effects have been reported with this protocol.

Additional research is warranted to determine whether lower doses will continue to provide good differentiation of neoplasms from healthy brain tissue. The timing of administration may also play an important role in fluorescein specificity. Since fluorescein permeates areas with compromised blood–brain barrier, it may continue to do so during surgery and therefore label nonneoplastic regions.[38] More research is required to determine whether fluorescein's sensitivity and specificity are altered during surgery.

## 10.6 Adverse Effect Profile

Fluorescein undergoes renal excretion and is associated with transient discoloration of skin and urine after administration. A limited number of patients have developed hypotension when administered fluorescein intravenously. These patients were administered doses of 20 mg/kg or higher and recovered after stays in the intensive care unit.[15,39] To date, no reports have been published in the neurosurgery field of anaphylactic shock or death after fluorescein administration at doses of 3 to 5 mg/kg for visualization of tumors. In specialties other than neurosurgery, fluorescein-mediated nephrotoxicity or injury to other organ systems has not been routinely reported or confirmed in the literature.[40]

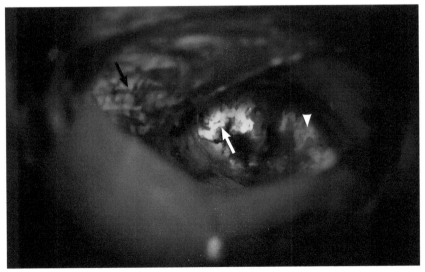

**Fig. 10.2** Intraoperative tumor fluorescence. An intraoperative image in yellow mode shows bright fluorescence centrally (*white arrow*), unlike an area of healthy brain (*white arrowhead*). Note fluorescence of dura visualized in the foreground (*black arrow*). (Reproduced with permission of Barrow Neurological Institute, Phoenix, Arizona.)

# 10.7 Fluorescence Surgical Microscope and Clinical Approval

## 10.7.1 Fluorescence Surgical Microscope

Fluorescein is a robust fluorescent contrast agent. Its characteristic yellow–green fluorescence can be visualized under the white light of standard surgical microscopes. However, studies investigating its clinical utility under white-light illumination required greater concentrations of the fluorophore. Optimally, fluorescein is excited at a wavelength of 494 nm, and its emission is detected at 514 nm. The introduction of the YE560 revitalized investigations into fluorescein's utility for neurosurgical applications by providing consistent visualization of the fluorophore. The introduction of additional fluorescence imaging technologies and refinement of the YE560 will lead to additional new applications for fluorescein and other intraoperative fluorescent agents.

## 10.7.2 Clinical Approval

In the United States, fluorescein is available for off-label use, as it is used in neurosurgery. This agent can be used for intraoperative guidance with institutional review board approval at some centers, and it can be used off-label with patient consent at others. Proposals submitted to the institutional review board typically include, at a minimum, the goal of tracking safety (e.g., noting adverse reactions) and, optimally, documenting the efficacy of the agent being used so that the use contributes to the greater body of knowledge about its best use.

# 10.8 Future Directions

In recent decades, fluorescence imaging has revolutionized the biological sciences. We are at the dawn of implementing these emerging technological advances in clinical neurosurgery. In its basic form, fluorescein indiscriminately localizes to regions of disrupted blood–brain barrier, much like gadolinium contrast. In the biological sciences, fluorescein has been conjugated to numerous molecular probes for the specific visualization of cell types and molecular processes. Neurosurgeons are beginning to embrace these concepts, and early reports suggest the clinical utility of conjugating this fluorophore, and similar fluorophores, to molecular probes for tumor-specific labeling.[41,42] As neurosurgical research continues with this organic compound, fluorescein may ultimately be used for intraoperative differentiation of specific tumors and visualization of infiltrative tumors outside the disrupted blood–brain barrier.

# 10.9 Conclusion

Intraoperative fluorescein imaging is a powerful neurosurgical tool for visualizing brain tumors and their margins. Multiple studies have interrogated the utility of fluorescein-guided resection of gliomas and metastases, and have shown that the use of intraoperative fluorescein contrast can increase GTR, EOR, and PFS. Additional work is being conducted to evaluate

the role of fluorescein in the resection of other lesions, such as meningiomas, skull base tumors, and abscesses. We will continue to witness further applications of fluorescein in neurosurgery with the development of new imaging technologies and fluorescein-conjugated molecular probes.

# References

[1] Schebesch KM, Brawanski A, Hohenberger C, Hohne J. Fluorescein sodium-guided surgery of malignant brain tumors: history, current concepts, and future project. Turk Neurosurg. 2016; 26(2):185–194

[2] Jakimovski D, Bonci G, Attia M, et al. Incidence and significance of intraoperative cerebrospinal fluid leak in endoscopic pituitary surgery using intrathecal fluorescein. World Neurosurg. 2014; 82(3–4):e513–e523

[3] Kirchner FR, Proud GO. Method for the identification and localization of cerebrospinal fluid, rhinorrhea and otorrhea. Laryngoscope. 1960; 70:921–931

[4] Moseley JI, Carton CA, Stern WE. Spectrum of complications in the use of intrathecal fluorescein. J Neurosurg. 1978; 48(5):765–767

[5] Stummer W, Pichlmeier U, Meinel T, Wiestler OD, Zanella F, Reulen HJ, ALA-Glioma Study Group. Fluorescence-guided surgery with 5-aminolevulinic acid for resection of malignant glioma: a randomised controlled multicentre phase III trial. Lancet Oncol. 2006; 7(5):392–401

[6] Butte PV, Mamelak A, Parrish-Novak J, et al. Near-infrared imaging of brain tumors using the tumor paint BLZ-100 to achieve near-complete resection of brain tumors. Neurosurg Focus. 2014; 36(2):E1

[7] Georges JF, Martirosyan NL, Eschbacher J, et al. Sulforhodamine 101 selectively labels human astrocytoma cells in an animal model of glioblastoma. J Clin Neurosci. 2014; 21(5):846–851

[8] Kim EH, Cho JM, Chang JH, Kim SH, Lee KS. Application of intraoperative indocyanine green videoangiography to brain tumor surgery. Acta Neurochir (Wien). 2011; 153(7):1487–1495, discussion 1494–1495

[9] Li Y, Rey-Dios R, Roberts DW, Valdés PA, Cohen-Gadol AA. Intraoperative fluorescence-guided resection of high-grade gliomas: a comparison of the present techniques and evolution of future strategies. World Neurosurg. 2014; 82(1–2):175–185

[10] Moore GE. Fluorescein as an agent in the differentiation of normal and malignant tissues. Science. 1947; 106(2745):130–131

[11] Shinoda J, Yano H, Yoshimura S, et al. Fluorescence-guided resection of glioblastoma multiforme by using high-dose fluorescein sodium: technical note. J Neurosurg. 2003; 99(3):597–603

[12] Cox IJ, Sheppard CJ. Scanning optical microscope incorporating a digital framestore and microcomputer. Appl Opt. 1983; 22(10):1474–1478

[13] Kuroiwa T, Kajimoto Y, Ohta T. Development of a fluorescein operative microscope for use during malignant glioma surgery: a technical note and preliminary report. Surg Neurol. 1998; 50(1):41–48, discussion 48–49

[14] Chen B, Wang H, Ge P, et al. Gross total resection of glioma with the intraoperative fluorescence-guidance of fluorescein sodium. Int J Med Sci. 2012; 9(8):708–714

[15] Acerbi F, Broggi M, Eoli M, et al. Fluorescein-guided surgery for grade IV gliomas with a dedicated filter on the surgical microscope: preliminary results in 12 cases. Acta Neurochir (Wien). 2013; 155(7):1277–1286

[16] Schebesch KM, Proescholdt M, Höhne J, et al. Sodium fluorescein-guided resection under the YELLOW 560 nm surgical microscope filter in malignant brain tumor surgery-a feasibility study. Acta Neurochir (Wien). 2013; 155 (4):693–699

[17] Diaz RJ, Dios RR, Hattab EM, et al. Study of the biodistribution of fluorescein in glioma-infiltrated mouse brain and histopathological correlation of intraoperative findings in high-grade gliomas resected under fluorescein fluorescence guidance. J Neurosurg. 2015; 122(6):1360–1369

[18] Acerbi F, Broggi M, Eoli M, et al. Is fluorescein-guided technique able to help in resection of high-grade gliomas? Neurosurg Focus. 2014; 36(2):E5

[19] Hamamcıoğlu MK, Akçakaya MO, Göker B, Kasımcan MO, Kırış T. The use of the YELLOW 560 nm surgical microscope filter for sodium fluorescein-guided resection of brain tumors: our preliminary results in a series of 28 patients. Clin Neurol Neurosurg. 2016; 143:39–45

[20] Höhne J, Hohenberger C, Proescholdt M, et al. Fluorescein sodium-guided resection of cerebral metastases—an update. Acta Neurochir (Wien). 2017; 159(2):363–367

[21] Höhne J, Brawanski A, Schebesch KM. Fluorescein sodium-guided surgery of a brain abscess: a case report. Surg Neurol Int. 2016; 7 suppl 39:S955–S957

[22] Höhne J, Brawanski A, Schebesch KM. Fluorescence-guided surgery of brain abscesses. Clin Neurol Neurosurg. 2017; 155:36–39

[23] Oppenlander ME, Wolf AB, Snyder LA, et al. An extent of resection threshold for recurrent glioblastoma and its risk for neurological morbidity. J Neurosurg. 2014; 120(4):846–853

[24] Sanai N, Polley MY, McDermott MW, Parsa AT, Berger MS. An extent of resection threshold for newly diagnosed glioblastomas. J Neurosurg. 2011; 115(1):3–8

[25] Behbahaninia M, Martirosyan NL, Georges J, et al. Intraoperative fluorescent imaging of intracranial tumors: a review. Clin Neurol Neurosurg. 2013; 115 (5):517–528

[26] Senders JT, Muskens IS, Schnoor R, et al. Agents for fluorescence-guided glioma surgery: a systematic review of preclinical and clinical results. Acta Neurochir (Wien). 2017; 159(1):151–167

[27] Kalkanis SN, Linskey ME. Evidence-based clinical practice parameter guidelines for the treatment of patients with metastatic brain tumors: introduction. J Neurooncol. 2010; 96(1):7–10

[28] Patchell RA, Tibbs PA, Walsh JW, et al. A randomized trial of surgery in the treatment of single metastases to the brain. N Engl J Med. 1990; 322(8): 494–500

[29] Schödel P, Schebesch KM, Brawanski A, Proescholdt MA. Surgical resection of brain metastases—impact on neurological outcome. Int J Mol Sci. 2013; 14 (5):8708–8718

[30] Rey-Dios R, Cohen-Gadol AA. Technical principles and neurosurgical applications of fluorescein fluorescence using a microscope-integrated fluorescence module. Acta Neurochir (Wien). 2013; 155(4):701–706

[31] Kamp MA, Fischer I, Bühner J, et al. 5-ALA fluorescence of cerebral metastases and its impact for the local-in-brain progression. Oncotarget. 2016; 7(41): 66776–66789

[32] Patchell RA, Tibbs PA, Regine WF, et al. Postoperative radiotherapy in the treatment of single metastases to the brain: a randomized trial. JAMA. 1998; 280(17):1485–1489

[33] Schackert G, Steinmetz A, Meier U, Sobottka SB. Surgical management of single and multiple brain metastases: results of a retrospective study. Onkologie. 2001; 24(3):246–255

[34] da Silva CE, da Silva VD, da Silva JL. Convexity meningiomas enhanced by sodium fluorescein. Surg Neurol Int. 2014; 5:3

[35] da Silva CE, da Silva JL, da Silva VD. Use of sodium fluorescein in skull base tumors. Surg Neurol Int. 2010; 1:70

[36] da Silva CE, da Silva VD, da Silva JL. Skull base meningiomas and cranial nerves contrast using sodium fluorescein: a new application of an old tool. J Neurol Surg B Skull Base. 2014; 75(4):255–260

[37] Schebesch KM, Hoehne J, Hohenberger C, et al. Fluorescein sodium-guided surgery in cerebral lymphoma. Clin Neurol Neurosurg. 2015; 139:125–128

[38] Pavlov V, Meyronet D, Meyer-Bisch V, et al. Intraoperative probe-based confocal laser endomicroscopy in surgery and stereotactic biopsy of low-grade and high-grade gliomas: a feasibility study in humans. Neurosurgery. 2016; 79(4):604–612

[39] Dilek O, Ihsan A, Tulay H. Anaphylactic reaction after fluorescein sodium administration during intracranial surgery. J Clin Neurosci. 2011; 18(3):430–431

[40] Alemzadeh-Ansari MJ, Beladi-Mousavi SS, Feghhei M. Effect of fluorescein on renal function among diabetic patients. Nefrologia. 2011; 31(5):612–613

[41] Georges JF, Liu X, Eschbacher J, et al. Use of a conformational switching aptamer for rapid and specific ex vivo identification of central nervous system lymphoma in a xenograft model. PLoS One. 2015; 10(4):e0123607

[42] Martirosyan NL, Georges J, Kalani MY, et al. Handheld confocal laser endomicroscopic imaging utilizing tumor-specific fluorescent labeling to identify experimental glioma cells in vivo. Surg Neurol Int. 2016; 7 suppl 40:S995–S1003

# 11 Fluorescein and High-Grade Gliomas

*Justin A. Neira, Randy S. D'Amico, and Jeffrey N. Bruce*

## Abstract

As use of 5-aminolevulenic acid (5-ALA) in guiding resection of malignant glioma has been popularized, the search for other fluorescent agents has ensued. In this context, fluorescein sodium has arisen as an alternative and, in some cases, adjunct to 5-ALA, especially in countries where 5-ALA use is not approved. Fluorescein is inexpensive, safe, and easily implemented in practice and can be used with or without a dedicated microscope. Thus far, fluorescein has mainly been applied to resection of malignant gliomas, and numerous studies have been conducted assessing fluorescein's utility in this context. This chapter will review fluorescein's presumed mechanism of action for labeling tumor, existing evidence in support of its use in malignant glioma surgery, and evolving new applications of its use in oncologic neurosurgery.

*Keywords:* high-grade glioma, glioblastoma, malignant, glioma, extent of resection, sodium fluorescein, fluorescein, 5-aminolevulenic acid

## 11.1 Introduction

The ability of 5-aminolevulinic acid (5-ALA) to provide safe and accurate, real-time identification of diffusely infiltrative glioblastoma (GBM) tumors, with associated improvements in extent of resection (EOR), has encouraged the investigation of additional fluorescent agents with similar capabilities.[1] This is particularly important as safe, maximal resection is widely accepted to be an independent predictor of prognosis in high-grade gliomas (HGGs).[2,3,4,5]

Fluorescein sodium is a green fluorescent compound that accumulates in areas of malignancy, vascular leaking defects, pooling defects, and abnormal vasculature or neovascularization.[6] Originally described as a method for intraoperative guidance during intracranial tumor resection in 1947 by George E. Moore,[6] the use of fluorescein has recently received renewed interest as its accumulation in regions of blood–brain barrier (BBB) breakdown can be used as an intraoperative, real-time method of accurately labeling tumor for resection.[7]

Compared with 5-ALA, fluorescein is inexpensive, easy to use, and associated with minimal side effects.[8] Furthermore, the recent introduction of operative microscopes fitted with fluorescein-specific filters has facilitated improved intraoperative visualization of fluorescein-stained tissue at lower doses than traditionally used, and, as a result, has accelerated interest in its use for the resection of HGGs with promising results.[9,10,11,12,13,14,15,16,17,18,19] However, definitive studies clearly outlining the benefits of fluorescein have not been performed.

This chapter will review the presumed mechanism of action of fluorescein for labeling tumor, specific technical considerations of its use, evidence supporting its use in HGGs, and potential future applications of fluorescein guidance for the resection of HGGs.

## 11.2 Molecular Mechanism of Fluorescein Staining in HGG

Fluorescein sodium ($NaC_{20}H_{10}Na_2O_5$; molecular weight = 376 g/mol) is a salt form of the synthetic organic fluorophore fluorescein.[8] Fluorescein's peak absorption spectrum occurs at 465 to 490 nm with an emission peak at 500 to 530 nm permitting autofluorescence in white light and easy observation by the naked eye.[9,15] In contrast to 5-ALA, which is metabolized within tumor cells into the fluorescent byproduct protoporphyrin IX (PpIX),[4] intravenously administered fluorescein is delivered systemically through the bloodstream where it nonpreferentially extravasates into regions of increased vascular permeability. Fluorescein then accumulates in the extracellular spaces of these regions of BBB breakdown caused by central nervous system (CNS) diseases such as HGGs.[7] Interestingly, while normal astrocytes have been shown to demonstrate some degree of intracellular fluorescein uptake, tumor cells have not.[12] This exclusion of fluorescein from glioma cells is believed to be the result of upregulation of organic anion efflux transporters such as multidrug resistance protein 1 (MRP1), of which fluorescein has been shown to be a substrate.[20,21,22]

Following the intravenous administration of fluorescein, circulating fluorescein is rapidly cleared from regions of normal healthy brain with intact vasculature. The resultant fluorescein-mediated identification of HGGs is derived from the differential identification of fluorescent drug in the extracellular space surrounding glioma pathology as compared with regions with a functional BBB (▶ Fig. 11.1).

## 11.3 Technical Considerations

The timing and dose of fluorescein administration remains nonstandardized, and the length of time before physical factors such as oxidation and drug metabolism affect fluorescence intensity remains poorly defined. Of particular concern is the length of time during which fluorescein is preferentially retained in pathologic tissues before it diffuses through and indiscriminately labels edematous peritumoral tissues, which also remains unknown.[23] The importance of timing is relevant as early surgical manipulation of normal tissue immediately following administration of intravenous fluorescein results in messy extravasation of the fluorescent dye if sufficient time for clearance by normal tissue is not provided.[24,25]

Currently, the most accepted protocol is to administer fluorescein following induction of anesthesia, just prior to incision, as this appears to allow excellent contrast between pathologic and normal tissue while avoiding extravasation of dye from surgically manipulated normal capillary beds in the period of time it takes an experienced surgeon to perform a craniotomy and expose a tumor.[11,12,14,24,25,26] Using this schedule, the sensitivity, specificity, and positive predictive value of fluorescein for identifying malignant glioma tissue is retained throughout a

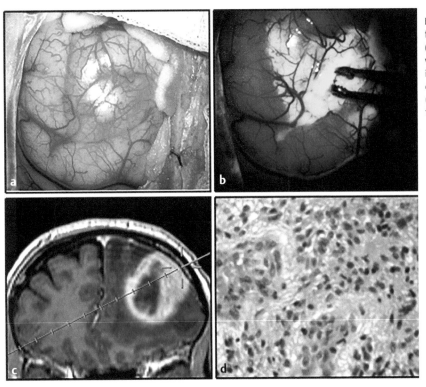

**Fig. 11.1** Intraoperative appearance of fluorescein under white light **(a)** and YELLOW 560 **(b)** during resection of GBM in patient treated with 3 mg/kg fluorescein following anesthesia induction. **(c)** Intraoperative neuronavigation correlates to region of fluorescence staining. **(d)** Representative tumor pathology from fluorescent region.

1- to 4-hour window postinjection and suggests that the administration of fluorescein prior to incision permits sufficient time for drug clearance from normal brain while permitting adequate extravasation within pathologic tissue and avoidance of unintentional extravasation through interrupted capillary beds.[14] Unfortunately, the effects of prolonged surgical procedures on the accuracy of fluorescein remain to be determined.

The optimal dose of fluorescein also remains poorly defined. Initial studies utilizing fluorescein relied on identification of tissue staining under operative white light with direct visualization of dyed tissue, and required higher doses of intravenous fluorescein up to 20 mg/kg. These higher doses are associated with common side effects such as nausea, vomiting, and urticaria in 0.01 to 9.24% of patients according to published series and serious adverse reactions such as bronchospasm and laryngeal edema occurring rarely.[15,16,17,27,28,29] Additionally, seizures have been reported with intrathecal fluorescein injection when used for identifying cerebrospinal fluid (CSF) leaks and therefore may be possible with extracellular extravasation of fluorescein into CSF spaces.[30,31,32]

The subsequent development and wide adoption of specialized microscopes with fluorescent filters that allow easy switching between white-light and fluorescence modes has permitted a reduction in dose to between 2 and 5 mg/kg, with subsequent reduced risk of dose-related adverse reactions. These doses permit identification of fluorescein staining that is imperceptible under white light.[24,25] Furthermore, available fluorescein filters are bright enough to provide adequate visualization of anatomy under fluorescent illumination, thus allowing the surgeon to perform tumor resection under the filter without the absolute need to switch to visible light.[14]

Despite advances in microscopy, there is currently no standardized way to view fluorescein. While fluorescent microscopy has facilitated lower doses and improved discrimination of fluorescent tissue, the ability to visualize fluorescein-stained tissue using white-light illumination is appealing, particularly in settings with limited resources. Even more variability exists when considering fluorescence microscopy. Various fluorescent filters have become commercially available, for example, the YELLOW 560 system (Carl Zeiss) or the FL560 System (Leica Microsystems), with variable wavelength absorption resulting in a lack of uniformity between existing and future studies. As a result, findings may not be generalizable depending on the fluorescence system used.

## 11.4 The Influence of Fluorescein-Guided Resection on Extent of Resection and Outcomes in High-Grade Glioma

Safe, maximal tumor resection improves symptoms, quality of life, progression-free survival (PFS), and overall survival (OS) in HGGs.[4] Given the success of 5-ALA for improving EOR, a number of studies have attempted to use fluorescein to improve EOR in malignant gliomas.[4,9,10,12,13,14,15,16,17,18,19]

The first modern studies describing fluorescein-guided resection of HGGs predated the popularization of intraoperative fluorescence microscopy (▶ Table 11.1).[15,16,17,18] These studies utilized high doses of intravenous fluorescein and relied on the ability to identify fluorescein-stained tissues under white light. In general, these studies all confirmed that fluorescein-guided resection of grossly visible, stained tissue under white-light illumination improved the surgeon's ability to completely resect regions of contrast-enhancing tumor as compared with conventional

**Table 11.1** Summary of existing trials of fluorescein use with white light illumination in glioma surgery, including the dosing protocol, fluorescein's effect on extent of resection in each trial.

| Author | Year | N (fluorescein) | N (control) | Light source | Dose (mg/kg) | Timing | Pathology | %GTR (fluorescein) | %GTR (control) | Sensitivity | Specificity |
|---|---|---|---|---|---|---|---|---|---|---|---|
| Shinoda[15] | 2003 | 32 | 73 | White light | 20 | Post dural opening | GBM | 84.4 | 30.1 | – | – |
| Koc[16] | 2008 | 47 | 33 | White light | 20 | Pre dural opening | GBM | 83 | 55 | – | – |
| Chen[17] | 2012 | 10 | 12 | White light | 15–20 | Post dural opening | II, III, IV | 80 | 33.3 | – | – |
| Liu[18] | 2013 | 56 | 27 | White light | ? | ? | I–IV | 80.4 | 40.7 | – | – |

**Table 11.2** Summary of fluorescein trials in which a specialized fluorescein microscope was used, including the dosing protocol, fluorescein's effect on extent of resection, and its sensitivity and specificity for identifying tumor in each trial

| Author | Year | N (fluorescein) | N (control) | Light source | Filter | Dose (mg/kg) | Timing | Pathology | %GTR (fluorescein) | %GTR (control) | Sensitivity (%) | Specificity (%) |
|---|---|---|---|---|---|---|---|---|---|---|---|---|
| Kuroiwa[9] | 1998 | 10 | – | | Filter | 8 | – | HGG | 80 | – | – | – |
| Schebesch[19] | 2013 | 35 | – | | YELLOW 560 | 3–4 | Predural opening | I–IV, mets | 80 | – | – | – |
| Acerbi[10] | 2014 | 20 | – | | BLU400 & YELLOW 560 | 5–10 | Postinduction | HGG | 80 | – | 94 | 89.5 |
| Rey-Dios[11] | 2014 | 3 | – | | YELLOW 560 | 3 | Postinduction | GBM | – | – | 79 | 100 |
| Diaz[12] | 2015 | 12 | – | | YELLOW 560 | 3 | Postinduction | HGG | 100 | – | 82.2 | 90.9 |
| Hamacioglu[13] | 2016 | 13* | – | | YELLOW 560 | 2–4 | Postinduction | HGG* | 69.2 | – | – | – |
| Neira[14] | 2016 | 32 | 32 | | YELLOW 560 | 4 | Postinduction | GBM | 93.1 | 77.3 | 75.6 | 75 |

*Subset of the study group in which diagnosis was GBM and not other CNS malignancies.

microsurgical techniques, with rates of gross total resection (GTR) ranging from 80 to 100% in regions amenable to GTR.[15,16,17,18]

The development of specialized surgical microscopes capable of identifying fluorescein-stained tissue further promoted interest in fluorescein guidance.[9] These microscopes originally utilized a xenon light source, a 450- to 490-nm excitation filter, and a barrier filter capable of only transmitting light greater than 510 nm.[9] This filter maximized fluorescein excitation (peak 450–490 nm), and observation of fluorescence emission (peak 500–530 nm) allowing improved discrimination of stained and unstained tissue with lower doses of fluorescein. Rates of GTR using newer technology fluorescence microscopy have ranged from 69.2 to nearly 100% in tumors arising within noneloquent regions considered amenable to GTR by the operating surgeon (▶ Table 11.2).[9,10,12,13,14,19]

# 11.5 Sensitivity and Specificity of Fluorescein Staining

The current evidence supporting the use of fluorescein guidance for the resection of HGGs remains limited to small published series and potential benefits of its use have been extrapolated from the success of 5-ALA in improving EOR and thus outcomes in the resection of HGGs. As the mechanisms of these fluorophores differ, a significant effort has been made to define the sensitivity and specificity of fluorescein guidance to better differentiate its utility as compared with 5-ALA, which, according to a recent meta-analysis of 20 studies, has sensitivity and specificity of 82.6 and 88.9%, respectively.[33] In addition, due to its nonspecific mechanism of action, well-justified concerns exist regarding the sensitivity and specificity of fluorescein, especially as diffusion through nonneoplastic areas of peritumoral edema can occur.[25,34] However, in studies using high-dose fluorescein and white-light illumination to guide resection in glioma patients, fluorescein staining has been shown to correlate well with the presence of pathologic features.[15,17] Importantly, this correlation is maintained with administration of low doses of sodium fluorescein as well. Acerbi et al[10] examined the sensitivity and specificity of fluorescent microscopy following administration of low-dose fluorescein by comparing biopsies taken from fluorescent and nonfluorescent tissue, and calculated the sensitivity to be 94% and the specificity to be 89.5%. However, interpretation of these results is limited as regions with tumor cell infiltration without clear morphologic features of GBM were considered "negative" for the purposes of simple analysis.

Given the diffusely infiltrative nature of malignant gliomas, attempts to circumvent the problem of infiltrated tumor by evaluating the degree of tumor involvement of fluorescent tissue have demonstrated the median tumor content of fluorescent tissue to be 95 versus 10% in nonfluorescent tissue.[12] Further, in at least one study, sensitivity-specificity analyses has demonstrated 2 false positives and 8 false negatives in 67 biopsies resulting in a sensitivity and specificity of 82.2 and 90.9%, respectively.[12] A subsequent study examining stereotactic needle biopsies of fluorescent and nonfluorescent peritumoral tissue similarly reported a sensitivity of 79% and a specificity of 100%.[11]

We recently reported our experience with 90 stereotactically guided open biopsies taken at the time of resection from both variably contrast-enhancing and fluorescent regions of HGGs.[14] Regions of fluorescence were categorized as no, low, medium, and high fluorescence, and these labels were correlated to quantified fluorescence. In an effort to circumvent the issues surrounding interpretation of fluorescent regions of tumor infiltration, histopathologic review considered specimens positive for tumor if there was frank tumor, glioma cell infiltration, or evidence of necrosis. The sensitivity and specificity of the presence of any florescence at all for the detection of tumor was 75.6 and 75%, respectively. In regions of contrast enhancement, sensitivity improved to 87.9% and specificity was not calculable due to a lack of true negatives, suggesting that in regions of contrast enhancement, fluorescein was very specific for the presence of tumor.[14] In regions of nonenhancing fluid-attenuated inversion recovery (FLAIR) positive tissue, sensitivity was 69.4% and specificity 66.7%, which suggested that fluorescein positivity may actually extend the ability of the surgeon to identify regions of tumor infiltration beyond the contrast-enhancing margin as determined by preoperative MRI.[14]

# 11.6 Future Directions

At the time of this writing, a large phase III clinical trial (FLUO-GLIO)[8,10] is underway, which may help clarify the role of fluorescein in the resection of malignant gliomas. In the meantime, given its low cost, ease of use, and safety profile, it offers a valuable adjunct to tumor surgeons. At least one group has begun investigations into the coadministration of fluorescein with 5-ALA in an effort to capitalize on the individual benefits of both agents such as the selectivity of 5-ALA, the background brightness of fluorescein fluorescence, and their ability to be visualized using the same fluorescent filter.[35] In this small study, fluorescein fluorescence was found in areas that were PpIX negative and reportedly did not contain tumor cells. While the authors felt fluorescein was not helpful in guiding the surgical resection, it provided enhanced background brightness to facilitate 5-ALA-guided discrimination and resection of pathologic tissue.[35]

Objective measurements of fluorescence eliminate subjectivity from assessments of fluorescence. Using digitally measured thresholds of fluorescence, our group defined a threshold above which there was 100% specificity for tumor beyond regions of contrast enhancement.[14] Nevertheless, the ability to quantify fluorescence was demonstrated and may represent an avenue for pursuit of automation of tumor detection based on objective fluorescence.

# 11.7 Conclusion

Fluorescein sodium provides a safe, affordable, and easy-to-use alternative to 5-ALA for fluorescence-guided glioma resection. While there is evidence that fluorescein guidance improves GTR, data are inconclusive regarding fluorescein's sensitivity and specificity and the effect of fluorescein guidance on outcomes in high-grade gliomas. Additionally, fluorescein dosing and methods of identification of fluorescence have not been optimized. Large-scale clinical trials to better elucidate these factors are still needed. As a result, fluorescence data must always be assessed within the context of all pertinent clinical information, including specific neuroanatomy, imaging, intraoperative navigation, functional mapping when necessary, and, above all, a surgeon's expertise and judgment.

# References

[1] Liu JT, Meza D, Sanai N. Trends in fluorescence image-guided surgery for gliomas. Neurosurgery. 2014; 75(1):61–71

[2] Lacroix M, Abi-Said D, Fourney DR, et al. A multivariate analysis of 416 patients with glioblastoma multiforme: prognosis, extent of resection, and survival. J Neurosurg. 2001; 95(2):190–198

[3] Sanai N, Polley MY, McDermott MW, Parsa AT, Berger MS. An extent of resection threshold for newly diagnosed glioblastomas. J Neurosurg. 2011; 115(1):3–8

[4] Stummer W, Pichlmeier U, Meinel T, Wiestler OD, Zanella F, Reulen HJ, ALA-Glioma Study Group. Fluorescence-guided surgery with 5-aminolevulinic acid for resection of malignant glioma: a randomised controlled multicentre phase III trial. Lancet Oncol. 2006; 7(5):392–401

[5] Stummer W, Reulen HJ, Meinel T, et al. ALA-Glioma Study Group. Extent of resection and survival in glioblastoma multiforme: identification of and adjustment for bias. Neurosurgery. 2008; 62(3):564–576, discussion 564–576

[6] Moore GE. Fluorescein as an agent in the differentiation of normal and malignant tissues. Science. 1947; 106(2745):130–131

[7] Kozler P, Pokorný J. Altered blood-brain barrier permeability and its effect on the distribution of Evans blue and sodium fluorescein in the rat brain applied by intracarotid injection. Physiol Res. 2003; 52(5):607–614

[8] Schebesch KM, Brawanski A, Hohenberger C, Hohne J. Fluorescein sodium-guided surgery of malignant brain tumors: history, current concepts, and future project. Turk Neurosurg. 2016; 26(2):185–194

[9] Kuroiwa T, Kajimoto Y, Ohta T. Development of a fluorescein operative microscope for use during malignant glioma surgery: a technical note and preliminary report. Surg Neurol. 1998; 50(1):41–48, discussion 48–49

[10] Acerbi F, Broggi M, Eoli M, et al. Is fluorescein-guided technique able to help in resection of high-grade gliomas? Neurosurg Focus. 2014; 36(2):E5

[11] Rey-Dios R, Hattab EM, Cohen-Gadol AA. Use of intraoperative fluorescein sodium fluorescence to improve the accuracy of tissue diagnosis during stereotactic needle biopsy of high-grade gliomas. Acta Neurochir (Wien). 2014; 156(6):1071–1075, discussion 1075

[12] Diaz RJ, Dios RR, Hattab EM, et al. Study of the biodistribution of fluorescein in glioma-infiltrated mouse brain and histopathological correlation of intraoperative findings in high-grade gliomas resected under fluorescein fluorescence guidance. J Neurosurg. 2015; 122(6):1360–1369

[13] Hamamcıoğlu MK, Akçakaya MO, Göker B, Kasımcan MO, Kırış T. The use of the YELLOW 560 nm surgical microscope filter for sodium fluorescein-guided resection of brain tumors: our preliminary results in a series of 28 patients. Clin Neurol Neurosurg. 2016; 143:39–45

[14] Neira JA, Ung TH, Sims JS, et al. Aggressive resection at the infiltrative margins of glioblastoma facilitated by intraoperative fluorescein guidance. J Neurosurg. 2017; 127(1):111–122

[15] Shinoda J, Yano H, Yoshimura S, et al. Fluorescence-guided resection of glioblastoma multiforme by using high-dose fluorescein sodium. Technical note. J Neurosurg. 2003; 99(3):597–603

[16] Koc K, Anik I, Cabuk B, Ceylan S. Fluorescein sodium-guided surgery in glioblastoma multiforme: a prospective evaluation. Br J Neurosurg. 2008; 22(1):99–103

[17] Chen B, Wang H, Ge P, et al. Gross total resection of glioma with the intraoperative fluorescence-guidance of fluorescein sodium. Int J Med Sci. 2012; 9(8):708–714

[18] Liu JG, Yang SF, Liu YH, Wang X, Mao Q. Magnetic resonance diffusion tensor imaging with fluorescein sodium dyeing for surgery of gliomas in brain motor functional areas. Chin Med J (Engl). 2013; 126(13):2418–2423

[19] Schebesch KM, Proescholdt M, Höhne J, et al. Sodium fluorescein-guided resection under the YELLOW 560 nm surgical microscope filter in malignant brain tumor surgery: a feasibility study. Acta Neurochir (Wien). 2013; 155(4):693–699

[20] Tivnan A, Zakaria Z, O'Leary C, et al. Inhibition of multidrug resistance protein 1 (MRP1) improves chemotherapy drug response in primary and recurrent glioblastoma multiforme. Front Neurosci. 2015; 9:218

[21] Sun H, Johnson DR, Finch RA, Sartorelli AC, Miller DW, Elmquist WF. Transport of fluorescein in MDCKII-MRP1 transfected cells and mrp1-knockout mice. Biochem Biophys Res Commun. 2001; 284(4):863–869

[22] Abe T, Hasegawa S, Taniguchi K, et al. Possible involvement of multidrug-resistance-associated protein (MRP) gene expression in spontaneous drug resistance to vincristine, etoposide and adriamycin in human glioma cells. Int J Cancer. 1994; 58(6):860–864

[23] McLaren JW, Brubaker RF. Measurement of fluorescein and fluorescein monoglucuronide in the living human eye. Invest Ophthalmol Vis Sci. 1986; 27(6):966–974

[24] Acerbi F, Broggi M, Broggi G, Ferroli P. What is the best timing for fluorescein injection during surgical removal of high-grade gliomas? Acta Neurochir (Wien). 2015; 157(8):1377–1378

[25] Stummer W. Factors confounding fluorescein-guided malignant glioma resections: edema bulk flow, dose, timing, and now: imaging hardware? Acta Neurochir (Wien). 2016; 158(2):327–328

[26] Rey-Dios R, Cohen-Gadol AA. Technical principles and neurosurgical applications of fluorescein fluorescence using a microscope-integrated fluorescence module. Acta Neurochir (Wien). 2013; 155(4):701–706

[27] Lira RP, Oliveira CL, Marques MV, Silva AR, Pessoa CdeC. Adverse reactions of fluorescein angiography: a prospective study. Arq Bras Oftalmol. 2007; 70(4):615–618

[28] Kwan AS, Barry C, McAllister IL, Constable I. Fluorescein angiography and adverse drug reactions revisited: the lions eye experience. Clin Experiment Ophthalmol. 2006; 34(1):33–38

[29] Butner RW, McPherson AR. Adverse reactions in intravenous fluorescein angiography. Ann Ophthalmol. 1983; 15(11):1084–1086

[30] Anari S, Waldron M, Carrie S. Delayed absence seizure: a complication of intrathecal fluorescein injection. A case report and literature review. Auris Nasus Larynx. 2007; 34(4):515–518

[31] Coeytaux A, Reverdin A, Jallon P, Nahory A. Non convulsive status epilepticus following intrathecal fluorescein injection. Acta Neurol Scand. 1999; 100(4):278–280

[32] Wallace JD, Weintraub MI, Mattson RH, Rosnagle R. Status epilepticus as a complication of intrathecal fluorescein. Case report. J Neurosurg. 1972; 36(5):659–660

[33] Eljamel S. 5-ALA fluorescence image guided resection of glioblastoma multiforme: a meta-analysis of the literature. Int J Mol Sci. 2015; 16(5):10443–10456

[34] Stummer W, Götz C, Hassan A, Heimann A, Kempski O. Kinetics of Photofrin II in perifocal brain edema. Neurosurgery. 1993; 33(6):1075–1081, discussion 1081–1082

[35] Suero Molina E, Wolfer J, Ewelt C, Ehrhardt A, Brokinkel B, Stummer W. Dual-labeling with 5-aminolevulinic acid and fluorescein for fluorescence-guided resection of high-grade gliomas: technical note. J Neurosurg. 201 8; 128:1:399–405

# 12 Second Window Indocyanine Green: Near-Infrared Optical Contrast for Intraoperative Identification of Brain Tumors

*Ryan D. Zeh, Ryan D. Salinas, Sunil Singhal, and John Y.K. Lee*

**Abstract**

While indocyanine green (ICG), an FDA-approved near-infrared contrast agent, has classically been used in neurosurgery for visualization of vasculature, new techniques can permit surgeons to use ICG to detect tumors in vivo.[1] Coined "second window" ICG (SWIG) in order to discriminate it from traditional videoangiography procedures that visualize the molecule within minutes of injection, this method relies on visualization 24 hours following high-dose intravenous infusion. A growing body of work has utilized this technique to visualize both primary and metastatic brain tumors. These preliminary findings suggest that SWIG has the potential for broad applications within the neurosurgical field as it can not only aid in localization intraoperatively, but also has promising features that can assist in margin detection.

*Keywords:* fluorescence imaging, indocyanine green, near-infrared, imaging, second window ICG

## 12.1 Introduction to Second Window Indocyanine Green

Indocyanine green (ICG, $C_{43}H_{47}N_2NaO_6S_2$) is a tricarbocyanine dye with a molecular mass of 751.4 Da that fluoresces in the near-infrared (NIR) range, with peak emission and excitation at 780 and 810 nm, respectively. ICG has been used in the medical field since the World War II era, and it was granted Food and Drug Administration (FDA) approval in 1959 for ophthalmologic applications.[1,2,3]

The most common purpose for ICG has traditionally been for angiographic procedures with some application for vascular studies in brain tumors.[4] Doses between 0.2 and 0.5 mg/kg are delivered to the patient intraoperatively; NIR light is then used to excite the dye, and an NIR camera is used to capture the emission of the molecule flowing through the vasculature for minutes following delivery of the bolus.

Early preclinical work with ICG has demonstrated that injection of ICG into rats can lead to persistence of signal an hour after injection. In 1996, Haglund et al found that ICG closely correlated with tumor margins in malignant rat tumors.[5] Preliminary studies in humans also demonstrated similar results. These studies, performed in the 1990s, were not studying the ICG signal in vivo. In these works, the tumor margins were analyzed after resection. This limited the researchers' ability to guide resection.

However, the use of ICG in human trials has only recently developed with the advent of novel endoscopes and open-field exoscopes that are able to facilitate intraoperative identification of ICG positive tissues following bolus injections of the molecule. A growing body of recent research has utilized ICG in a different manner from investigations of the vasculature. New techniques have been developed that can help surgeons localize tumors intraoperatively. This technique has been coined second window ICG (SWIG).[6] In this procedure, doses as high as 5.0 mg/kg are delivered to the patient up to 24 hours in advance of imaging.

By delivering these high doses with injections nearly 24 hours prior to imaging, it is presumed that the ICG becomes subject to the enhanced permeability and retention (EPR) effect, the mechanism by which very small molecules (e.g., nanoparticles) can accumulate in tumors, or other places with similarly unique pathophysiological characteristics.[7] While the exact mechanism is not entirely clear, it is believed that ICG reversibly binds to serum albumin. Potential contributing factors to its subsequent deposition in tumors include defective endothelial cells, fenestrations in the vasculature, disorganized draining (e.g., lymphatic system), and otherwise altered permeability.[6,7,8] SWIG has demonstrated the capacity to identify solid tumors in subcutaneous animal models, canine, and in human clinical trials. Furthermore, studies of ICG in human tumors have been applied in numerous different cancer types not limited to lung, prostate, breast, ovarian, colorectal, pancreatic, esophageal, metastatic, and brain cancers.

## 12.2 Preclinical Work

Jiang et al demonstrated the value of delayed, high-dose SWIG in a rodent model, thus providing the basis for administering ICG to human patients 24 hours in advance of their surgery. In this study, ICG was administered to mice with subcutaneous tumors grafted from metastatic lung cancer cell lines, mesothelioma cell lines, and esophageal carcinoma cell lines. Varying doses of ICG ranging from 0.7 to 10.0 mg/kg were administered via tail vein injection to the mice. The tumors were then imaged serially at time points up to 72 hours later. In doing this, it was determined that 5.0 mg/kg doses were superior to lower doses, and the best signal-to-background ratio (SBR) occurred 24 hours after delivery of the ICG.[9,10] For these reasons, 5.0 mg/kg doses are delivered to patients enrolled in human clinical trials the day prior to surgery.

Further work has been performed to evaluate murine models of other types of cancer outside of the brain. In particular, studies of breast cancer, esophageal cancer, prostate cancer, and lung cancer in murine and large animal (canine) models have been performed.[6,10,11,12,13,14,15,16,17,18,19] These studies demonstrated the capacity of ICG to localize to primary tumors in vivo using SWIG. Further, SWIG has also been found to have the ability to detect residual disease in the wound bed after tumor resection in a mouse and canine model.[18]

Our group has also investigated value of SWIG in a rodent model of intracranial brain tumors using the U251-Luc-GFP cell line (not yet published). Two doses were administered, and although peak SBR appears to be seen just an hour after administration, there is a long plateau period from 6 to 72 hours. In this plateau, the SBR remains relatively stable, thus allowing for a broad time window for visualization. Our human clinical studies with SWIG have been performed 24 hours after systemic administration of ICG.

## 12.3 Peer-Reviewed Studies of SWIG in Other Body Systems

SWIG has successfully been used to identify tumors in multiple other cancer types in humans. Keating et al,[16] Newton et al,[19] and Okusanya et al[20] showed SWIG could be used to identify pulmonary nodules and various lung cancers. Xia et al showed SWIG could be used to identify metastatic lymph nodes from seminoma and prostate cancer.[10,21] Keating et al showed SWIG could be used to detect thymoma, breast cancer, and lung metastases.[14,15,17]

All of these studies demonstrated ICG accumulation in these various tumor types when administered with the SWIG technique. However, one of the major limitations to SWIG in these settings is background fluorescence due to nonspecific accumulation. ICG is delivered heterogeneously to various organs following high-dose delivery due to its presence in the systemic circulation. ICG is also metabolized hepatically, and thus accumulates largely within the liver and bowel. Nonspecific accumulation can lead to potential high background fluorescence in areas near the nodule of interest.

The use of ICG in brain tumors is unique in that the brain has a relatively impermeable blood–brain barrier (BBB) and, additionally, is isolated from these other tissues that can accumulate ICG. Thus, brain tumors are ideal candidates for SWIG, as background fluorescence remains minimal in the intracranial environment. Indeed, in a publication by Lee et al,[6] the SBR is extremely high in the order of 7 to 10, as the adjacent brain parenchyma reveals minimal fluorescence, as shown in ▶ Fig. 12.1 and ▶ Fig. 12.2.

## 12.4 General Findings in Brain Tumors

One of the important findings using SWIG is the ability to localize tumors at depths beyond the view of the unaided eye. Due to the fact that NIR can penetrate brain tissue up to 2 cm, this can permit visualization of brain tumors through the dura, which can aid in the intraoperative planning at the time of the dural opening (▶ Fig. 12.1c, d). Furthermore, the NIR signal emanating from deep tissues can also assist in planning the corticectomy (▶ Fig. 12.1e, f; ▶ Fig. 12.2c, d). This can help minimize damage to normal adjacent brain structures. This feature is remarkable, as laser excitation of the fluorophore can allow for visualization of the tumor even before the dural opening and before corticectomy (▶ Fig. 12.2).

SWIG for intraoperative localization does not rely on stereotactic imaging and utilization of surface landmarks, which can be inaccurate due to a variety of factors. One concern is baseline inaccuracy due to shifting of brain surface landmarks during

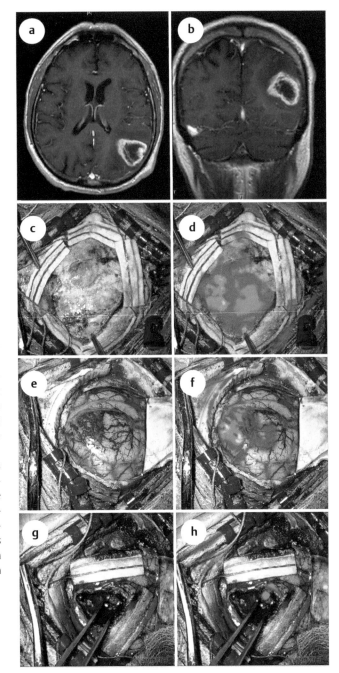

**Fig. 12.1** Second window indocyanine green (SWIG) localizes to glioma. Newly diagnosed glioblastoma. **(a)** T1-weighted gadolinium-enhanced axial MRI. **(b)** T1-coronal MRI. **(c)** Visible light view prior to opening dura. **(d)** Near-infrared (NIR) signal overlay prior to dural opening. **(e)** Visible light view upon dural opening. **(f)** NIR signal overlay after dural opening. Note, the tumor can be visualized through parenchyma. **(g)** Visible light postresection surgical margin. **(h)** Residual NIR signal in the resection cavity.

patient positioning and placement of cranial pins. Furthermore, brain shift during tumor resection can render stereotactic navigation unreliable. The real-time intraoperative localization of SWIG has led to further analysis of its ability to study tumor margins.

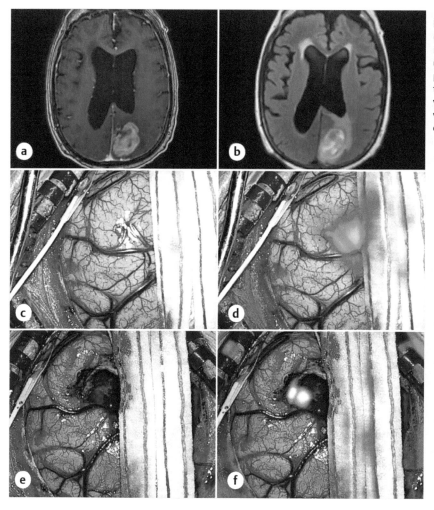

**Fig. 12.2** Second window indocyanine green (SWIG) localizes to metastases. Newly diagnosed metastatic adenocarcinoma. **(a)** Axial T1 MRI. **(b)** Axial FLAIR MRI. **(c)** Visible light view through parenchyma. **(d)** Near-infrared signal overlay through parenchyma. Note, the tumor can be visualized through parenchyma. **(e)** Visible light view of surgical resection cavity. **(f)** NIR signal overlay in surgical resection cavity.

In order to study SWIG's utility in defining surgical margins for tumors, we have compared SWIG to the unaided eye of the surgeon. Each biopsy specimen was coded as either pathologically positive or negative by the senior surgeon using white light only. Immediately after this was recorded, the NIR camera was brought into the field, and the specimen was coded as positive or negative for NIR fluorescence.

It is important to note that in these studies, the extent of resection did not change due to NIR fluorescence findings; biopsies were only taken if deemed safe by the senior surgeon. Using final pathology of the specimen as the gold standard, diagnostic testing for sensitivity, specificity, positive predictive value, and negative predictive value was performed.

## 12.5 Second Window Indocyanine Green for Brain Tumors

### 12.5.1 Second Window Indocyanine Green for Glioma

The first published study on SWIG for brain tumors included all gliomas of all WHO grades I to IV.[6] Fifteen patients (10 glioblastoma [GBM], 1 WHO grade III anaplastic astrocytoma [AA], 2 WHO grade II astrocytomas, and 1 WHO grade I juvenile pilocytic astrocytoma [JPA]) were enrolled in a phase I clinical trial. On average, NIR fluorescence imaging took place 22.8 hours after infusion of 5.0 mg/kg ICG. The tumors had a mean SBR of 9.5 ± 0.8, and were able to be identified with NIR fluorescence through the dura to a maximum depth of 13 mm.

Of the 15 gliomas analyzed, 12 of them demonstrated positive NIR fluorescence (▶ Fig. 12.1). Interestingly, the three gliomas that did not demonstrate NIR fluorescence all also did not enhance after gadolinium administration on the preoperative MRI. No association was found between positive fluorescence with tumor size and volume, histology, or injection time.

Surgical margins were analyzed at the completion of the resection (▶ Fig. 12.1g, h). The NIR imaging device was used to scan the resection cavity and areas of residual fluorescence were biopsied if deemed safe by adjacent anatomy by the senior surgeon. Diagnostic test characteristics on 71 specimens were taken from the 12 patients with positive NIR fluorescence; 51 (71.8%) were characterized as positive for glioma by pathology, while 61 (85.9%) were positive for NIR fluorescence. Using final pathology as the gold standard, the sensitivity, specificity, positive predictive value, and negative predicted values were calculated based on the surgeon's impression and NIR fluorescence (▶ Table 12.1).

This study was the first work to demonstrate the practicality of SWIG as a tool for the detection and resection of gliomas.

**Table 12.1** Diagnostic characteristics of second window indocyanine green for glioma

|  | Visible light vs. pathology (%) | Near-infrared positivity vs. pathology (%) |
| --- | --- | --- |
| Sensitivity | 84.3 | 98.0 |
| Specificity | 80.0 | 45.0 |
| Positive predictive value | 91.5 | 82.0 |
| Negative predictive value | 66.7 | 90.0 |

**Table 12.3** Diagnostic characteristics of second window indocyanine green for WHO grade II atypical meningiomas

|  | Visible light vs. pathology (%) | Near-infrared positivity vs. pathology (%) |
| --- | --- | --- |
| Sensitivity | 81.8 | 90.4 |
| Specificity | 100 | 55.6 |
| Positive predictive value | 100 | 71.4 |
| Negative predictive value | 81.8 | 83.3 |

**Table 12.2** Diagnostic characteristics of second window indocyanine green for all meningioma

|  | Visible light vs. pathology (%) | Near-infrared positivity vs. pathology (%) |
| --- | --- | --- |
| Sensitivity | 82.1 | 96.4 |
| Specificity | 100 | 38.9 |
| Positive predictive value | 100 | 71.1 |
| Negative predictive value | 78.3 | 87.5 |

Gadolinium-enhancing tumors were shown to have detectable NIR fluorescence contrast in the operating room that could be visualized in real time during surgery. The sensitivity of NIR fluorescence using this technique was found to be superior to the unaided eye, although this came at the expense of specificity. Although the specificity appears to be low, perhaps due to the nonspecific accumulation of ICG within tumors via the EPR effect, we believe the hematoxylin and eosin (H&E) can oftentimes underestimate the presence of tumor in the biopsied sample, and as such, we believe that the true rate of false positives is lower than presented.[22] SWIG has become a promising tool for identifying gliomas both through the dura and through limited brain parenchyma. Its utility for margin detection and determination of extent of resection warrants further investigation.

## 12.5.2 Second Window Indocyanine Green for Meningioma

A second published study of SWIG analyzed 18 patients (13 females and 5 males) with meningioma.[23] The mean age of the patients was 55 years (range 20–74 years). Eleven patients had convexity meningiomas, 1 had a parasagittal frontal meningioma, and the remaining 6 had intraventricular or skull base meningiomas (olfactory groove, cerebellopontine angle, and medial sphenoid wing). Final pathology revealed 15 WHO grade I meningiomas and 3 WHO grade II meningiomas. The pathological subtypes of these tumors were as follows: 12 meningothelial, 3 transitional, 1 psammomatous, and 2 either lacking or inconclusive of any further pathological grading.

Using the SWIG protocol, NIR fluorescence was able to positively identify 14/18 (78%) meningiomas intraoperatively. The tumors in these patients on average had an SBR of 5.6 ± 1.7. The NIR signal was observable in all 14 of these patients prior to opening the dura (▶ Fig. 12.3).

The four patients who did not have fluorescent tumors displayed a peculiar "inverse" fluorescence pattern. In these cases, adjacent brain parenchyma had a higher NIR signal than the tumor (SBR = 0.31 ± 0.1). This inversion pattern did not have a correlation with gender, WHO grade, and history of prior surgery or radiation. All of the inversions occurred in women with WHO grade I meningiomas who had no prior surgical or radiation history. Furthermore, maximum tumor diameter, age, presence of peritumoral T2/fluid-attenuated inversion recovery (FLAIR) signal on pre-op MRI, T1 signal intensity, tumor location, BMI, Ki-67, and pathological subtype all did not predict inversion via logistical regression. Only one variable approached statistical significance ($p < 0.25$) for predicting inversions: time from infusion to imaging. The average time from infusion to tumor visualization in the NIR positive patients was 22.4 hours, whereas in the four inversion patients the average time from infusion to imaging was 24.4 hours. One possible explanation for this is the fact that the nonspecifically and extracellularly accumulated ICG diffuses out of the tumor space into the adjacent brain after an extended period of time.

Interestingly, all four tumors in the fluorescence inversion cases still contained measurable traces of ICG. These tumors demonstrated the inversion pattern in vivo; however, when the tumor was removed and imaged ex vivo, the fluorescent signal was still significantly stronger than the adjacent dura. Thus, these tumors still demonstrated ICG accumulation, and the lack of NIR signal in vivo could also be due to saturation of ICG within the tumor.

Using the previously described mechanism for margin detection, 46 total specimens from the 14 patients with positive tumor fluorescence were analyzed (▶ Table 12.2). Twenty-three of these were coded as positive for tumor using only white light, and 38 of the specimens were positive for NIR fluorescence. Ultimately, pathology revealed 28 specimens to be positive pathologically for tumor.

An independent analysis was also performed on atypical meningiomas, as this type of tumor is more likely to have residual disease in the margins and has higher recurrence rates. ▶ Table 12.3 shows the characteristics for the 20 specimens biopsied from atypical WHO grade II meningiomas.

This study was the first work to demonstrate the practicality of SWIG as a tool for the detection and resection of meningiomas. Using SWIG to determine extent of resection in real time for meningiomas is a very sensitive technique, but comes at the cost of specificity. For higher-grade meningiomas, the specificity improves; however, it is still not as good as a surgeon's impression using visible light only. Its utility for margin detection warrants further investigation.

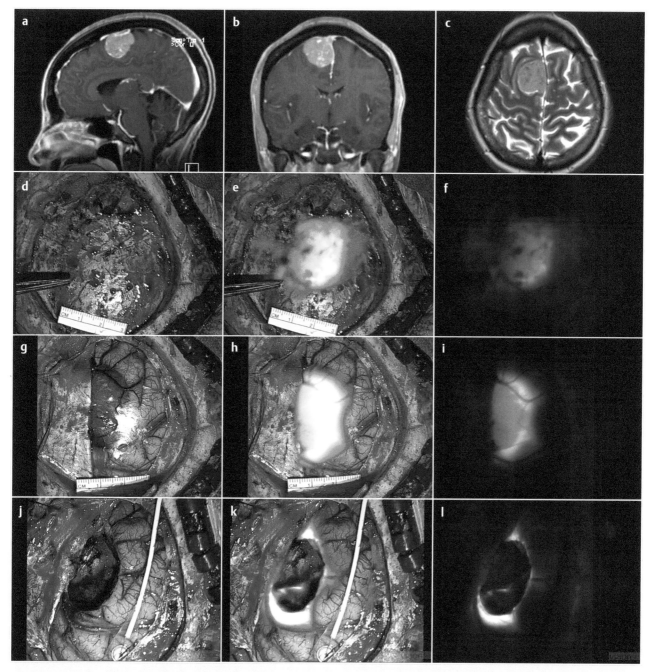

Fig. 12.3 Second window indocyanine green (SWIG) localizes to intracranial meningioma. Patient demonstrating intracranial meningioma. (a–c) Sagittal, coronal, and axial postcontrast MRI. (d–f) View prior to opening dura. From left to right: visible light view, fused near-infrared (NIR) overlay, NIR light-only image. (g–i) View after opening dura. (j–l) Margin following resection of gross tumor.

## 12.5.3 Second Window Indocyanine Green for Brain Metastases

The following data was presented as a poster at American Association of Neurological Surgeons conference in 2017. It is currently under peer review for publication.

SWIG can be used to identify intraparenchymal brain metastases (▶ Fig. 12.2; Video 12.1). Data were analyzed from the first 13 patients (4 males and 9 females) between the ages of 36 and 73 years (mean = 59 years) enrolled in the clinical trial presenting with intraparenchymal brain metastases. Primary cancer pathologies consisted of lung ($n = 4$), melanoma ($n = 2$), colon ($n = 2$), breast ($n = 2$), ovarian ($n = 1$), kidney ($n = 1$), and esophageal ($n = 1$). The average SBR of these lesions was 6.62 ± 1.6. In contrast to what was found in the glioma analysis, the T1 signal intensity on the preoperative MRI did not correlate with the intraoperative signal intensity of brain metastases.

Of all the metastatic brain cancers included in this analysis, melanoma had the weakest SBR. Specifically, melanoma metastasis did not show any fluorescence until the cyst contents

**Table 12.4** Diagnostic characteristics of second window indocyanine green for brain metastases

|  | Visible light vs. pathology (%) | Near-infrared positivity vs. pathology (%) |
| --- | --- | --- |
| Sensitivity | 82.1 | 96.4 |
| Specificity | 90.9 | 27.3 |
| Positive predictive value | 95.8 | 77.1 |
| Negative predictive value | 66.7 | 75.0 |

**Table 12.5** Types of tumors detected with second window indocyanine green

|  | Number |
| --- | --- |
| Glioma | 44 |
| • Glioblastoma (GBM) | 34 |
| • Other gliomas | 10 |
| Meningioma | 47 |
| • WHO grade I | 40 |
| • WHO grade 2 | 7 |
| Metastases | 30 |
| • Melanoma | 4 |
| • Lung (NSCLC and carcinoma) | 7 |
| • Breast | 4 |
| • Colorectal | 4 |
| • Other | 11 |
| Pituitary adenoma | 13 |
| Craniopharyngioma | 3 |
| Chordoma | 5 |
| Other histopathology | 15 |

Abbreviation: NSCLC, non–small cell lung cancer.

were opened. The authors hypothesize that this is due to melanin's light-absorbing physical characteristics.

Using previously described methods, the ability of SWIG to detect residual tumor in the surgical margins was analyzed (▶ Table 12.4). There were 39 total specimens in this analysis, including 13 main tumor specimens. Using visible light only, 23 of these specimens were coded as positive for tumor. In contrast, NIR fluorescence was noted in 27 of these specimens. On final pathology, 28 of these specimens came back as tumor. ▶ Table 12.4 shows the diagnostic characteristics.

Since the time of this analysis, SWIG has been successfully utilized to visualize other metastatic cancers including prostate, lymphoma, intracranial solitary fibrous tumor, and sarcoma of gluteus muscle (unpublished data). This study was the first work to demonstrate the practicality of SWIG as a tool for the detection and resection of intraparenchymal metastases. Similarly to gliomas and meningiomas, SWIG for metastasis resection is more sensitive than the naked eye, but this comes at the cost of specificity. SWIG also appears to be a very applicable tool for identifying metastases both through the dura and through limited brain parenchyma (▶ Fig. 12.2c, d). Its utility for margin detection and determination of extent of resection warrants further investigation (▶ Fig. 12.2e, f).

### 12.5.4 Second Window Indocyanine Green for Other Brain Tumors

In addition to gliomas, meningiomas, and metastasis, we have explored the utility of SWIG in a variety of histopathologies. Early unpublished work has shown great variety in the ability to localize ICG to different types of brain tumors (▶ Table 12.5). NIR fluorescent signal can be "perfectly" confined to some types of lesions. Other times, fluorescence can be observed from normal structures that would otherwise contrast enhance on MRI such as the pituitary gland, radiation changes, and sinus mucosa. The variety in types of ICG localization specifically in tumors may be attributable to differences in tumor growth patterns, location, and perfusion patterns—specifically in light of BBB disruptions in these regions.

## 12.6 Potential Advantages of Second Window Indocyanine Green

The use of NIR signaling to localize brain tumors can facilitate tumor visualization with the intraoperative approach. Current intraoperative neuronavigation technologies primarily utilize

stereotactic mechanisms through recognition of surface landmarks. These surface landmarks, which are normally established through a preoperative MRI scan, can become altered prior to surgery through skin movement based on positioning or even from fixation of the head using Mayfield pins. These MRI-based localization techniques are furthermore based off of preoperative scans that may become inaccurate with brain shift as a tumor is resected.

Unlike MRI-based navigation, SWIG appears to correlate with contrast enhancement both live and in vivo. This allows for the potential of the surgeon to assess the extent of resection in real time in the operating room.

## 12.7 Limitations of Second Window ICG

### 12.7.1 Camera Gain

Although all camera systems for visualizing NIR fluorescence have different features, one of the main sources of limitation with the camera system used has been the dynamic autoexposure feature. In the absence of strong signals, the system boosts exposure. This causes spots to fluoresce that normally would not, and is likely contributing to false-positive biopsies. Hence, we believe that the false-positive rate (specificity) can be improved by optimization of camera settings.

### 12.7.2 Specificity

ICG is nonspecific. Pathologic slides of ICG positive margins would oftentimes be negative for tumor by pathology. However, this may be due to sampling error. The authors' own correlations with pathology, as published by Lee et al[6,23] suggest that the sensitivity of this technique for margin detection is high but the specificity is low. Indeed, ICG is not receptor bound, and we do not believe it is necessarily internalized into the cell, as it is generally bound to plasma albumin. Hence, SWIG may not be a specific dye. Despite these limitations, SWIG may be valuable in determination of extent of resection as a proxy for gadolinium enhancement.

### 12.7.3 Science of the Enhanced Permeability and Retention Effect

Earlier research has demonstrated that ICG can distinguish cancer from normal tissue but not from inflammation.[11] Indeed, in many studies of ICG in human brain tumors, enhancement from radiation necrosis is also positive for ICG. ICG is not receptor bound, so its location in the tumor environment is not precisely understood. Further work into understanding how or why ICG will accumulate in tissues in the brain would be helpful in leveraging this tool in a more efficacious manner.

## 12.8 Conclusion

In conclusion, SWIG has emerged has a powerful tool to help detect and resect both primary and metastatic brain tumors. SWIG can be used to visualize tumors through both intact dura and limited brain parenchyma. These features provide assistance in surgical planning prior to corticectomy, thus allowing for minimal sacrifice to normal tissue. SWIG is also advantageous in that it does not rely on stereotactic imaging or utilization of normal tissue surface landmarks, which can be inaccurate due to a range of variables such as inaccurate registration and brain shift during tumor resection.

SWIG has also demonstrated value in maximizing clearance of surgical margins following resection of the gross tumor specimen. Based on preliminary results in a phase I clinical trial, SWIG appears to be more sensitive than the unaided surgeon's eye in detecting residual disease in the wound bed, although this comes at the cost of specificity.

SWIG is a technique that can be readily and easily performed in virtually every operating room, allowing for tumor visualization in real time without delay. A growing body of work suggests that this technique has broad applications for both early and accurate identification of brain tumors within the operating room.

## References

[1] Vahrmeijer AL, Hutteman M, van der Vorst JR, van de Velde CJ, Frangioni JV. Image-guided cancer surgery using near-infrared fluorescence. Nat Rev Clin Oncol. 2013; 10(9):507–518

[2] Cherrick GR, Stein SW, Leevy CM, Davidson CS. Indocyanine green: observations on its physical properties, plasma decay, and hepatic extraction. J Clin Invest. 1960; 39:592–600

[3] Reinhart MB, Huntington CR, Blair LJ, Heniford BT, Augenstein VA. Indocyanine green: historical context, current applications, and future considerations. Surg Innov. 2016; 23(2):166–175

[4] Kim EH, Cho JM, Chang JH, Kim SH, Lee KS. Application of intraoperative indocyanine green videoangiography to brain tumor surgery. Acta Neurochir (Wien). 2011; 153(7):1487–1495, discussion 1494–1495

[5] Haglund MM, Hochman DW, Spence AM, Berger MS. Enhanced optical imaging of rat gliomas and tumor margins. Neurosurgery. 1994; 35(5):930–940, discussion 940–941

[6] Lee JY, Thawani JP, Pierce J, et al. Intraoperative near-infrared optical imaging can localize gadolinium-enhancing gliomas during surgery. Neurosurgery. 2016; 79(6):856–871

[7] Singhal S, Nie S, Wang MD. Nanotechnology applications in surgical oncology. Annu Rev Med. 2010; 61:359–373

[8] Iyer AK, Khaled G, Fang J, Maeda H. Exploiting the enhanced permeability and retention effect for tumor targeting. Drug Discov Today. 2006; 11(17–18):812–818

[9] Jiang JX, Keating JJ, Jesus EM, et al. Optimization of the enhanced permeability and retention effect for near-infrared imaging of solid tumors with indocyanine green. Am J Nucl Med Mol Imaging. 2015; 5(4):390–400

[10] Xia L, Zeh R, Mizelle J, et al. Near-infrared intraoperative molecular imaging can identify metastatic lymph nodes in prostate cancer. Urology. 2017; 106: 133–138

[11] Holt D, Okusanya O, Judy R, et al. Intraoperative near-infrared imaging can distinguish cancer from normal tissue but not inflammation. PLoS One. 2014; 9(7):e103342

[12] Holt D, Parthasarathy AB, Okusanya O, et al. Intraoperative near-infrared fluorescence imaging and spectroscopy identifies residual tumor cells in wounds. J Biomed Opt. 2015; 20(7):76002

[13] Keating J, Judy R, Newton A, Singhal S. Near-infrared operating lamp for intraoperative molecular imaging of a mediastinal tumor. BMC Med Imaging. 2016; 16:15

[14] Keating J, Newton A, Venegas O, et al. Near-infrared intraoperative molecular imaging can locate metastases to the lung. Ann Thorac Surg. 2017; 103(2): 390–398

[15] Keating J, Tchou J, Okusanya O, et al. Identification of breast cancer margins using intraoperative near-infrared imaging. J Surg Oncol. 2016; 113(5):508–514

[16] Keating JJ, Kennedy GT, Singhal S. Identification of a subcentimeter pulmonary adenocarcinoma using intraoperative near-infrared imaging during video-assisted thoracoscopic surgery. J Thorac Cardiovasc Surg. 2015; 149(3):e51–e53

[17] Keating JJ, Nims S, Venegas O, et al. Intraoperative imaging identifies thymoma margins following neoadjuvant chemotherapy. Oncotarget. 2016; 7 (3):3059–3067

[18] Madajewski B, Judy BF, Mouchli A, et al. Intraoperative near-infrared imaging of surgical wounds after tumor resections can detect residual disease. Clin Cancer Res. 2012; 18(20):5741–5751

[19] Newton AD, Kennedy GT, Predina JD, Low PS, Singhal S. Intraoperative molecular imaging to identify lung adenocarcinomas. J Thorac Dis. 2016; 8 suppl 9:S697–S704

[20] Okusanya OT, Holt D, Heitjan D, et al. Intraoperative near-infrared imaging can identify pulmonary nodules. Ann Thorac Surg. 2014; 98(4):1223–1230

[21] Xia L, Venegas OG, Predina JD, Singhal S, Guzzo TJ. Intraoperative molecular imaging for post-chemotherapy robot-assisted laparoscopic resection of seminoma metastasis: a case report. Clin Genitourin Cancer. 2017; 15(1): e61–e64

[22] Yano H, Nakayama N, Ohe N, Miwa K, Shinoda J, Iwama T. Pathological analysis of the surgical margins of resected glioblastomas excised using photodynamic visualization with both 5-aminolevulinic acid and fluorescein sodium. J Neurooncol. 2017; 133(2):389–397

[23] Lee JY, et al. Near-infrared fluorescent image-guided surgery for intracranial meningioma. J Neurosurg. 2018; 128:380–390

# 13 Cancer-Targeted Alkylphosphocholine Analogs for Intraoperative Visualization

*Ray R. Zhang, Paul A. Clark, Jamey P. Weichert, and John S. Kuo*

**Abstract**

Within the last decade, several clinical trials pairing targeted fluorophores for cancer with their detection instrumentation have emerged in an effort to improve resection outcomes and survival. This rapidly expanding field of fluorescence-guided surgery (FGS) is ready to revolutionize the way oncological surgeries are performed in the operating room. Alkylphosphocholine (APC) analogs are a group of versatile small molecules that can be attached to different "diapeutic" moieties for targeted diagnostic imaging and therapy of cancer. They work by a unique mechanism in multiple kinds of cancers, through selective uptake through lipid rafts that are overexpressed in cancer cells, and prolonged retention by decreased catabolism in cancer cells. Several APC agents are in clinical trial testing, and the fluorescent APC analogs 1501 and 1502 have successfully demonstrated selective uptake and retention in several orthotopic and xenograft rodent models of human cancer, including orthotopic human-derived cancer stem cell models of glioblastoma multiforme. 1501 carries a green fluorescent BODIPY (boron-dipyrromethene) tag for subcellular localization studies, and 1502 (with a near-infrared fluorophore IR-775) was validated for FGS in multiple preclinical rodent models of cancer with high tumor-to-normal tissue contrast. Dual-labeled PET/fluorescent APC analogs have also been synthesized and validated in order to better characterize and understand the new modality of fluorescence. With an armamentarium of several APC analogs of different diagnostic and therapeutic moieties at our disposal that target cancer by the same purported mechanism, we are able to preoperatively image, intraoperatively resect, and postoperatively treat and follow multiple types of cancers, offering a level of synergy that may improve cancer care and outcomes.

*Keywords:* alkylphosphocholine analogs, fluorescence-guided surgery, targeted fluorophores, near-infrared fluorophores, glioblastoma multiforme, surgical oncology

## 13.1 Introduction

Surgical resection remains a primary treatment of cancer, and the extent of tumor resection has prognostic impact on patient survival.[1,2,3] In most cancer types, patients who have microscopic residual and positive tumor margins experience cancer recurrence and significantly shorter long-term survival compared to patients with complete resections and negative tumor margins.[4,5,6,7] In the case of brain malignancies, gross total resection (GTR) is associated with improved long-term survival compared to patients with subtotal resections (13 vs. 8 months for high-grade gliomas and 15 vs. 9.9 years for low-grade gliomas).[4,5,8] Furthermore, microscopically positive margins have been reported in up to 65% high-grade glioma resections, highlighting the need for better intraoperative distinction between malignant and nonmalignant tissues.[8] At the same time, while positive margins are associated with increased rates of recurrence and worse survival compared with GTR, overzealous resection can compromise adjacent vital tissue, resulting in poor neurological functional outcomes.[2,3] Fluorescence-guided surgery (FGS) could achieve better resection margins and also improve functional outcomes of patients undergoing surgeries by providing a superimposable and real-time field of visualization (FOV) that distinguishes malignant tissue from benign tissue.

Traditionally, surgeons rely on subjective assessments during resection and ablative procedures including subtle tactile and visual tissue differences to intraoperatively distinguish cancer from adjacent tissues. Improvements in cancer imaging technology are now aiding surgeons in visualizing cancer in the operating room. Several intraoperative modalities including ultrasound, fluoroscopy, CT, and MRI have all been harnessed to improve and facilitate cancer removal. These intraoperative imaging modalities can be used to provide additional information about anatomical localization of abnormal lesions, adjacent vital structures, and tissue shift during an operation. However, these intraoperative imaging modalities rely on general characteristics such as abnormal perfusion or tissue consistency, lack cancer specificity, are limited in their contrast detection sensitivities, and offer distinctly different and nonsuperimposable FOV from the surgical cavity. Fluorescence imaging has several favorable characteristics that are conducive for clinical implementation. These include real-time detection capabilities with a superimposable FOV, an abundance of cancer-targeted fluorophores, high detection sensitivity compared to other imaging modalities, an excellent safety record with clinically used probes,[9,10,11,12] lack of ionizing radiation exposure, lower costs, and markedly less cumbersome detection instrumentation compared with other intraoperative imaging modalities.[13,14,15,16] Importantly, fluorophores can be attached to a variety of available targeting molecules, enabling the application of this modality to many cancer types.

Fluorescence-guided imaging usually involves the administration of a cancer-selective fluorophore, followed by excitation and detection of its fluorescence at an optimal time point to achieve contrast. Near-infrared (NIR) fluorophores with excitation and emission spectra in the NIR wavelength range (700–900 nm) exhibit improved depth penetration and lower in vivo background compared to fluorophores that excite and emit fluorescence at shorter wavelengths. NIR fluorophores have attracted the most attention because of their favorable characteristics and improved contrast.[17,18]

## 13.2 Fluorescent Alkylphosphocholine Analogs 1501 and 1502

Weichert et al has recently expanded the repertoire of cancer-targeting alkylphosphocholines (APCs; small molecule platform agents) for cancer imaging by creating fluorescent APC analogs

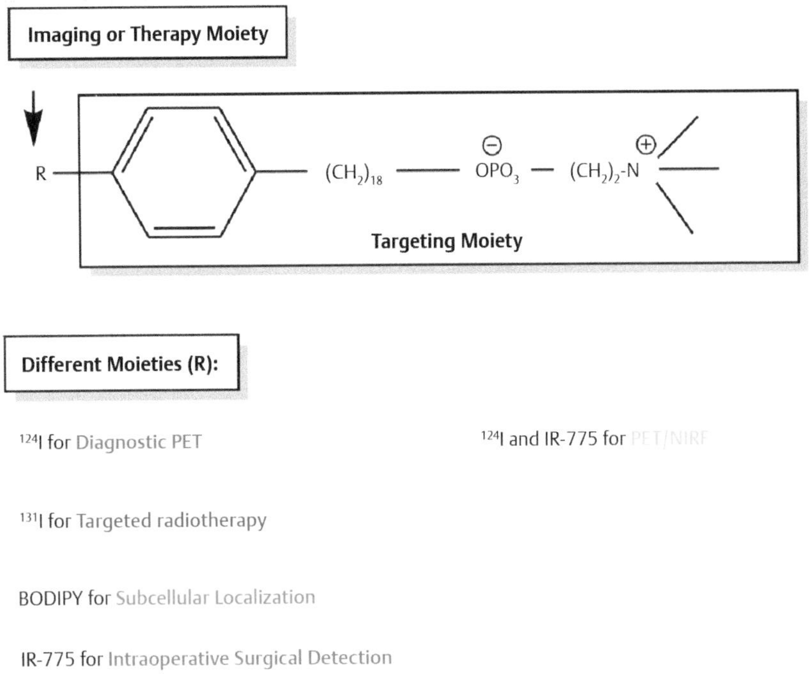

**Imaging or Therapy Moiety**

R —
(CH$_2$)$_{18}$ — OPO$_3^{\ominus}$ — (CH$_2$)$_2$-N$^{\oplus}$

**Targeting Moiety**

**Different Moieties (R):**

$^{124}$I for Diagnostic PET

$^{124}$I and IR-775 for PET/NIRF

$^{131}$I for Targeted radiotherapy

BODIPY for Subcellular Localization

IR-775 for Intraoperative Surgical Detection

**Fig. 13.1** Alkylphosphocholine (APC) analogs for multimodality cancer imaging and therapy. APC analogs are composed of a phosphocholine head, a C18 alkyl chain, and an aromatic ring, which together comprise the targeting moiety and an imaging or therapy moiety. $^{124}$I is used for PET imaging, $^{131}$I is used for targeted radiotherapy, the fluorophore BODIPY (boron-dipyrromethene) is used for subcellular localization and mechanistic studies, and the fluorophore IR-775 for near-infrared imaging. Other imaging and therapy moieties can also be added to the APC targeting backbone for multimodality cancer imaging and therapy.

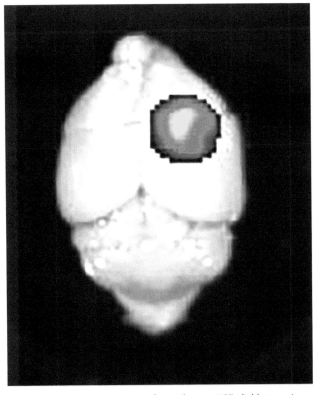

**Fig. 13.2** Fluorescence imaging of an orthotopic U87 glioblastoma in a mouse brain with the near-infrared alkylphosphocholine analog 1502.

for intraoperative surgical illumination of cancer margins. In 2014, Weichert et al reported APC analogs, a new class of small synthetic phospholipid ether molecules for PET imaging and targeted radiotherapy, that demonstrate broad-spectrum tumor-targeting potential in over 60 preclinical cancer models and in

early human clinical studies.[19] Through extensive structure activity relationship studies, NM404 was selected from 30 related phospholipid ether and APC compounds as the optimal tumor-imaging agent.[20] The PET compound $^{124}$I-NM404 can be used for noninvasive localization and staging of cancer, and $^{131}$I-NM404 (a companion radioisotope) can be used for cancer-targeted radiotherapy (▶ Fig. 13.1).[19,21,22] Due to the broad tumor-targeting potential of NM404, two fluorescent APC analogs (1501 and 1502) were created by labeling the same APC-targeting backbone with different fluorophores; these fluorescent APC agents were synthesized for subcellular localization studies and FGS, respectively (▶ Fig. 13.1). 1501 carries a green fluorescent boron-dipyrromethene (BODIPY) tag for subcellular localization studies and 1502 (with an NIR fluorophore [NIRF] IR-775) was validated for FGS in multiple preclinical rodent models of cancer. Other APC analogs are also being synthesized and tested for multimodality cancer imaging and therapy (▶ Fig. 13.1).

Subcellular localization studies with 1501 offered insight into the mechanism of APC's cancer specificity.[19] In co-culture with normal cells, cancer cells demonstrated more uptake of 1501 compared to normal fibroblasts. As found with other APC analogs, methyl-beta-cyclodextrin disruption of cell membrane lipid rafts prior to addition of 1501 to tumor cells markedly decreased 1501 uptake and fluorescence by over 60%. These key studies suggest an APC-selective uptake in cancer cells through cell membrane lipid rafts, and many groups have also reported that lipid rafts are overexpressed on cancer cells.[23,24,25] These results are consistent with mechanistic studies using multiple other APC analogs.[23,24,25]

In a study that compared the properties of fluorescent analogs 1501, 1502, and 5-ALA in mice with stereotactically implanted glioblastoma (GBM) xenografts, both 1501 and 1502 demonstrated high tumor-to-normal brain contrast ratios of 7.23 and 9.28, respectively. The observed tumor-to-normal brain contrast ratio of 9.28 for 1502 is significantly higher than that observed for 5-ALA at 4.81 (▶ Fig. 13.2).[26] This illustrates

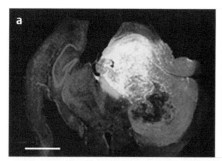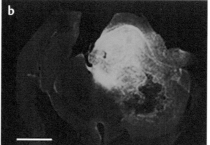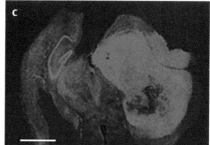

**Fig. 13.3** Confocal microscopy images of a glioblastoma stem cell–derived xenograft with 1501 and ToPro3 nuclear stain. **(a)** Overlay of 1501 and ToPro fluorescence, **(b)** 1501 fluorescence, and **(c)** ToPro3 nuclear stain in an orthotopic glioma stem cell xenograft brain section.

that 1502 offers superior contrast than the clinically approved FGS fluorophore, 5-ALA, recently approved for FGS of GBM in the United States and already clinically used worldwide. In the mice with orthotopic GBM xenografts treated with 1501, flow cytometry analysis of normal brain cells and tumor cells demonstrated that tumor-associated 1501 fluorescence was 14.8 times higher than the background signal in normal brain cells.[26] Histological analysis of the tumor margins illustrated that 1501 fluorescence was localized to the tumor, and not beyond the tumor margins (▶ Fig. 13.3). These studies illustrate the cancer selectivity of 1501 and 1502 in GBMs, and the potential of 1502 as a viable and sensitive intraoperative fluorescent agent.

In other studies, 1502 demonstrated higher uptake in colon and breast adenocarcinoma tumor xenografts compared to adenomas and surrounding normal tissue.[27,28] 1502 was also able to detect regional hyperplastic lymph nodes surrounding the sites of adenocarcinoma, which is important for disease staging and prognosis in both colon and breast cancer. Moreover, fluorescence intensities in the tumor and regional lymph nodes of the breast adenocarcinoma were highest in mice after about 1.5 days after 1502 injection into the bloodstream. Single photon emission CT with the [131]I-tagged radioisotope [131]I-NM404 detected colorectal cancer metastases in the lung of a human colorectal cancer patient, highlighting the multimodality imaging and staging potential of regional and disseminated disease with these APC analogs.[28]

## 13.3 Alkylphosphocholines: Mechanism of Action

APC analogs are a novel group of small molecules that target a broad spectrum of different cancers.[19] They act through a two-part mechanism of cancer selective uptake and retention by cancer cells. APCs are taken up by lipid rafts, which are cellular plasma membrane subdomains that contain high concentrations of cholesterol, glycosphingolipids, and important transmembrane proteins involved in signal transduction and cell adhesion.[19,29] It is reported that cancer cells and cancer stem cells overexpress lipid rafts.[23] Once taken up, these synthetic APC compounds are retained due to a deficiency of catabolic enzymes in cancer cells. It remains unknown which enzymes or enzymatic isoforms are involved in the metabolism of these synthetic molecules.[30,31] However, the phosphate carbon ether

linkage in APCs and structurally related analogs are more slowly cleaved in cancer cells compared to normal tissues.

The broad-spectrum tumor-targeting properties of APC analogs are retained even with the addition of bulkier diagnostic imaging and therapy moieties. Substitution of the iodine with BODIPY or the cyanine fluorophore IR-775 did not alter the broad-spectrum tumor-targeting ability.[21,26] Continued synthesis, testing, and validation of next-generation APC analogs broaden the diagnostic and therapeutic applications of this interesting class of small cancer-targeting molecules. Another significant advantage of these analogs is their high positive specificity for tumor, and discriminating avoidance of inflammatory foci.[19] Other imaging and therapy agents often cross-react with inflammatory foci and result in false-positive signals, therefore decreasing diagnostic accuracy and therapeutic efficacy.[32]

Interestingly with these APC analogs, the kinetics of tumor uptake are consistent in many tumor types, but differ slightly between the different APC analogs. With the fluorescent compounds 1501 and 1502, tumor uptake can be appreciated within 1 hour after administration, and generally peaks between 24 and 48 hours. Ongoing studies looking at the partitioning of these compounds to different blood components are lending insight into how the functional moieties impact binding to plasma proteins, and how that influences their kinetics of uptake and elimination.

## 13.4 Multimodality Imaging Using Dual-Labeled Iodo-1502 Analog

Since imaging modalities all have unique strengths and limitations, combining multiple imaging modalities is a possible strategy to overcome the limitations of single modalities via synergism of both modalities. Combining fluorophores with radioactive tracers could achieve the potential advantages of quantitative detection, unlimited depth of detection, and high spatial resolution and functional molecular imaging ideal for in vivo applications. This enables careful characterization of the NIRF modality using PET as a quantitative gold standard. Additionally, gross fluorescence behavior can be complicated by phenomena such as quenching at high concentrations in tissues, and issues with photostability of fluorophores in vivo and over time. The knowledge acquired with this unique dual-labeled agent would be of substantial novelty and interest,

Table 13.1 The combination of PET and near-infrared fluorescence (NIRF) into one analog overcomes the main limitations of the NIRF modality: quantitation and depth penetration

| Advantages | NIRF | PET | NIRF/PET |
|---|---|---|---|
| Sensitivity | X | X | X |
| Real-time detection | X | | X |
| Quantitation | | X | |
| Depth penetration | | X | X |

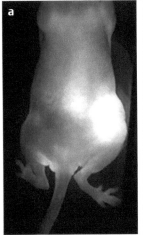
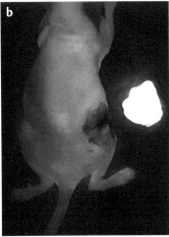

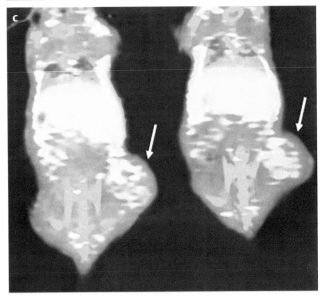

because very little research on NIRF quantitation and its limitations has been performed as this new modality is still in its infancy.

Also of clinical importance, the dual-modality agent with both NIRF and PET imaging capabilities would permit detection of nonsuperficial cancers and metastases, greatly enhancing prospective clinical indications. This agent would also allow primary localization of these lesions for staging and diagnoses, and depending on the context, surgical excision of these tumor lesions without additional anatomical imaging except for PET/CT. Furthermore, the same pharmacokinetics, biodistribution, and toxicity profiles greatly simplify the administration and use of a tandem-labeled APC agent. Because of these potential benefits, the dual-modality approach proves a synergistic means to not only study and better understand the limitations of NIRF, but also start the development process for an agent that successfully overcomes NIRF's limitations, positioning this multimodality APC analog for future clinical application (▶ Table 13.1).

An iodine on the aromatic ring of 1502 was appended to create the dual-labeled compound Iodo-1502. The Iodo-1502 compound was synthesized, purified, and radiolabeled. Preliminary studies with the novel dual-labeled agent, Iodo-1502, successfully demonstrate tumor targeting in a rodent flank xenograft model of cancer. Both fluorescence and PET signals are detectable in the U87 GBM flank tumor on imaging at 48 hours post-administration of Iodo-1502 (▶ Fig. 13.4). Imaging of an orthotopic glioma stem cell–derived xenograft model confirmed both fluorescence and PET activity in the orthotopic brain tumor (▶ Fig. 13.5). These preliminary in vivo experiments validate the hypothesis that addition of an ortho-iodine on the aromatic

Fig. 13.4 Fluorescence and PET imaging of U87 flank glioblastoma (GBM) xenografts using Iodo-1502. **(a,b)** Fluorescence imaging before and after resection of a flank U87 GBM with Iodo-1502. **(c)** PET/CT imaging of the flank U87 xenograft reveals PET activity in the flank tumor, denoted by white arrows.

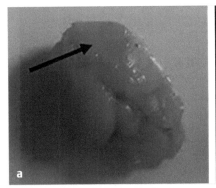
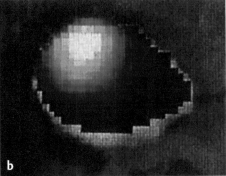
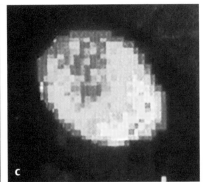

Fig. 13.5 Fluorescence and Cherenkov imaging of an orthotopic glioblastoma stem cell model using Iodo-1502. **(a)** White light, **(b)** fluorescence, and **(c)** Cherenkov (from $^{124}$I decay) of a GSC orthotopic tumor ex vivo with the dual-modality Iodo-1502 analog.

ring does not significantly impact the in vivo tumor-targeting ability and pharmacokinetics of these APC analogs. These studies demonstrate the feasibility of studying NIRF agents with the dual-labeled APC analog Iodo-1502.

These proof-of-concept studies illustrate the feasibility of harnessing PET and NIRF in one compound for synergistic diagnostic detection of cancer. Future quantitative studies with Iodo-1502 will address some of the key limitations of the NIRF modality. A deeper understanding of some of the unique behaviors of fluorophores (such as quenching at very high concentrations) will yield important insights into and caveats to using these fluorescent technologies for clinical applications. Additionally, the combination of NIRF and PET into one dual-labeled APC agent will help overcome the issue of depth penetration and lack of quantitation of the NIRF modality, permitting more diagnostic accuracy as well as localization and staging of deep tumors and lymph nodes. As the FGS becomes more accepted and standardized, appropriate thresholding of tumor to background signals may help differentiate tumor from adjacent vital tissue, which will maximize extent of resection without compromising functional outcomes for patients. The creation of the dual-labeled analog will hopefully lend insights and better understanding into the discrimination of tumor from nontumor tissues.

## 13.5 Other APC Analogs for Personalized Diagnosis and Treatment of Multiple Cancers

There are several APC analogs that can be used for multimodality imaging and therapy. [124]I-NM404 and [131]I-NM404 are companion radioisoteres that can be used for noninvasive PET imaging and targeted radiotherapy, respectively.[21] Currently, NM404 is being evaluated in numerous clinical trials for several different cancers. 1502 was created for fluorescence-guided surgical detection of cancerous tissues. Future analogs will expand the versatility of these compounds for multimodality imaging and targeted therapies, including cancer-targeted MRI.

Due to the same purported mechanism of uptake across all APC analogs, this diagnostic and therapeutic repertoire may offer a level of synergy in each stage of patient management.[21] To illustrate the powerful potential advantage of these multimodality agents, consider a patient with cancer: [124]I-NM404 is administered initially for whole body or global for initial diagnostic assessment of cancer lesion(s) and staging. 1502 can be used for FGS to optimize and safely maximize the extent of tumor resections. Postoperative uptake of APC PET imaging tracer can be used to calculate personalized dosimetry for the targeted radiotherapy agent [131]I-NM404. Follow-up APC PET imaging may further inform clinical patient management by detection of possible tumor recurrence. As this example demonstrates, due to the identical cancer-targeting mechanism of APCs, this suite of synthetic phospholipid ether analogs can be used at multiple phases of clinical cancer management, potentially maximizing effectiveness and simultaneously minimizing complications during surgery and radiotherapy on an individualized patient basis. We have advanced the multimodality imaging and therapy potential of these APCs to include APCs for

PET imaging, fluorescent APCs for FGS, and APCs for targeted radiotherapy. Creation and testing of next-generation APCs that significantly expand the potential for multimodality cancer imaging and therapy are currently underway.

## 13.6 Conclusion and Future Directions

Because 1502's excitation and emission are in the NIR range, higher tissue penetrance and improved tumor-to-normal contrast can be achieved using this newer generation NIR-labeled APC rather than 1501 and 5-ALA. Importantly, 1502 represents a broad-spectrum cancer-selective NIRF agent that has tremendous potential to improve surgical resections in multiple types of cancer. The 1502 APC have been tested and validated in GBM, breast, and colon cancers, and its PET companion analog, [124]I-NM404, has been tested and validated in over 60 preclinical cancer models and is already in clinical trials.

The simplicity and low cost of manufacturing for this small molecule APC platform offers some important comparative advantages to other larger carriers, better extravasation, and improved uptake and retention by cancer cells compared with agents such as antibodies. In addition, the near-universal uptake in cancers is striking, and current work to investigate APC's cancer-selective uptake and retention mechanism of action may lead to new cancer-targeting strategies and cancer-targeted drugs.

Finally, there are multiple APC analogs that can be used for multimodality cancer imaging and therapy. Due to the same uptake mechanism for APCs, this diagnostic and therapeutic repertoire of APC analogs may offer a level of utility in each stage of clinical cancer management. Clinical trials with some of these APC analogs are already underway, and many more of these APC analogs for multimodality imaging and therapy are continually being developed. Targeted magnetic resonance imaging APC analogs for cancer and targeted radiotherapies with other radioisotopes are currently being developed and tested. Continued synthesis, testing, and validation of these agents will hopefully allow for a more personalized and multimodal approach to diagnostic imaging and therapy of many types of cancers in the future.

## 13.7 Cancer-Selective Fluorophores in Clinical Trials Testing

The field of FGS has progressed rapidly in the last decade. Recently, 5-ALA was approved in the United States for FGS of GBM after a successful phase III study (BALANCE study), after having been approved in the last decade in Europe and Japan for the same indication. With the emergence of brighter, deeper penetrating fluorophores, and targeted ligands specific for cancer, the field of FGS has also witnessed the advent of new clinical trials with higher specificity and improved tumor-to-background ratios. These new targeted fluorophores utilize primarily cyanine fluorophores that have excitation and emission in the NIR window (700–900 nm). IRDye-800CW (Li-COR,

Lincoln, NE) has been the most popular cyanine fluorophore due to its commercial availability, safety, overlap of spectrum with its predecessor cyanine green (and thus available clinical instrumentation for detection), and ease of conjugation.

The indications of these targeted agents have been extended from GBMs to include other cancer types. Scientists and physicians have selected targetable and highly expressed cancer subtypes for FGS indications that include vascular endothelial growth factor expressing breast, colorectal, rectal and esophageal cancers, prostate-specific membrane antigen (PSMA) prostate cancers, folate receptor positive cancers, and carbonic anhydrase 9 expressing renal cell cancers, among others. The strategies to target these different cancers include antibodies (Bevacizumab, cetuximab), small peptides (PSMA), and small molecules (folate). Additionally, because of the ability to quench fluorescence, new strategies in clinical trials testing also incorporate "activatable" fluorophores that are cleaved by enzymes present in the tumor microenvironment, which activate or turn on the fluorescence at the site of tumor. This novel strategy drastically enhances tumor-to-background ratios and may improve the sensitivity of tumor detection. Multimodal agents have also initiated clinical trial testing for renal cell carcinoma.

With the emergence of FGS in clinical trial testing, instrumentation to detect these fluorophores are also being developed in tandem. As new fluorophores emerge with better properties, concurrent detection instrumentation must also be developed as these fluorophores do not have the same spectral overlap. The challenge of approving both the targeted fluorophore and its camera counterpart may impose regulatory barriers in which regulatory agencies such as the Food and Drug Administration (FDA) may require pairing of both the targeted fluorophore and its detection device (combination product). In an effort to facilitate preclinical-to-clinical translation of new targeted agents, the FDA has allowed exploratory investigational new drug (eIND) processes, which allows imaging agents given at subpharmaceutical doses to be tested in 10 to 15 patients for demonstration of feasibility before a more time-consuming and costly IND process is initiated. Several new clinical trials with targeted fluorophores have initiated eIND testing.

# References

[1] Zhang RR, Schroeder AB, Grudzinski JJ, et al. Beyond the margins: real-time detection of cancer using targeted fluorophores. Nat Rev Clin Oncol. 2017; 14 (6):347–364

[2] Rosenthal EL, Warram JM, de Boer E, et al. Successful translation of fluorescence navigation during oncologic surgery: a consensus report. J Nucl Med. 2016; 57(1):144–150

[3] Rosenthal EL, Warram JM, Bland KI, Zinn KR. The status of contemporary image-guided modalities in oncologic surgery. Ann Surg. 2015; 261(1):46–55

[4] McGirt MJ, Chaichana KL, Gathinji M, et al. Independent association of extent of resection with survival in patients with malignant brain astrocytoma. J Neurosurg. 2009; 110(1):156–162

[5] McGirt MJ, Chaichana KL, Attenello FJ, et al. Extent of surgical resection is independently associated with survival in patients with hemispheric infiltrating low-grade gliomas. Neurosurgery. 2008; 63(4):700–707, author reply 707–708

[6] Yossepowitch O, Briganti A, Eastham JA, et al. Positive surgical margins after radical prostatectomy: a systematic review and contemporary update. Eur Urol. 2014; 65(2):303–313

[7] McMahon J, O'Brien CJ, Pathak I, et al. Influence of condition of surgical margins on local recurrence and disease-specific survival in oral and oropharyngeal cancer. Br J Oral Maxillofac Surg. 2003; 41(4):224–231

[8] Stummer W, Pichlmeier U, Meinel T, Wiestler OD, Zanella F, Reulen HJ, ALA-Glioma Study Group. Fluorescence-guided surgery with 5-aminolevulinic acid for resection of malignant glioma: a randomised controlled multicentre phase III trial. Lancet Oncol. 2006; 7(5):392–401

[9] Hope-Ross M, Yannuzzi LA, Gragoudas ES, et al. Adverse reactions due to indocyanine green. Ophthalmology. 1994; 101(3):529–533

[10] Marshall MV, Draney D, Sevick-Muraca EM, Olive DM. Single-dose intravenous toxicity study of IRDye 800CW in Sprague-Dawley rats. Mol Imaging Biol. 2010; 12(6):583–594

[11] Marshall MV, Rasmussen JC, Tan IC, et al. Near-infrared fluorescence imaging in humans with indocyanine green: a review and update. Open Surg Oncol J. 2010; 2(2):12–25

[12] Obana A, Miki T, Hayashi K, et al. Survey of complications of indocyanine green angiography in Japan. Am J Ophthalmol. 1994; 118(6):749–753

[13] Zhu B, Sevick-Muraca EM. A review of performance of near-infrared fluorescence imaging devices used in clinical studies. Br J Radiol. 2015; 88 (1045):20140547

[14] Mondal SB, Gao S, Zhu N, Liang R, Gruev V, Achilefu S. Real-time fluorescence image-guided oncologic surgery. Adv Cancer Res. 2014; 124:171–211

[15] Nguyen QT, Tsien RY. Fluorescence-guided surgery with live molecular navigation–a new cutting edge. Nat Rev Cancer. 2013; 13(9):653–662

[16] Hong G, Antaris AL, Dai H. Near-infrared fluorophores for biomedical imaging. Nature Biomedical Engineering. 2017; 1:10

[17] Frangioni JV. In vivo near-infrared fluorescence imaging. Curr Opin Chem Biol. 2003; 7(5):626–634

[18] Vahrmeijer AL, Hutteman M, van der Vorst JR, van de Velde CJ, Frangioni JV. Image-guided cancer surgery using near-infrared fluorescence. Nat Rev Clin Oncol. 2013; 10(9):507–518

[19] Weichert JP, Clark PA, Kandela IK, et al. Alkylphosphocholine analogs for broad-spectrum cancer imaging and therapy. Sci Transl Med. 2014; 6(240): 240ra75

[20] Pinchuk AN, Rampy MA, Longino MA, et al. Synthesis and structure-activity relationship effects on the tumor avidity of radioiodinated phospholipid ether analogues. J Med Chem. 2006; 49(7):2155–2165

[21] Zhang RR, Swanson KI, Hall LT, Weichert JP, Kuo JS. Diapeutic cancer-targeting alkylphosphocholine analogs may advance management of brain malignancies. CNS Oncol. 2016; 5(4):223–231

[22] Grudzinski JJ, Titz B, Kozak K, et al. A phase 1 study of 131I-CLR1404 in patients with relapsed or refractory advanced solid tumors: dosimetry, biodistribution, pharmacokinetics, and safety. PLoS One. 2014; 9(11):e111652

[23] Mollinedo F, Gajate C. Lipid rafts as major platforms for signaling regulation in cancer. Adv Biol Regul. 2015; 57:130–146

[24] Gajate C, Mollinedo F. Edelfosine and perifosine induce selective apoptosis in multiple myeloma by recruitment of death receptors and downstream signaling molecules into lipid rafts. Blood. 2007; 109(2):711–719

[25] Gajate C, Mollinedo F. The antitumor ether lipid ET-18-OCH(3) induces apoptosis through translocation and capping of Fas/CD95 into membrane rafts in human leukemic cells. Blood. 2001; 98(13):3860–3863

[26] Swanson KI, Clark PA, Zhang RR, et al. Fluorescent cancer-selective alkylphosphocholine analogs for intraoperative glioma detection. Neurosurgery. 2015; 76(2):115–123, discussion 123–124

[27] Korb ML, Warram JM, Grudzinski J, Weichert J, Jeffery J, Rosenthal EL. Breast cancer imaging using the near-infrared fluorescent agent, CLR1502. Mol Imaging. 2014; 13:1–9

[28] Deming DA, Maher ME, Leystra AA, et al. Phospholipid ether analogs for the detection of colorectal tumors. PLoS One. 2014; 9(10):e109668

[29] Hilgard P, Klenner T, Stekar J, Unger C. Alkylphosphocholines: a new class of membrane-active anticancer agents. Cancer Chemother Pharmacol. 1993; 32 (2):90–95

[30] Snyder F, Blank M, Morris HP. Occurrence and nature of O-alkyl and O-alk-1-enyl moieties of glycerol in lipids of Morris transplanted hepatomas and normal rat liver. Biochimica et Biophysica Acta. 1969; 176:502–510

[31] Snyder F, Wood R. The occurrence and metabolism of alkyl and alk-1-enyl ethers of glycerol in transplantable rat and mouse tumors. Cancer Res. 1968; 28(5):972–978

[32] Chao ST, Suh JH, Raja S, Lee S-Y, Barnett G. The sensitivity and specificity of FDG PET in distinguishing recurrent brain tumor from radionecrosis in patients treated with stereotactic radiosurgery. Int J Cancer. 2001; 96(3):191–197

# 14 Tozuleristide Fluorescence-Guided Surgery of Brain Tumors

*Harish Babu, Dennis M. Miller, Julia E. Parrish-Novak, David Scott Kittle, Pramod Butte, and Adam N. Mamelak*

## Abstract

Tozuleristide is a near-infrared (NIR) tumor-targeting molecule. The tozuleristide molecule is a combination of the tumor-targeting peptide chlorotoxin and the NIR fluorophore indocyanine green. Tozuleristide demonstrates excellent binding to multiple tumor types including high- and low-grade gliomas. It has been tested in a number of human phase I trials, with no appreciable toxicity or side effects. Tozuleristide is now being tested for its capacity for fluorescence-guided removal of gliomas. In conjunction with a novel highly sensitive NIR imaging device (Synchronized InfraRed Imaging System [SIRIS]), which is required to detect the low levels of NIR light generated from tumor-specific targeting of tozuleristide in the brain, phase I trials demonstrated reliable uptake and the ability to differentiate tumor from normal brain tissue. Surgeon acceptance of the drug/device combination has also been very good. This chapter describes the preclinical and clinical experience with tozuleristide for gliomas and the associated imaging devices.

*Keywords:* fluorescence, near-infrared, tumor specific, intraoperative, imaging, chlorotoxin, tozuleristide, glioma, imaging device, surgery

## 14.1 Introduction

An estimated 25,000 surgical resections or biopsies are performed for brain tumors each year in the United States. Several studies have shown that the extent of resection is the single most important factor in determining survival.[1,2] Balancing maximal tumor cytoreduction with preservation of adjacent brain parenchyma is often limited due to the invasive nature of gliomas and their spread along the connection between cortical and subcortical structures within the brain. As gliomas recur locally at the edge of the previous resection margin, efforts to maximize the extent of resection correlates with increased tumor control and improved survival and quality of life. Current use of the operating microscope relies on visual inspection of the subjective tumor margin, but often tumor deposits are not appreciated with these methods. MRI-based frameless neuronavigation assists in evaluating the tumor margins, but accuracy is lost once a surgical resection leads to "brain shift."[3] Advanced technologies such as confocal microscopy,[4] MRI spectroscopy, time-resolved fluorescence spectroscopy,[5] and Raman spectroscopy[6,7] remain research tools at present.

Imaging techniques can be divided between those that work on untreated tissue (endogenous contrast) and those requiring administration of extrinsic contrast agents. Endogenous contrast can be achieved through modifications in autofluorescence, infrared reflectivity, Raman scattering, and microanatomical cytoarchitecture. Exogenous contrast agents allow improved contrast between diseased and normal tissue. Fluorescence-guided neurosurgery requires agents that not only specifically target glioma tissue, but also can do so while the tissue is within the living patient, rather than following tissue excision. Simultaneous evolution of imaging technologies along with fluorescent dyes has generated a powerful tool that allows a surgeon to easily identify and remove tumor while sparing normal tissue. Fluorescent-labeled probes with unique molecular targets can provide intraoperative real-time distinction of cellular edge between glioma and adjacent normal brain. This technique of "fluorescence-guided surgery" (FGS) could revolutionize glioma surgery, allowing better delineation of tumor and thus improved extent of resection.

## 14.2 Agents for Fluorescence-Guided Glioma Surgery

There are three principal approaches used to generate a relatively strong fluorescent signal in brain tumors to guide resection: (1) passive—labeling occurs when the damaged blood–brain barrier allows exogenous agents to accumulate at the tumor site (e.g., fluorescein, indocyanine green [ICG], etc.); (2) metabolic—endogenous fluorescent agents are internalized, metabolized, and accumulated intracellularly within the tumor cells (e.g., 5-aminolevulinic acid [5-ALA]); and (3) molecular—targeted agents that bind to molecules on the cell surface of the tumor cell or are internalized into tumor cells (e.g., chlorotoxin [CTX]).

Here we focus on the specific imaging properties of tozuleristide, a promising tumor-specific fluorescent probe for FGS, and related imaging device requirements. Approaches for tumor resection using other fluorescent agents, such as the use of 5-ALA, and unconjugated fluorophores like sodium fluorescein and ICG will be addressed in other chapters in the book.

## 14.3 Advantages of Near-Infrared Imaging for Fluorescence-Guided Surgery

Fluorescent probes that emit light in the near-infrared (NIR; 700- to 1,000-nm excitation and emission) range offer several unique advantages over agents that fluoresce in the ultraviolet or visible light ranges. These include less scatter of emitted light, low tissue autofluorescence, and superior penetration of incident photons. The emission in the NIR spectrum allows for better visualization of deeper structures than seen using the visible or ultraviolet wavelength range. This spectral window does not interfere with other tissue components such as water, hemoglobin, and deoxyhemoglobin that can autofluoresce, making it ideal for fluorescence imaging of living tissue. Several NIR fluorophores are commercially available, including ICG, IRDye800 (Licor), Alexa800, and Cy5.5. At present only ICG is Food and Drug Administration (FDA) approved for clinical use in humans. ICG has a peak excitation of 780 nm and it emits at 805 to 825 nm in human tissues. ICG fluorescence angiography has been used in vascular neurosurgery to identify and characterize vessel integrity. Tumors induce neoangiogenesis that lead to angiogenic hot spots. This property of gliomas can be exploited, allowing angiogenic hot spots to be visualized through ICG fluorescence angiography. The dye accumulates in glioma due to the enhanced permeability and retention (EPR) effect. This accumulation in tumor tissue is enhanced because of the hypoxic environment[8] in most gliomas. Studies have shown direct correlation between gadolinium enhancement and ICG fluorescence.[8] It was recently shown that intensity of intraoperative fluorescence was directly proportional to the amount of tumor cells.[9] Similar to other nonspecific fluorophores, ICG-based detection is far superior in high-grade tumors, and typically absent in low-grade gliomas. It has also demonstrated some utility for meningioma.[10]

## 14.4 Targeted Fluorescence

Targeted NIR fluorescence imaging is performed by conjugating a ligand that binds to tumor cells with a fluorophore to generate a fluorescent signal to guide surgical removal. Examples include a cathepsin-activated tumor ligand conjugated to ICG,[11,12] an NIR fluorescent alkylphosphocholine analog,[13] and modified integrin receptor ligands conjugated to an NIR dye.[14,15] This strategy is appealing as the fluorescent signal is specific to the tumor cells themselves. Such specificity should theoretically lead to better and more confident delineation of tumor margins and regions of infiltrating tumor, while avoiding unintended removal of adjacent brain tissue. In exchange for this increased specificity, targeted fluorescence signals are often several orders of magnitude less bright than those generated by free, unbound fluorophores such as ICG or sodium fluorescein, and therefore require specialized instrumentation to reliably detect the fluorescence. To date, the most appealing strategy for glial tumor is tozuleristide (Blaze Bioscience), a covalent conjugate of a tumor-targeting peptide CTX and ICG.

## 14.5 Chlorotoxin

CTX, a peptide initially isolated from the venom of the scorpion *Leiurus quinquestriatus*, preferentially binds to gliomas and other tumors of neuroectodermal origin.[16] CTX is a 36-amino acid peptide (4.7 kD) with four disulfide bridges. It has been shown to indirectly inhibit the $ClC_3$ chloride ion channel,[17] and to bind matrix metalloproteinase 2 (MMP-2),[18] and annexin A2.[19] Annexin A2 when combined with S100A10 is the putative primary binding target. Upon binding, CTX is internalized into the cell via clathrin-mediated endocytosis (and possibly other mechanisms[20,21,22]) in glioma cells. In normal cells, annexin A2 is generally expressed as an intracellular protein, but in cancerous cells is phosphorylated and combines with S100A10 to be expressed on the cell surface.[23] There are also reports of increased annexin A2 expression in gliomas.

The extent of CTX binding to glioma cells, as measured by immunohistochemistry, has been shown to correlate with histological grade. Essentially complete and uniform binding occurs with all WHO grade IV (glioblastoma [GBM]) tumors,

90% binding in WHO grade III tumors, and only 40 to 45% binding in WHO grade I to II (low-grade glioma).[24] This is likely attributable to the observation that the number of cell surface receptors increases with grade, but nonetheless does appear to be present in all gliomas to an extent. In mouse xenograft and genetically modified spontaneous tumor models, pathological tissues tagged as cancer using a CTX:Cy5.5 fluorescence conjugate were confirmed to be cancerous, while adjacent nonfluorescent tissues were histologically normal.[25] This was true for a variety of cancers in mouse models. Interestingly, in these mouse models, glioma tissue was distinguishable from normal tissue 14 days after injection of CTX-Cy5.5.[25] Negative imaging (i.e., no fluorescence signal) was seen in mice in which tumors failed to implant, indicating that the effect is tumor specific and not related to local blood–brain barrier disruption alone. Intravenously administered radioactive Iodine ([131]I) labeled CTX had a high concentration in tumor compared to surrounding normal tissue.[26] In a phase I clinical trial, a single dose of CTX labeled with radioactive iodine (TM601; Transmolecular Industries), delivered directly into the patient's brain via an intracavitary Ommaya reservoir after surgical resection of glioma, was shown to be well tolerated.[27] While unbound TM601 was eliminated from the body within 24 to 48 hours after delivery,[27,28] the drug that bound to the tumor cavity could be detected up to 7 days after administration, with a dose indicating long-term binding. Comparison of tumor volumes as determined by single-photon emission computed tomography (SPECT) imaging and MRI showed that tumor volumes obtained by [131]I-CTX closely paralleled the T2-, but not T1-weighted gadolinium contrast volume with MRI.[28] Unfortunately, these studies and subsequent phase II studies failed to demonstrate sufficient survival advantage to justify further trials. In vivo animal studies using systemically injected fluorescent dyes (Cy5.5, IRDye800) conjugated to CTX have confirmed the specific binding of CTX to GBM.[25,29,30]

MRI-compatible contrast agents or nanoparticles conjugated to CTX have been used both for advanced imaging and as a therapeutic molecule in animal model.[31,32] CTX-conjugated nanoparticles have been used to deliver chemotherapeutic drugs to glioma cells.[33] Importantly, all reported human clinical trials of CTX have demonstrated negligible toxicity in humans.

## 14.6 Tozuleristide

Tozuleristide is a conjugate of a modified CTX covalently attached to ICG. Tozuleristide is a drug candidate being developed for the specific purpose of FGS in many tumors types, with an initial focus on brain cancers, including gliomas (▶ Fig. 14.1). Tozuleristide has undergone extensive preclinical toxicity testing in both small and large animal models, as well as testing in animals harboring tumors. These data demonstrated that to date tozuleristide has minimal toxicity, even at very high doses, and can reliably detect a variety of tumors.[34,35] Tozuleristide is administered as a single intravenous (IV) injection, and tumor imaging is typically performed the same day or the next day (~ 24 hours) after IV administration, unlike traditional ICG imaging performed minutes after injection. Tozuleristide imaging is more similar to the technique of "second window" ICG imaging, in which tumors such as meningioma or glioma can be detected

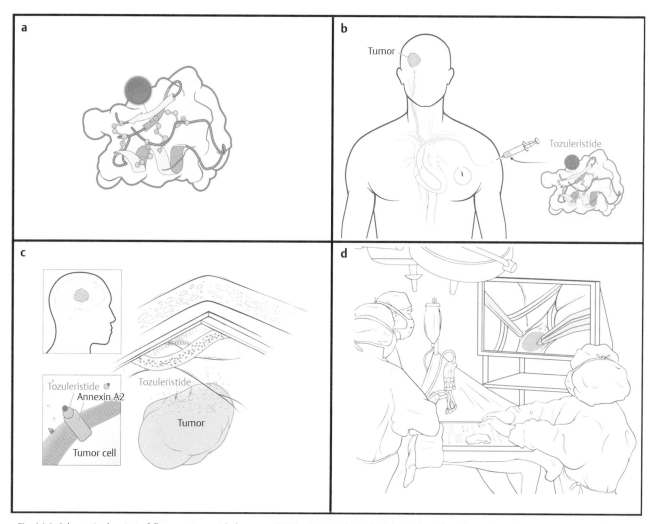

**Fig. 14.1** Schematic drawing of fluorescence-guided surgery (FGS) using tozuleristide. **(a)** Tozuleristide is formed by covalent bond of the *knottin* peptide chlorotoxin to a single indocyanine green (ICG; *red dot*). The chlorotoxin binds the tumor, while the ICG provides a fluorescent signal. **(b)** Tozuleristide is administered intravenously and travels through the blood stream to the tumor, where it is taken up. **(c)** The chlorotoxin moiety on tozuleristide binds to the extracellular membrane of glioma cells via annexin A2 receptors and is then internalized. **(d)** Excitation of the covalently bound ICG with a near-infrared (NIR) light source produced emission fluorescence that can be visualized with a sensitive NIR camera and used to guide tumor detection and removal.

18 hours or more after initial ICG injection, by taking advantage of the EPR effect.[10] Delayed imaging allows time for unbound tozuleristide in the circulation to be washed out, with specifically bound drug accumulating in the tumor tissue (accumulation in ancillary tissues such as dura do not affect its potential utility). This unique feature of targeted FGS results in a very low concentration (50 pM–50 nM) of the fluorophore to be visualized during surgical resection. These concentrations are typically 100 to 1,000 times less than is seen in typical vascular applications of ICG imaging. Tozuleristide is capable of binding to both low-grade glioma (LGG) and high-grade glioma (HGG) with no appreciable uptake in normal brain tissue.

The ability of tozuleristide to target brain tumors in vivo was evaluated using nude mice with an intracranial implanted glioblastoma cell line. Eighteen days after implantation, the mice received a single dose of tozuleristide. Two days after injection of tozuleristide into the tail veins, they were sacrificed and the brain was sectioned and mounted on glass slides. Fluorescence

signal was determined using quantitative NIR scanning methods (Odyssey CLx, Licor). Histology confirmed the presence of tumor in tozuleristide fluorescent regions. No uptake was observed in surrounding brain tissue.[29,36] Similar results were observed in studies on dogs[34] containing a variety of tumors, for which tozuleristide was administered prior to tumor excision and fluorescence uptake compared to tumor histology. Tozuleristide could also reliably detect squamous cell carcinoma in a hamster model of dysplasia and carcinogenesis, and also differentiate high-grade from low-grade dysplasia.[37] These studies reliably demonstrated tumor-specific uptake by tozuleristide as detected by quantitative NIR scanning. In situ imaging in these dogs was carried out using a prototype NIR detection camera (Denali—a prototype of the Solaris, Perkin-Elmer). This system demonstrated that in vivo detection during surgical resection was indeed feasible and that tozuleristide fluorescence signal could provide contrast between tumor tissue and surrounding normal tissues in many tumor types. Taken as a whole, the tumor selective uptake of tozuleristide provided the clear motivation to move tozuleristide into phase I clinical trials in humans.

## 14.6.1 Use of Tozuleristide in Human Subjects

A phase I dose escalation study in patients with suspected skin cancers (squamous cell carcinoma, basal cell carcinoma, and melanoma) was carried out to determine safety, tolerability, and pharmacokinetic (PK) distribution of escalating doses of tozuleristide (NCT02097875, Blaze Bioscience).[38] In situ imaging was feasible as all suspected lesions were on the skin. In situ imaging on patients was performed with the Fluobeam 800 (Fluoptics, Grenoble, France) hand-held NIR imaging system. Doses of 1 to 18 mg of tozuleristide were administered to 21 patients. Neither dose-limiting toxicity nor severe adverse events were observed. PK data indicated peak levels of drug in serum within 30 minutes after injection, with a sharp fall off between hours 2 and 4 and almost complete elimination of serum drug within 12 to 24 hours. Tumor-specific uptake was documented by serial imaging at 2 to 24 hours after injection. At doses with adequate signal and contrast (3–12 mg), fluorescence correlated with the presence of tumor (based on subsequent pathology) approximately 90% of the time. These data suggested that tozuleristide was well tolerated up to 18 mg and adequate tumor fluorescence for imaging could be achieved. The subsequent experience with Fluobeam 800 in brain cancer (NCT02234297) pointed to a key need for clinical trials with tumor-specific FGS for glioma (as opposed to skin cancer). A surgeon-friendly, microscope-integrated yet highly sensitive imaging device to detect fluorescence in situ would be a critical feature required for clinical success. Subsequently, significant effort was directed toward developing such an imaging unit.

## 14.6.2 Development of Imaging System with Adequate Sensitivity for Tozuleristide Detection In Vivo

To successfully advance a molecule like tozuleristide through human trials for glioma tumors, a surgically relevant yet sufficiently sensitive fluorescence imaging unit is required. Several imaging systems have been developed for intraoperative detection of fluorescence.[39,40,41,42,43,44,45,46,47] These include NIR imaging modes in several commercial surgical microscopes, such as IR800 incorporated into the Zeiss Pentero microscopes, or FL800 incorporated into Leica microscopes, and stand-alone devices such as the Fluobeam 800 (Fluoptics), Artemis (Quest), and SPY Elite (Novadaq) systems, as well as several endoscope-based systems. Each of these other systems was designed to primarily detect intravascular ICG, which has a typical concentration of 100 nM to 50 μM in blood during fluorescence angiography. Systems such as the Fluobeam 800 can detect low nanomolar concentrations of ICG, but cannot do so at real-time video rate, or overlay those images on a color visible light background. Finally, none of the systems with potentially adequately sensitive fluorescence detection capabilities are integrated into the surgical microscopes traditionally used for glioma surgery. The absence of such an imaging device motivated us to design and build such a device in anticipation of clinical trials of tozuleristide for glioma surgery.

To address the need for a practical way to perform FGS for glioma with tozuleristide and similar targeted fluorophores, we developed a prototype device that can detect very low concentrations of NIR fluorophores in tissue.[29,48] Our system has a small profile and allows the surgeon to use the operating microscope separate from the NIR imaging system. Traditional NIR systems use two separate sensors for visible and NIR channels. Although this allows for the use of high-sensitivity infrared camera, it also adds to the weight and size of the device. We designed a clinical prototype system (Synchronized InfraRed Imaging System [SIRIS]) that uses the same sensor for both visible and NIR channels.[29] We use a single high-definition (HD) charged-couple device camera for both channels. Both NIR and visible light are delivered to the surgical field from a custom-built light source that is programmed to deliver synchronized pulses of NIR and visible light. The NIR and visible light sources (Lumencor ASTRA light engine, Beaverton, OR) are alternatively pulsed and synchronized with frame capture rates of 300 frames per second. A fixed focal length lens (35 mm) is attached to a C-mount. The NIR light (785 nm) is pulsed from the laser (Coherent, Santa Clara, CA), while four LEDs (blue, cyan, green, and red) deliver cool balanced white light.[36] The pulse rate, fluency, timing, and width of the laser pulse are controlled via software. A 785-nm notch filter is attached to the front of the lens to filter out the excitation light from the return image. The 785-nm laser wavelength is near peak absorption spectrum for tozuleristide and ICG in Intralipid[49,50] and far away from the peak emission spectrum curves. The collected light is transmitted to a graphics processing unit (GPU) via a CameraLink cable for image processing. A GPU is required due to high data rate (718 Mb/s) and real-time requirements. The resultant HD quality visible light images are superimposed on pseudocolored fluorescent maps of tozuleristide distribution (▶ Fig. 14.2).

The system is draped during surgical procedure for sterile operating room environments. Our custom-built SIRIS system was found to detect tozuleristide fluorescence down to 50 pM at video frame rates (< 30 millisecond NIR exposures), enabling imaging of targeted fluorescent probes in the surgical setting. It was also found to provide 25 to 1,000 times greater NIR sensitivity than current commercially available systems for intraoperative NIR detection (▶ Fig. 14.3).

## 14.6.3 Clinical Results from Phase I Trials of Tozuleristide

Four phase I clinical trials with tozuleristide in humans have been initiated and as of February 2017 over 80 patients have received different doses of tozuleristide. Three trials (NCT02097875, NCT02234297, and NCT02496065) have been completed with one trial (NCT02462629 in pediatric central nervous system [CNS] tumor subjects) ongoing.

NCT02097875 was the first in human trial of tozuleristide in adult subjects with suspected skin cancers. Blaze Bioscience then initiated NCT02234297, a dose escalation study in adults with new or recurrent gliomas[51] and a similar trial in pediatric CNS tumors (NCT02462629). Trial NCT02496065 initially examined tozuleristide in several solid tumor types, but ultimately focused on adult subjects with breast cancer. The

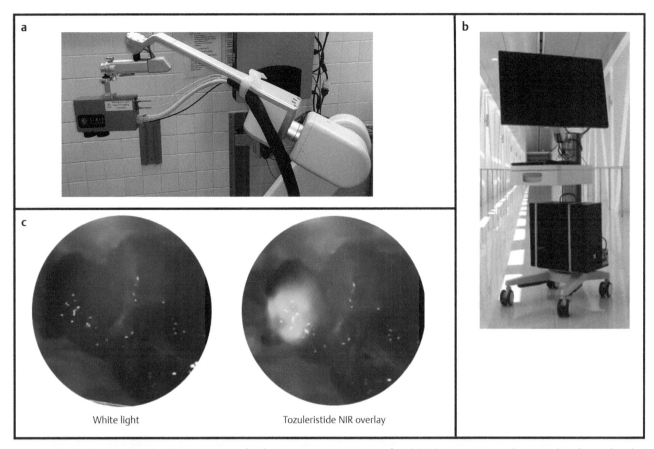

**Fig. 14.2** **(a,b)** The optical head and imaging station for the prototype sensitive near-infrared (NIR) imaging system device used in phase I clinical studies of tozuleristide. The camera was held over the operative field for in situ imaging and over tissue specimens for ex vivo imaging. **(c)** A screenshot of an excised low-grade glioma (oligodendroglioma grade II) with white-light imaging only and superimposed NIR imaging of tozuleristide.

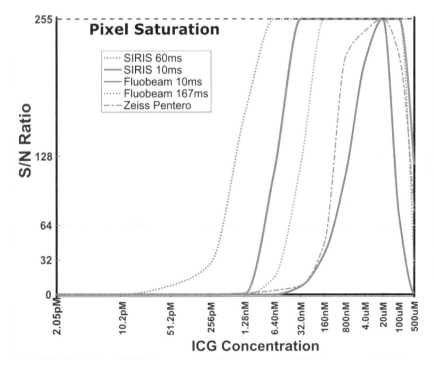

**Fig. 14.3** Comparison of indocyanine green (ICG) detection sensitivity (signal-to-noise ratio [SNR]) of Synchronized Infra-Red Imaging System (SIRIS) with two commercial near-infrared (NIR) devices, the Fluobeam 800 and the IR800 mode of the Zeiss Pentero 900 microscope. SIRIS was operated at 35 mW/cm² fluence, which is a typical energy for clinical use, while the other devices were tested at maximal sensitivity settings. SIRIS was 25 times more sensitive and 3 to 30 times faster. The flat horizontal portion of each curve represents ICG concentrations for which the device exceeded the dynamic range of the device. Note that as ICG concentrations increase above the 20-μM range the SNR diminishes due to the well-known quenching effects of ICG at higher concentrations. For tumor-specific fluorescence-guided surgery detection, sensitivity in the range of 50 pM to 50 nM is optimal.

endpoints of these dose escalation trials included safety, PK, and tumor fluorescence. Fluobeam 800 was initially used alone and then the SIRIS was incorporated into ongoing studies following institutional review board's (IRB's) approval. To date, over 80 patients have received tozuleristide in doses ranging from 3 to 30 mg, with no dose-limiting toxicity observed. SIRIS has been used for ex situ imaging in 52 patients and for in situ use in 30 patients. As the studies progressed, Fluobeam 800 was replaced by SIRIS at all trial sites. PK results from the adult glioma study paralleled the first-in-human data, with rapid fall off in serum levels a few hours after dosing. For the initial three dose levels, surgery was performed approximately 24 hours after injection. Subsequent dosing cohorts permitted surgery as early as 2 hours after injection.

In 17 adult subjects with glioma, ex vivo evidence of tozuleristide uptake into tumor tissue was both dose and time related. There were nine HGG and eight LGG cases. At doses below 9 mg, imaging signal intensity was low, likely due to lower dose used and more than 24-hour interval between injection and surgery. At doses of 9 mg and above, clear evidence of tozuleristide uptake into tumor was observed in 9 of 14 cases (64%). HGG was consistently positive for fluorescence signal as well as one low-grade pilocytic astrocytoma. Three of eight oligodendroglioma cases displayed fluorescence following tozuleristide dosing. Detection of fluorescence correlated with presence of tumor on pathological evaluation in every case (i.e., no false positives). Importantly, fluorescence was not observed in normal brain tissue in situ (i.e., no false-positive fluorescence). Representative in situ and ex vivo images are shown in ▸ Fig. 14.4.

In a phase I study of pediatric brain tumors, imaging was performed within 4 to 24 hours of tozuleristide injection. Among the 15 cases treated in the dose escalation portion of the study, 13 have shown ex vivo fluorescent signal from pathology-verified tumor tissue. Likewise, in a study in adult subjects with breast cancer, in which imaging was performed as soon as 2 hours after injection of tozuleristide, ~ 90% of cases showed ex vivo fluorescent signal from the tumor with SIRIS imaging.

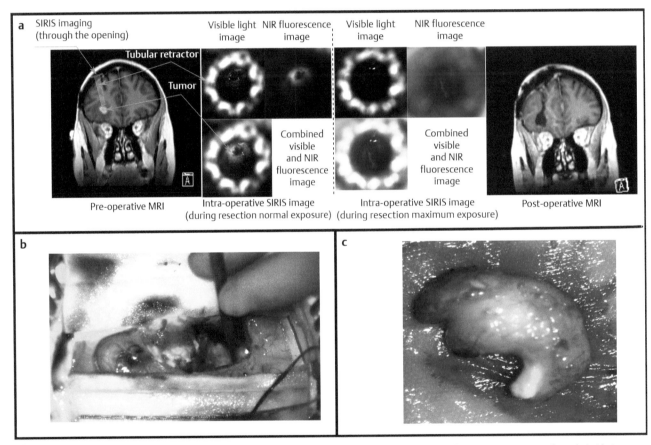

**Fig. 14.4** Representative in situ and ex vivo imaging of tozuleristide-labeled tumors. **(a)** Intraoperative fluorescence imaging of tozuleristide in a patient with suspected glioma using the Synchronized InfraRed Imaging System (SIRIS) prototype. The patient received a dose of 24-mg tozuleristide 4 hours prior to surgery. The tumor was approached using frameless navigation and a Brain Path (Nico Corp.) dilator/retractor. White-light imaging down the dilator demonstrated normal-appearing tissue, while fluorescence imaging indicated tumor in a portion of the cavity. Surgical resection was performed and repeated fluorescence imaging revealed no residual fluorescence signal. A postoperative MRI confirmed a gross total removal. Pathology of the resected tissue consisted of high-grade glioma (WHO grade III). **(b)** Intraoperative image of tozuleristide fluorescence after resection of a glioma invading motor cortex. Stimulation mapping confirmed the location of motor cortex and fluorescence was not resected. Note bright fluorescence signal from surrounding dura, which is a ubiquitous finding, whereas uptake in normal bran or brain vasculature is absent. **(c)** Excised low-grade glioma imaged ex vivo. Note the sharp demarcation in fluorescence. Absence of fluorescence correlated with normal tissue on histology, indicating the tumor-specific nature of tozuleristide uptake.

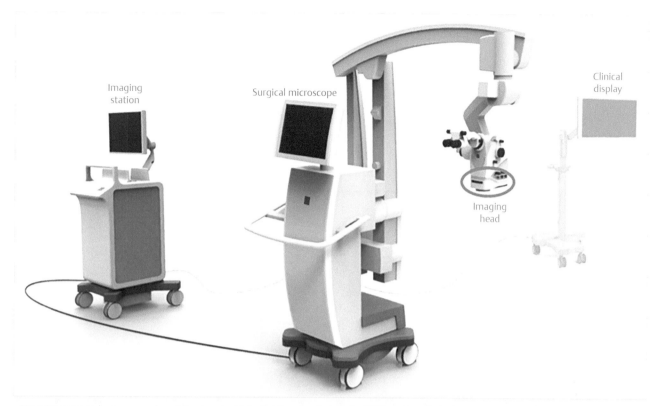

**Fig. 14.5** Proposed microscope-based Synchronized InfraRed Imaging System (mSIRIS) version of a high-sensitivity near-infrared (NIR) detecting system, designed for studies of tozuleristide-guided FGS of glioma and other tumors.

To quantify the accuracy of tozuleristide fluorescence in the adult glioma study, biopsy specimens from surgery were sectioned on a cryostat, plated on glass slides, and then reviewed by an independent pathologist. Regions of tumor defined by the pathologist were outlined. The specimens were then scanned on an Odyssey NIR scanner and compared with pathology and SIRIS imaging. As shown in ▶ Fig. 14.4, regions of bright fluorescence (▶ Fig. 14.4a, b, with white-light overlay) corresponded well to regions of documented tumor (▶ Fig. 14.4c). In contrast, no tumor was detected in regions without SIRIS or Odyssey NIR (▶ Fig. 14.4a). These data validate the tumor detection capabilities of tozuleristide when imaged with SIRIS, and the overall feasibility of the approach. Importantly, while these studies demonstrate a correlation between SIRIS fluorescence and pathology, they do not indicate the exact tissue concentrations of tozuleristide. At present, this value can only be estimated by comparison with fluorescence signal measured in Intralipid tissue phantoms that mimic the tissue being studied. Such phantom standards are currently being developed, using a combination of Intralipid 20% and India Ink to closely replicate biological tissues for future studies.[49]

## 14.7 Next Steps

At present, several trials are being planned or initiated to more definitely determine the utility of tozuleristide in FGS. These larger multicenter trials will hopefully provide the data to support routine clinical use of tozuleristide for FGS of gliomas and other tumors. As the imaging device used to detect tozuleristide is of critical significance for surgeon acceptance of this method, we are modifying our original SIRIS prototype design so that it is directly integrated with the surgical microscope, allowing the surgeon real-time visualization of tozuleristide fluorescence in situ, with white-light image overlay. The microscope-integrated SIRIS system (Teal Light Surgical, Inc., Seattle, WA) should provide even better detection sensitivity than its prototype (▶ Fig. 14.5). The system will contain a user-friendly interface, and many other features. Future brain tumor studies in both children and adults will utilize the microscope-based device. At the same time, expansion of tozuleristide FGS to non-CNS tumor surgery is underway.

## 14.8 Outlook for Tozuleristide-Guided Tumor Surgery

Fluorescence-guided surgical resection with neuronavigation and/or multimodal functional imaging will likely become the standard of treatment for glioma. FGS could be applied for other cerebral tumor types such as meningioma, or metastases.[52,53] While evaluation of tozuleristide-guided resection is underway to show similar or better improvements in extent of resection as seen with 5-ALA,[54] early clinical trial data are promising in suggesting such improvement to be a realistic possibility.

# References

[1] Eyüpoglu IY, Buchfelder M, Savaskan NE. Surgical resection of malignant gliomas-role in optimizing patient outcome. Nat Rev Neurol. 2013; 9(3):141–151

[2] Sanai N, Berger MS. Glioma extent of resection and its impact on patient outcome. Neurosurgery. 2008; 62(4):753–764, discussion 264–266

[3] Benveniste RJ, Germano IM. Correlation of factors predicting intraoperative brain shift with successful resection of malignant brain tumors using image-guided techniques. Surg Neurol. 2005; 63(6):542–548, discussion 548–549

[4] Martirosyan NL, Georges J, Kalani MYS, et al. Handheld confocal laser endomicroscopic imaging utilizing tumor-specific fluorescent labeling to identify experimental glioma cells in vivo. Surg Neurol Int. 2016; 7 Suppl 40: S995–S1003

[5] Butte PV, Fang Q, Jo JA, et al. Intraoperative delineation of primary brain tumors using time-resolved fluorescence spectroscopy. J Biomed Opt. 2010; 15(2):027008

[6] Bentley JN, Ji M, Xie XS, Orringer DA. Real-time image guidance for brain tumor surgery through stimulated Raman scattering microscopy. Expert Rev Anticancer Ther. 2014; 14(4):359–361

[7] Pointer KB, Zhang RR, Kuo JS, Dempsey RJ. Detecting brain tumor with Raman scattering microscopy. Neurosurgery. 2014; 74(2):N12–N14

[8] Wu JB, Shao C, Li X, et al. Near-infrared fluorescence imaging of cancer mediated by tumor hypoxia and HIF1α/OATPs signaling axis. Biomaterials. 2014; 35(28):8175–8185

[9] Eyüpoglu IY, Hore N, Fan Z, et al. Intraoperative vascular DIVA surgery reveals angiogenic hotspots in tumor zones of malignant gliomas. Sci Rep. 2015; 5: 7958

[10] Lee JYK, Pierce JT, Thawani JP, et al. Near-infrared fluorescent image-guided surgery for intracranial meningioma. J Neurosurg. 2018; 128(2):380–390

[11] Eward WC, Mito JK, Eward CA, et al. A novel imaging system permits real-time in vivo tumor bed assessment after resection of naturally occurring sarcomas in dogs. Clin Orthop Relat Res. 2013; 471(3):834–842

[12] Mito JK, Ferrer JM, Brigman BE, et al. Intraoperative detection and removal of microscopic residual sarcoma using wide-field imaging. Cancer. 2012; 118 (21):5320–5330

[13] Swanson KI, Clark PA, Zhang RR, et al. Fluorescent cancer-selective alkylphosphocholine analogs for intraoperative glioma detection. Neurosurgery. 2015; 76(2):115–123, discussion 123–124

[14] Moore SJ, Leung CL, Norton HK, Cochran JR. Engineering agatoxin, a cystine-knot peptide from spider venom, as a molecular probe for in vivo tumor imaging. PLoS One. 2013; 8(4):e60498

[15] van Dam GM, Themelis G, Crane LMA, et al. Intraoperative tumor-specific fluorescence imaging in ovarian cancer by folate receptor-α targeting: first in-human results. Nat Med. 2011; 17(10):1315–1319

[16] Lyons SA, O'Neal J, Sontheimer H. Chlorotoxin, a scorpion-derived peptide, specifically binds to gliomas and tumors of neuroectodermal origin. Glia. 2002; 39(2):162–173

[17] DeBin JA, Maggio JE, Strichartz GR. Purification and characterization of chlorotoxin, a chloride channel ligand from the venom of the scorpion. Am J Physiol. 1993; 264(2 Pt 1):C361–C369

[18] Deshane J, Garner CC, Sontheimer H. Chlorotoxin inhibits glioma cell invasion via matrix metalloproteinase-2. J Biol Chem. 2003; 278(6):4135–4144

[19] Kesavan K, Ratliff J, Johnson EW, et al. Annexin A2 is a molecular target for TM601, a peptide with tumor-targeting and anti-angiogenic effects. J Biol Chem. 2010; 285(7):4366–4374

[20] Wiranowska M, Colina LO, Johnson JO. Clathrin-mediated entry and cellular localization of chlorotoxin in human glioma. Cancer Cell Int. 2011; 11:27

[21] Dardevet L, Rani D, Aziz TA, et al. Chlorotoxin: a helpful natural scorpion peptide to diagnose glioma and fight tumor invasion. Toxins. 2015; 7(4): 1079–1101

[22] Stroud MR, Hansen SJ, Olson JM. In vivo bio-imaging using chlorotoxin-based conjugates. Curr Pharm Des. 2011; 17(38):4362–4371

[23] Lokman NA, Ween MP, Oehler MK, Ricciardelli C. The role of annexin A2 in tumorigenesis and cancer progression. Cancer Microenvironment. 2011; 4: 199–208

[24] Ullrich N, Bordey A, Gillespie GY, Sontheimer H. Expression of voltage-activated chloride currents in acute slices of human gliomas. Neuroscience. 1998; 83(4):1161–1173

[25] Veiseh M, Gabikian P, Bahrami S-B, et al. Tumor paint: a chlorotoxin:Cy5.5 bioconjugate for intraoperative visualization of cancer foci. Cancer Res. 2007; 67(14):6882–6888

[26] Shen S, Khazaeli MB, Gillespie GY, Alvarez VL. Radiation dosimetry of 131I-chlorotoxin for targeted radiotherapy in glioma-bearing mice. J Neurooncol. 2005; 71(2):113–119

[27] Mamelak AN, Jacoby DB. Targeted delivery of antitumoral therapy to glioma and other malignancies with synthetic chlorotoxin (TM-601). Expert Opin Drug Deliv. 2007; 4(2):175–186

[28] Hockaday DC, Shen S, Fiveash J, et al. Imaging glioma extent with 131I-TM-601. J Nucl Med. 2005; 46(4):580–586

[29] Butte PV, Mamelak A, Parrish-Novak J, et al. Near-infrared imaging of brain tumors using the Tumor Paint BLZ-100 to achieve near-complete resection of brain tumors. Neurosurg Focus. 2014; 36(2):E1

[30] Kovar JL, Curtis E, Othman SF, Simpson MA, Olive DM. Characterization of IRDye 800CW chlorotoxin as a targeting agent for brain tumors. Anal Biochem. 2013; 440(2):212–219

[31] Fu Y, An N, Li K, Zheng Y, Liang A. Chlorotoxin-conjugated nanoparticles as potential glioma-targeted drugs. J Neurooncol. 2012; 107(3):457–462

[32] Meng XX, Wan JQ, Jing M, Zhao SG, Cai W, Liu EZ. Specific targeting of gliomas with multifunctional superparamagnetic iron oxide nanoparticle optical and magnetic resonance imaging contrast agents. Acta Pharmacol Sin. 2007; 28(12):2019–2026

[33] Mu Q, Lin G, Patton VK, Wang K, Press OW, Zhang M. Gemcitabine and chlorotoxin conjugated iron oxide nanoparticles for glioblastoma therapy. J Mater Chem B Mater Biol Med. 2016; 4(1):32–36

[34] Fidel J, Kennedy KC, Dernell WS, et al. Preclinical validation of the utility of BLZ-100 in providing fluorescence contrast for imaging spontaneous solid tumors. Cancer Res. 2015; 75(20):4283–4291

[35] Parrish-Novak J, Byrnes-Blake K, Lalayeva N, et al. Nonclinical profile of BLZ-100, a tumor-targeting fluorescent imaging agent. Int J Toxicol. 2017; 36:104–112

[36] Kittle DS, Mamelak MDA, Parrish-Novak JE, et al. Fluorescence-guided tumor visualization using the tumor paint BLZ-100. Cureus. 2017; 6:1–19

[37] Baik FM, Hansen S, Knoblaugh SE, et al. Fluorescence identification of head and neck squamous cell carcinoma and high-risk oral dysplasia with BLZ-100, a chlorotoxin-indocyanine green conjugate. JAMA Otolaryngol Head Neck Surg. 2016; 142(4):330–338

[38] Miller DM, Yamada M, Lowe M, et al. First in human phase 1 safety study of BLZ-100 in subjects with skin cancer. E-poster presented at the 2015 annual meeting of the American Academy of Dermatology, March 20–24, 2015. https://www.aad.org/eposters/Submissions/getFile.aspx?id=1389&type=sub

[39] Cahill RA, Anderson M, Wang LM, Lindsey I, Cunningham C, Mortensen NJ. Near-infrared (NIR) laparoscopy for intraoperative lymphatic road-mapping and sentinel node identification during definitive surgical resection of early-stage colorectal neoplasia. Surg Endosc. 2012; 26(1):197–204

[40] Crane LMA, Themelis G, Pleijhuis RG, et al. Intraoperative multispectral fluorescence imaging for the detection of the sentinel lymph node in cervical cancer: a novel concept. Mol Imaging Biol. 2011; 13(5):1043–1049

[41] Gotoh K, Yamada T, Ishikawa O, et al. A novel image-guided surgery of hepatocellular carcinoma by indocyanine green fluorescence imaging navigation. J Surg Oncol. 2009; 100(1):75–79

[42] Hirche C, Engel H, Kolios L, et al. An experimental study to evaluate the Fluobeam 800 imaging system for fluorescence-guided lymphatic imaging and sentinel node biopsy. Surg Innov. 2013; 20(5):516–523

[43] Mieog JSD, Hutteman M, van der Vorst JR, et al. Image-guided tumor resection using real-time near-infrared fluorescence in a syngeneic rat model of primary breast cancer. Breast Cancer Res Treat. 2011; 128(3):679–689

[44] Themelis G, Yoo JS, Soh K-S, Schulz R, Ntziachristos V. Real-time intraoperative fluorescence imaging system using light-absorption correction. J Biomed Opt. 2009; 14(6):064012

[45] van der Poel HG, Buckle T, Brouwer OR, Valdés Olmos RA, van Leeuwen FWB. Intraoperative laparoscopic fluorescence guidance to the sentinel lymph node in prostate cancer patients: clinical proof of concept of an integrated functional imaging approach using a multimodal tracer. Eur Urol. 2011; 60 (4):826–833

[46] Yamashita S, Tokuishi K, Anami K, et al. Video-assisted thoracoscopic indocyanine green fluorescence imaging system shows sentinel lymph nodes in non-small-cell lung cancer. J Thorac Cardiovasc Surg. 2011; 141(1):141–144

[47] Yamauchi K, Nagafuji H, Nakamura T, Sato T, Kohno N. Feasibility of ICG fluorescence-guided sentinel node biopsy in animal models using the HyperEye Medical System. Ann Surg Oncol. 2011; 18(7):2042–2047

[48] Kittle DS, Vasefi F, Patil CG, Mamelak A, Black KL, Butte PV. Real time optical biopsy: time-resolved fluorescence spectroscopy instrumentation and validation. Sci Rep. 2016; 6:38190

[49] Jacques SL. Optical properties of biological tissues: a review. Phys Med Biol. 2013; 58(11):R37–R61

[50] Yuan B, Chen N, Zhu Q. Emission and absorption properties of indocyanine green in Intralipid solution. J Biomed Opt. 2004; 9(3):497–503

[51] Patil C, Walker D, Miller DM, et al. Phase 1 safety, PK, and fluorescence imaging study of tozuleristide (BLZ-100) in adults with newly diagnosed or recurrent gliomas. Neurosurgery, in review (2018).

[52] Kamp MA, Grosser P, Felsberg J, et al. 5-aminolevulinic acid (5-ALA)-induced fluorescence in intracerebral metastases: a retrospective study. Acta Neurochir (Wien). 2012; 154(2):223–228, discussion 228

[53] Valdes PA, Bekelis K, Harris BT, et al. 5-Aminolevulinic acid-induced protoporphyrin IX fluorescence in meningioma: qualitative and quantitative measurements in vivo. Neurosurgery. 2014; 10 suppl 1:74–82, discussion –82–83

[54] Stummer W, Pichlmeier U, Meinel T, Wiestler OD, Zanella F, Reulen H-J, ALA-Glioma Study Group. Fluorescence-guided surgery with 5-aminolevulinic acid for resection of malignant glioma: a randomised controlled multicentre phase III trial. Lancet Oncol. 2006; 7(5):392–401

# Suggested Readings

[1] Liu Q, Xu S, Niu C, et al. Distinguish cancer cells based on targeting turn-on fluorescence imaging by folate functionalized green emitting carbon dots. Biosens Bioelectron. 2015; 64:119–125

[2] Miller DM, Yamada M, Lowe M, et al. Phase 1 dose escalation and expansion safety study of BLZ-100 in subjects with skin cancer. J Clin Oncol. 2017; 33 suppl 15

[3] Stummer W, Tonn J-C, Mehdorn HM, et al. ALA-Glioma Study Group. Counterbalancing risks and gains from extended resections in malignant glioma surgery: a supplemental analysis from the randomized 5-aminolevulinic acid glioma resection study. Clinical article. J Neurosurg. 2011; 114(3):613–623

# 15 Confocal Endomicroscopy

*Christina E. Sarris and Nader Sanai*

## Abstract

Fluorescence image-guided surgery is rapidly demonstrating its ability to improve brain tumor resections. However, there are still a number of limitations inherent to all wide-field fluorescence imaging techniques, such as limited sensitivity to detect glioma infiltration at the margins and ambiguous image contrast. Confocal endomicroscopy is a complimentary technology to targeted fluorescence in tumor resection, and it is certain that as our technology for fluorescent probes continues to evolve, the confocal microscope will continue to be refined. Recent work suggests that intraoperative high-resolution microscopy, a real-time alternative to invasive biopsy and histopathology, has the potential to better quantify tumor burden at the final stages of surgery and ultimately to improve patient outcomes when combined with wide-field imaging approaches. Additional studies are needed to further elucidate the clinical benefits of these new technologies for brain tumor patients.

*Keywords:* confocal endomicroscopy, high-resolution microscopy, fluorescence, extent of resection, histopathology, brain tumor

## 15.1 Introduction

Postoperative patient survival for brain tumor surgery is largely dependent on extent of resection. However, surgeons continue to face challenges in intraoperative differentiation of healthy brain parenchyma from pathologic tissue. Improvements in microscope technology, along with development of novel fluorescent agents, are helping neurosurgeons overcome these challenges as we become better able to characterize these boarder zones in tumor resection. Wide-field fluorescence image-guided surgery (FIGS) has been reported to have many benefits in glioma resection, but it does have several challenges that limit its utility. High-resolution confocal endomicroscopy has recently been introduced to the neurosurgical armamentarium and is demonstrating benefit in brain tumor resection. As this technology continues to improve and neurosurgeons become more comfortable with its incorporation into operative workflow, confocal endomicroscopy may contribute significantly to better tumor resections and patient outcomes.

## 15.2 Wide-Field Microscopy and Tumor Surgery

Visualization in fluorescence microscopy relies on fluorescence and phosphorescence rather than reflection of light as in conventional white-light microscopy. In fluorescence microscopy, the specimen is instead illuminated by a particular wavelength of light. The development of fluorescence microscopy has been motivated by the observation that reflectance imaging does not provide sufficient and reliable image contrast to distinguish between healthy and pathologic tissues. It has been well established that fluorescence can aid in this distinction.

One such type of fluorescence microscopy is wide-field fluorescence imaging. Utilization involves a low-powered surgical microscope, which continuously acquires the entire specimen on the microscope stage through the use of an eyepiece, and/or at a rapid frame rate with a digital detector array. Innately, the resolution of this technology is assumed to be low, as the field of view ranges from tens to hundreds of millimeters along any given lateral dimension, with a spatial resolution of tens to hundreds of microns. The most popular commercially available surgical microscopes for wide-field FIGS have been the Zeiss Pentero BLUE400 and the Leica FL400 microscopes, both utilized in numerous clinical studies and approved for routine use in the United States and Europe.

FIGS, however, suffers from a number of challenges[1]:

- *Angle and working distance:* When utilizing wide-field microscopy, one should attempt to maintain a perpendicular angle to the field and a constant working distance between the microscope and the tissue. This becomes challenging as tumor cavities are often out of range for the fixed working distance of the standard fluorescence microscopes used for FIGS, and often side walls are difficult to visualize because of their steep angle with respect to the illumination source. Finally, tumors located within sulci and behind bends are inaccessible without a miniature imaging probe.[2]

- *Ambiguity at margins:* Wide-field imaging does not allow for qualitatively or reproducibly defining margins for gliomas. For example, visualization of 5-aminolevulinic acid (5-ALA) induced protoporphyrin IX (PpIX) contrast is effective at revealing regions of bulk tumor (deep red), but fluorescence intensities decay near the margins (lighter pink) and vanish entirely as the tumor cell density continues to decline. On histopathological examination, however, all three territories demonstrate glioma cell infiltration.[3]

- *Sensitivity:* Unfortunately, visible fluorescence is not always captured with wide-field FIGS. For low-grade gliomas (LGGs), wide-field FIGS with 5-ALA remains ineffective, as it does not produce visible fluorescence for the majority of low-grade tumors. In some cases, heterogeneous fluorescence has been noted in focal areas of anaplastic transformation. However, the vast majority of LGGs are invisible with 5-ALA.[4,5,6,7,8,9,10] Interestingly, PpIX fluorescence can be measured ex vivo in LGG tissue following 5-ALA administration.[7,8] In these analyses, the resultant fluorescence intensity of the tumor tissue is significantly higher than in similarly treated normal tissue[8] and increases with both tumor grade and proliferative index.[3,7,11]

- *Quantification:* The ultimate goal of these novel technologies is to reliably distinguish between pathologic and normal tissues via use of a contrast agent and to accurately quantify the concentration of that contrast agent at each resolvable tissue location. This is not, however, easily done as the image pixel is complicated by background and variations in tissue optical properties. Thus, recent research efforts have been spent with attempts to advance the FIGS systems and correct these issues such that image intensities correlate directly with fluorophore concentration (▶ Fig. 15.1). For example,

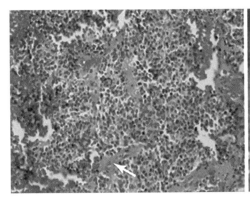 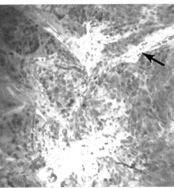

**Fig. 15.1** Comparison of traditional hematoxylin and eosin stained tumor section (*left*) and confocal view (*right*) of an anaplastic oligodendroglioma. Both images demonstrate hypercellular tumor with pleomorphic nuclei. Prominent vascular channels (*arrows*) are seen with both techniques.

advanced FIGS systems are now utilizing multispectral imaging. This involves the illumination and/or detection of fluorophores and backscattered illumination light at various optical wavelengths, which helps correct for tissue optical properties as well as nonspecific accumulation of molecular contrast agents.[12,13,14] These methods typically utilize proportional imaging (normalization), either between fluorescence measurements[12,13,14,15] or a combination of fluorescence and light attenuation images.[16,17] The SurgOptix T3-platform is based on one such multispectral imaging technology. Another system under development is the FLARE system,[18,19,20] which has incorporated color imaging with dual-band fluorescence imaging. This system utilizes an automated background subtraction algorithm in its operation, similar to the Zeiss OPMI Pentero system. This allows for isolation of fluorescence from other sources of background light in the operating room.

While improvements in FIGS technology are ongoing, its innate limitations have allowed clinician scientists to explore other means by which to improve tumor surgery.

## 15.3 High-Resolution Intraoperative Microscopy

The reported rates of gross total tumor resection continue to remain low despite use of imaging technologies such as intraoperative MRI and wide-field FIGS. As discussed earlier, a major reason for this is that these wide-field imaging techniques lack the resolution, and hence the sensitivity, to detect the disseminated tumor cells at the margins of such diffuse tumors. Thus, the neurosurgeon is faced with the challenge of interpreting subjective image intensities to determine an appropriate surgical margin. This process is neither quantitative nor reproducible for one surgeon or between multiple surgeons. For some extra-axial lesions, the gross appearance of the tumor is sufficient to establish the tumor-brain tissue planes with microdissection techniques. Other lesions, however, are less easily distinguished, particularly in the setting of prior treatment effect, cerebral edema, or microscopic infiltration. This is particularly true for gliomas and higher-grade meningiomas, where defining extent of resection on the basis of gross tissue characteristics is insufficient and neuronavigation can be unreliable due to brain shift.

Beyond identifying tumor margins, the opportunity to intraoperatively define tumor grade and histologic subtype is of critical importance, particularly for intracranial gliomas, where tumor grade is not reliably predicted with either preoperative MRI[21] or stereotactic biopsy.[22] Some have thus advocated for the use of frozen-section pathology to confirm tissue status during glioma resection,[2] which unfortunately is time consuming and relies on the invasive removal of biopsies. Intraoperative frozen-section analysis can be misleading or nondiagnostic, particularly in cases of mechanical tissue disruption from the resection process.[23,24] Such diagnostic unpredictability is further complicated by the inherent heterogeneity of gliomas, which can contain high-grade populations nested within a low-grade stroma.[25] Others have suggested the need for quantitative measurements of PpIX fluorescence, such as with spectral measurement probes.[4,8,26]

To overcome these persistent challenges in the resection of complex intra- and extra-axial brain tumors, recent work has been directed toward adapting routine postoperative neuropathology methods into a real-time intraoperative technique. Overwhelmingly, this has led to development of a potentially powerful complement to wide-field FIGS–intraoperative high-resolution optical-sectioning microscopy, or confocal microscopy. Confocal microscopy is an optical imaging technique that uses point illumination and a spatial pinhole to eliminate out-of-focus light in specimens that are thicker than the focal plane, thereby enhancing optical resolution beyond light microscopy and detecting light produced by fluorescence very close to the focal plane. Intraoperative confocal microscopy has miniaturized this approach to enable visualization of live tissue cytoarchitecture with spatial resolution on a cellular level.[27,28,29,30] Ultimately, this allows the physician to have biopsy images displayed in real time to aid in immediate operative decision-making. This microscope can be placed directly in contact with tissues to quantify the presence of labeled cells in real time without the need for excisional biopsy and time-consuming histopathology. While late to become part of the neurosurgical armamentarium, the technology has been widely utilized and has proved feasible in various bodily regions outside the central nervous system, including the colon, pancreas, stomach, and alveoli.[31,32,33,34,35,36] In neurosurgery, the ability to resolve and detect sparse subpopulations of labeled cells, such as tumors cells at the diffuse margins of a glioma, could provide a standardized quantitative metric by which neurosurgeons may eventually be able to optimize their resections as well as to objectively determine an unambiguous "extent of resection" for their surgeries (▶ Fig. 15.1).

## 15.3.1 Confocal Microscope Evolution

Marvin Minsky, American scientist and inventor, first introduced confocal microscopy in 1955 with demonstration that it was possible to obtain optical sections via aid of a pinhole and detector combination.[37] Since that time, the last sixty years have seen development of numerous confocal microscopes based off the principle that a pinhole equivalent blocks out-of-focus light.[38] The usability of confocal endomicroscopy has been limited by instrument size and ease of surgical incorporation for the neurosurgeon. Until recently, the size of the requisite apparatus limited the technology to examination of excised tissue samples or isolated cells in a bench-top setting. Newer technology, however, features fiberoptic and microscopic miniaturization, substantially expanding its portability and applicability in an in vivo clinical setting.[39,40,41,42] These systems now consist of a miniature handheld probe and movable workstation with an LCD screen. Using a single optical fiber as both the illumination point source and detection pinhole, high-resolution images are acquired and combined with miniaturized scanning and optical systems.[43] Thus, the widespread use of confocal endomicroscopy in the gastrointestinal tract has been largely because of the ease of incorporating the technology into the distal tip of conventional video endoscopes. The bladder mucosa, skin, and eye have similarly been studied with in vivo confocal microscopy.[44,45,46,47] Even more recently, in vivo confocal microscopy has been utilized in robotic-assisted radical prostatectomy.[48]

Microscope designs have undergone numerous modifications to achieve optical sectioning such as multiphoton excitation,[49] single-axis confocal microscopy,[50,51] dual-axis confocal (DAC) microscopy,[52] and structured illumination.[53,54,55] Designs have also differed in their scanning mechanisms, including proximally scanned coherent fiber bundles,[56,57,58,59,60,61,62,63,64,65] distally scanned fiber tips,[66,67,68,69,70] and microelectromechanical systems (MEMS) scanners.[52,71,72,73,74,75,76,77,78] There are several commercially available confocal microscopy systems, including the Cellvizio (Mauna Kea Technologies, Paris, France) and Optiscan FIVE 1—both of which have been utilized in neurosurgery.[79,80] The first microscope used in vivo for brain tumor resection in humans was the Optiscan system utilized by researchers at the Barrow Neurological Institute (BNI) in Phoenix, AZ.[5,81,82] The Optiscan has a 475 × 475 μm field of view and focal plane depth to 250 μm. As a result of the unique resonant-scanning mechanism used for imaging, this microscope is somewhat limited by a slow frame rate (0.8 frames/s) that leads to motion artifacts and makes the clinical use of the device less effective. The Cellvizio (Mauna Kea Technologies) is a miniature microscope based on coherent fiber-bundle technologies.[57,58,60,61,62,64,83] These confocal microscopes treat each fiber within the bundle as a separate confocal pinhole for spatial filtering of out-of-focus and scattered light for high-contrast imaging of tissues at modest depths. Proximal scanning allows the distal tip of the device to be extremely small (0.5–3 mm) and flexible. One disadvantage of these technologies is that they often do not allow for axial adjustment of the focal plane since the mechanisms for doing so would significantly increase the size of the distal tip of these devices. While the ability to image deeply is

not a fundamental necessity for intraoperative determinations of tissue status, there are practical advantages for being able to adjust the focal plane of an optical-sectioning device during surgery. For example, adjustment of the axial imaging depth allows the surgeon to search for an optimal imaging plane in which the tissues show minimal signs of surgical disruption, and at which signal levels and contrast are optimal. Another limitation to fiber-bundle-based approaches is that current fiber-bundle manufacturers utilize ion-doped glass fibers that create large autofluorescence backgrounds when excited at 405 nm.[84] This is less of an issue at other excitation wavelengths, such as at 488 nm, but the autofluorescence background limits the ability of these technologies to be utilized for imaging 5-ALA-induced PpIX, in which the optimal absorption peak is at 405 nm. Both the Optiscan and Cellvizio use a 488-nm excitation light, and Cellvizio additionally has a 660-nm single-band excitation light.[80] The EndoMAG1 by Karl Storz Company has also been evaluated for use in neurosurgery, with a circular scanning field covering 300 × 300 μm and an 80-μm scanning depth.[85]

In addition to miniature optical-sectioning devices that utilize conventional single-axis confocal approaches, recent efforts have been made to develop intraoperative microscopes using an alternative confocal architecture called a DAC microscope or a divided-pupil confocal microscope.[52,86,87,88,89,90,91,92,93] In the DAC architecture, the illumination and collection beam paths are spatially separated, as opposed to the common-path configuration of typical microscopes. Simulations and experiments have shown that the DAC configuration provides certain benefits in terms of optical-sectioning contrast in tissues, including the ability to image at deeper depths compared to conventional single-axis confocal microscopes.[88,91,94,95] In addition, dual-axis designs, which utilize low-numerical-aperture (NA; weakly focusing) beams as opposed to the high-NA beams preferred for conventional confocal microscopy, have been shown to be scalable in portable devices with diameters ranging from 3 to 10 mm.[90,92,96] These devices have utilized miniature MEMS scanning mirrors to scan an image within tissues. MEMS-scanned microscopes have been shown to enable high frame rate imaging (up to 30 Hz),[92] which is beneficial in clinical settings to reduce motion artifacts and image blur during handheld use.

## 15.3.2 Feasibility and Results in Neurosurgery

There are numerous reasons for introducing confocal endomicroscopy to neurosurgery. Aggressive resection with cleaner, near-normal tissue margins is often acceptable in areas that are not adjacent to eloquent brain. However, in certain localized regions near eloquent brain, a real-time high-resolution "optical biopsy" could potentially provide the surgeon with an accurate calibration measurement that, in combination with intraoperative neuronavigation and other surgical cues, may allow significant improvement in extent of resection. In LGGs, the need for intraoperative optical-sectioning microscopy is especially compelling due to the fact that 5-ALA-induced PpIX fluorescence is often not detectable with wide-field FIGS.[4,5,7,8,9,10] Since the metabolic conversion of 5-ALA to fluorescent PpIX is associated with highly proliferative and mitotic tumor cells, only a small subset of tumor cells are fluorescent in LGGs. As a result, wide-field imaging, in which each resolvable pixel represents an average signal from thousands of cells, lacks the sensitivity to detect the presence of these sparse tumor cell populations. On the contrary, it has recently been demonstrated that intraoperative high-resolution microscopy is able to visualize and quantify the presence of sparsely scattered fluorescent cells in LGGs.[5] Recent work illustrates the ability of intraoperative high-resolution microscopy to detect and quantify sparse cell populations where wide-field imaging fails.

Bringing the confocal microscope to neurosurgery remained challenging until recent years because of the difficulty of safely introducing such instrumentation to the brain in vivo. The first results of use of confocal endomicroscopy in neurosurgery were published in 2010.[30] Using the Optiscan FIVE 1 system, this study demonstrated the feasibility of performing in vivo confocal microscopy in an animal brain tumor model and compared this imaging with conventional histologic images from the same tissue. Using intravenous fluorescein and topical acriflavine dye, handheld confocal imaging produced suitable images that correlated well with corresponding histologic sections, effectively distinguishing tumor versus nontumor with readily identifiable margins by observers without prior neuropathology training (▶ Fig. 15.2).

The first human feasibility study of confocal microscopy for brain tumor resection was published shortly after.[82] Thirty-three patients with brain tumors received intravenous sodium fluorescein, followed by confocal imaging with the Optiscan FIVE 1 system probe. Initial examination of tissue integrity during confocal visualization demonstrated good tissue preservation, with intact parenchyma and vasculature on the surface and as deep as 500 μm. Also, areas of neovascularization from tumor-induced angiogenesis could distinguish pathologic from normal parenchyma. Specific confocal features of high-grade glioma—dense cellularity, irregular cellular phenotypes, and neovascularization—were defined. This study established the technology's potential value during the microsurgical resection of both intra- and extra-axial tumors. For a variety of tumor histologies, including gliomas, meningiomas, hemangioblastomas, and central neurocytomas, the handheld device generated a real-time, fluorescein-enhanced pathological image of sufficient resolution for a neuropathologist to establish a preliminary diagnosis. This preliminary analysis of intraoperative confocal microscopy not only suggested a correlation between imaging and tumor grade, but also demonstrated a capacity to distinguish tumor margins from adjacent parenchyma.

Subsequent work in a series of 50 microsurgical tumor resections with confocal microscopy[81] compared confocal microscopy images with corresponding biopsy samples. The pathologist in a blinded fashion reviewed the images to evaluate their usefulness as a diagnostic tool, and ultimately had a diagnostic accuracy rate of 92.9%. This study further characterized the confocal microscopic features of various tumor types, including gliomas of various grades, meningiomas, schwannomas, and a hemangioblastoma. The fluorescein-contrasted pathological images were found to be of sufficient resolution for a neuropathologist to establish a preliminary diagnosis without a frozen-section sample, as well as the technology's potential for in vivo identification of infiltrating tumor edge to help maximize resection. A later fluorescein study of intracranial neoplasms in

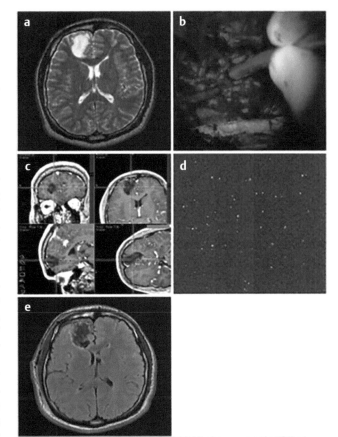

**Fig. 15.2** Microscopic detection of 5-aminolevulinic acid (5-ALA) tumor fluorescence in a WHO grade II glioma with confocal microscopy. **(a)** Axial MRI of a 21-year-old patient with suspected right frontal low-grade glioma. **(b)** Intraoperative view of use of the handheld confocal microscope. **(c)** Intraoperative neuronavigation confirming localization of the confocal imaging within the tumor mass. **(d)** Multiple fluorescent cells in tumor bed, corresponding with 5-ALA metabolism. **(e)** Postoperative MRI demonstrating a 98% volumetric extent of resection.

74 patients demonstrated confocal endomicroscopy specificity and sensitivity were, respectively, 94 and 91% for gliomas and 93 and 97% for meningiomas.[97]

A separate group, utilizing the EndoMAG1 endomicroscope, demonstrated their series of 100 consecutive confocal endomicroscopy patients.[85] In this study, investigators utilized previously established criteria for structural patterns of tumors seen on confocal endomicroscopy scans and applied them to their series. They demonstrated sensitivity for correct diagnosis in 82 to 90% of high-grade gliomas, LGGs, schwannomas, and meningiomas. Only 37% sensitivity was found for metastases.

The initial neurosurgical study with the Cellvizio system reported the largest series of confocal endomicroscopy in neurosurgery to date, and analyzed 150 patients with brain or spinal cord tumors and compared them for accuracy with the standard histology.[98] The microscope was used for immediate ex vivo imaging after fluorescein-guided resection. The confocal images demonstrated features similar to the histological images of the same tissue, and surgeons found its use was easily integrated into daily routine. Still pending comparison with standard histological staining in validation assessments, clinical trials with the Cellvizio are currently underway in Europe.[99,100]

## 15.3.3 Clinical Workflow

The workflow of confocal endomicroscopy is of utmost importance to the neurosurgeon. It is well known that intraoperative histopathology has numerous shortcomings—tissue alteration during specimen preparation, sampling errors, and, even more importantly, the wait time for frozen section results, often nearing 30 minutes to 1 hour. However, recent reports using intraoperative handheld microscopy[5,30,81,82] and portable spectroscopy[3,4,26] have suggested the clinical utility of performing a real-time "optical biopsy" of select regions of the resection cavity considered to be at high risk for residual tumor. The success of the neurosurgeon introducing new technology to the operating room relies on the ability to incorporate such tools with safety and ease. One example of a clinical workflow model is outlined below:

- Standard neurosurgical techniques are used to debulk the central portions of a glioma.
- As the radiographic boundaries of the tumor are approached, regions adjacent to noneloquent brain may be resected more aggressively to assure maximal extent of resection.
- Ambiguous regions at critical locations (e.g., near eloquent brain) may be probed with high-resolution microscopy of the exposed tissue, enabling quantitative measurement of tumor burden to calibrate operative decision-making.

Several neurosurgical studies have outlined their intraoperative workflow with use of confocal endomicroscopy. With use of the Optiscan system, surgeons have utilized a foot pedal remote intraoperatively to control the imaging plane depth from the surface to a depth of 0 to 500 μm.[97] This group acquired in vivo images 5 minutes after injection of 5 mL 10% FNa, and the majority of their images were obtained by attaching the microscope probe to a Greenberg retractor arm. The probe was also co-registered with the image-guided surgical system to allow for precise intraoperative localization. The probe was then moved gently along the surface of the tissue to obtain images from several biopsy locations. The probe is able to be used in a free-hand fashion, as well. The total time of use of the device in the operating room was 5.8 minutes per patient (range 1.4–17.0 minutes).

With this technology, surgeons can choose to perform imaging in vivo and ex vivo. For ex vivo imaging, tissue samples suspicious for tumor can be harvested from the surgical field and imaged on a separate workstation away from the patient but still within the operating room.[97] This allows for immediate review of tissue without the probe distracting the surgical field. While our current technology limits us to a precision of no better than approximately 0.5 cm, each high-resolution microscope image provides a real-time, noninvasive alternative to biopsy that facilitates a rapid risk–benefit assessment of further resection. Thus, in the context of daily neurosurgical workflow, comprehensive high-resolution imaging over the entire tumor cavity is neither necessary nor practical to perform in the operating room. Instead, an "optical biopsy" can assess tumor burden within high-risk regions during the terminal stages of glioma resection. Real-time image-processing algorithms will

ultimately need to be developed to quantify fluorescence expression and to display this information to surgeons.

## 15.3.4 Limitations of Confocal Endomicroscopy

We have now discussed the initial promising findings of confocal microscopy in human brain tumor surgery, but several areas still are in need of technical refinement. One obvious trade-off for high-resolution microscopy is the small field of view (0.5 mm in diameter), as well as the need to visualize the obtained images on a separate monitor. The interpretation of results relies on the surgeon's knowledge of histopathology, as the resultant images differ from the stained histopathological slides and a learning curve does exist for interpretation.[80] Inherently, the technology also relies on the laser excitation spectrum and corresponding detection power. Due to its reliance on optics, confocal endomicroscopy is susceptible to erythrocyte contamination of the probe, which can obscure the field of view. Contamination can be addressed by elevating the probe from the tissue surface and manually cleaning it with gentle irrigation.[82] Future versions of the device may benefit from an auto-irrigation mechanism, similar to the endoscope.[57] Furthermore, while fluorescein contrast allows for detailed assessment of overall tissue cellularity, the ability to discern cellular cytoplasm remains limited, as does its specificity for nuclear morphology. Since tumor cell nucleus-to-cytoplasm ratios are critical to histopathological diagnosis, other contrasting agents should be investigated. Fluorescein also has a relatively high rate of photobleaching.[101] One alternative candidate agent is 5-ALA, which allows highly specific localization of tumor cells.

## 15.3.5 Future Directions

Confocal microscopes continue to improve alongside development of more reliable contrast agents and better wide-field FIGS technology. Furthermore, the ability of the device to scan as much as 500 μm through the visible tissue surface permits analysis of an even broader spectrum of tissue. It is therefore likely that confocal endomicroscopy may be of use in examining subependymal regions through an intraventricular corridor, allowing detection of pockets of subependymal tumor migration that are radiographically undetectable and remote from the primary tumor site. It has been postulated that subependymal spread is both a negative prognostic sign and a primary route of glioma migration.[102] The ability to detect its occurrence at an early stage may permit anticipatory and focused interventions, as well as lead to insight into basic mechanisms of gliomagenesis.[103]

Also, confocal microscopy allows us the opportunity to observe active blood flow through tumor capillaries, providing a unique visual dimension to tissue assessment. It remains unclear what impact antiangiogenic agents may have the ability to identify tumor neovascularization, although angioarchitecture is one of several distinguishing features enhanced with confocal microscopy. The probe can also quickly survey the visible extent of a tumor with the potential to detect disconnected, cell-dense islands that may portend worse histologic grade and heterogeneity. Additional pilot studies not only will enhance

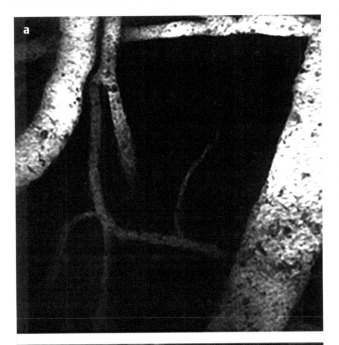

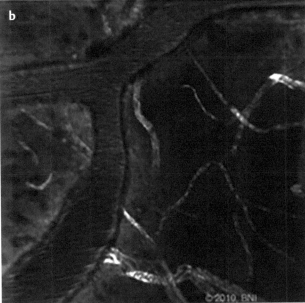

**Fig. 15.3** Intraoperative confocal images of normal and tumor microvasculature. **(a)** Normal brain arteriole and capillary systems highlighted with intravascular fluorescein. **(b)** Multiple branch points are evident and real-time flow is seen.

landmarks no longer co-localize with preoperatively obtained MR images. In these circumstances, confocal microscopy can confirm the presence of tumor when the reliability of neuronavigation is in doubt. Future studies comparing the predictive value of confocal microscopy to intraoperative MRI and intraoperative ultrasound techniques may be of value as well.

## 15.4 Conclusion

Confocal endomicroscopy is a complimentary technology to targeted fluorescence in tumor resection, and it is certain that as our technology for fluorescent probes continues to evolve, the confocal microscope will continue to be refined. FIGS is emerging as a valuable technology to improve glioma resections while minimizing accompanying neurological deficits. Numerous contrast agents are in various stages of preclinical and clinical development. 5-ALA-induced PpIX, in particular, has been shown to be a reliable biomarker for gliomas. However, there are still a number of limitations inherent to all wide-field (low-resolution) imaging techniques with FIGS and standard-of-care MRI, such as limited sensitivity to detect glioma infiltration at the margins and ambiguous image contrast. Recent work suggests that intraoperative high-resolution microscopy, a real-time alternative to invasive biopsy and histopathology, has the potential to better quantify tumor burden at the final stages of surgery and ultimately to improve patient outcomes when combined with wide-field imaging approaches. Additional studies are needed to further elucidate the clinical benefits of these new technologies for brain tumor patients.

## References

[1] Liu JT, Meza D, Sanai N. Trends in fluorescence image-guided surgery for gliomas. Neurosurgery. 2014; 75(1):61–71

[2] Tonn J-C, Stummer W. Fluorescence-guided resection of malignant gliomas using 5-aminolevulinic acid: practical use, risks, and pitfalls. Clin Neurosurg. 2008; 55:20–26

[3] Valdés PA, Kim A, Brantsch M, et al. δ-aminolevulinic acid-induced protoporphyrin IX concentration correlates with histopathologic markers of malignancy in human gliomas: the need for quantitative fluorescence-guided resection to identify regions of increasing malignancy. Neuro-oncol. 2011; 13(8):846–856

[4] Valdés PA, Leblond F, Kim A, et al. Quantitative fluorescence in intracranial tumor: implications for ALA-induced PpIX as an intraoperative biomarker. J Neurosurg. 2011; 115(1):11–17

[5] Sanai N, Snyder LA, Honea NJ, et al. Intraoperative confocal microscopy in the visualization of 5-aminolevulinic acid fluorescence in low-grade gliomas. J Neurosurg. 2011; 115(4):740–748

[6] Valdés PA, Kim A, Leblond F, et al. Combined fluorescence and reflectance spectroscopy for in vivo quantification of cancer biomarkers in low- and high-grade glioma surgery. J Biomed Opt. 2011; 16(11):116007

[7] Floeth FW, Sabel M, Ewelt C, et al. Comparison of (18)F-FET PET and 5-ALA fluorescence in cerebral gliomas. Eur J Nucl Med Mol Imaging. 2011; 38(4): 731–741

[8] Ishihara R, Katayama Y, Watanabe T, Yoshino A, Fukushima T, Sakatani K. Quantitative spectroscopic analysis of 5-aminolevulinic acid-induced protoporphyrin IX fluorescence intensity in diffusely infiltrating astrocytomas. Neurol Med Chir (Tokyo). 2007; 47(2):53–57, discussion 57

[9] Widhalm G, Wolfsberger S, Minchev G, et al. 5-Aminolevulinic acid is a promising marker for detection of anaplastic foci in diffusely infiltrating gliomas with nonsignificant contrast enhancement. Cancer. 2010; 116(6): 1545–1552

[10] Stockhammer F, Misch M, Horn P, Koch A, Fonyuy N, Plotkin M. Association of F18-fluoro-ethyl-tyrosin uptake and 5-aminolevulinic acid-induced fluorescence in gliomas. Acta Neurochir (Wien). 2009; 151(11):1377–1383

our familiarization with this technique, but also may demonstrate an extent of correlation with frozen section findings that could allow its eventual replacement of conventional intraoperative diagnostic methods. This modernized approach to intraoperative diagnosis would also lend itself to remote, internet-based analyses, expanding the accessibility of diagnostic expertise beyond centers with dedicated tumor neuropathologists.

Beyond its utility for tumor diagnosis, intraoperative confocal microscopy also provides a real-time alternative to neuronavigation in identifying abnormal tissue (▶ Fig. 15.3). This is particularly useful in cases of brain shift, where the parenchymal

[11] Stummer W, Stepp H, Möller G, Ehrhardt A, Leonhard M, Reulen HJ. Technical principles for protoporphyrin-IX-fluorescence guided microsurgical resection of malignant glioma tissue. Acta Neurochir (Wien). 1998; 140(10):995–1000

[12] Liu JTC, Helms MW, Mandella MJ, Crawford JM, Kino GS, Contag CH. Quantifying cell-surface biomarker expression in thick tissues with ratiometric three-dimensional microscopy. Biophys J. 2009; 96(6):2405–2414

[13] Tichauer KM, Samkoe KS, Sexton KJ, Gunn JR, Hasan T, Pogue BW. Improved tumor contrast achieved by single time point dual-reporter fluorescence imaging. J Biomed Opt. 2012; 17(6):066001

[14] Tichauer KM, Samkoe KS, Sexton KJ, et al. In vivo quantification of tumor receptor binding potential with dual-reporter molecular imaging. Mol Imaging Biol. 2012; 14(5):584–592

[15] Bogaards A, Sterenborg HJCM, Trachtenberg J, Wilson BC, Lilge L. In vivo quantification of fluorescent molecular markers in real-time by ratio imaging for diagnostic screening and image-guided surgery. Lasers Surg Med. 2007; 39(7):605–613

[16] van Dam GM, Themelis G, Crane LM, et al. Intraoperative tumor-specific fluorescence imaging in ovarian cancer by folate receptor-α targeting: first in-human results. Nat Med. 2011; 17(10):1315–1319

[17] Themelis G, Yoo JS, Soh KS, Schulz R, Ntziachristos V. Real-time intraoperative fluorescence imaging system using light-absorption correction. J Biomed Opt. 2009; 14(6):064012

[18] Keereweer S, Kerrebijn JDF, van Driel PBAA, et al. Optical image-guided surgery–where do we stand? Mol Imaging Biol. 2011; 13(2):199–207

[19] Troyan SL, Kianzad V, Gibbs-Strauss SL, et al. The FLARE intraoperative near-infrared fluorescence imaging system: a first-in-human clinical trial in breast cancer sentinel lymph node mapping. Ann Surg Oncol. 2009; 16(10): 2943–2952

[20] Gioux S, Choi HS, Frangioni JV. Image-guided surgery using invisible near-infrared light: fundamentals of clinical translation. Mol Imaging. 2010; 9(5): 237–255

[21] Kondziolka D, Lunsford LD, Martinez AJ. Unreliability of contemporary neurodiagnostic imaging in evaluating suspected adult supratentorial (low-grade) astrocytoma. J Neurosurg. 1993; 79(4):533–536

[22] Muragaki Y, Chernov M, Maruyama T, et al. Low-grade glioma on stereotactic biopsy: how often is the diagnosis accurate? Minim Invasive Neurosurg. 2008; 51(5):275–279

[23] Tilgner J, Herr M, Ostertag C, Volk B. Validation of intraoperative diagnoses using smear preparations from stereotactic brain biopsies: intraoperative versus final diagnosis–influence of clinical factors. Neurosurgery. 2005; 56 (2):257–265, discussion 257–265

[24] Uematsu Y, Owai Y, Okita R, Tanaka Y, Itakura T. The usefulness and problem of intraoperative rapid diagnosis in surgical neuropathology. Brain Tumor Pathol. 2007; 24(2):47–52

[25] Dowling C, Bollen AW, Noworolski SM, et al. Preoperative proton MR spectroscopic imaging of brain tumors: correlation with histopathologic analysis of resection specimens. AJNR Am J Neuroradiol. 2001; 22(4):604–612

[26] Valdés PA, Leblond F, Jacobs VL, Wilson BC, Paulsen KD, Roberts DW. Quantitative, spectrally-resolved intraoperative fluorescence imaging. Sci Rep. 2012; 2:798

[27] Becker DE, Ancin H, Szarowski DH, Turner JN, Roysam B. Automated 3-D montage synthesis from laser-scanning confocal images: application to quantitative tissue-level cytological analysis. Cytometry. 1996; 25(3):235–245

[28] Khoshyomn S, Penar PL, McBride WJ, Taatjes DJ. Four-dimensional analysis of human brain tumor spheroid invasion into fetal rat brain aggregates using confocal scanning laser microscopy. J Neurooncol. 1998; 38(1):1–10

[29] Tadrous PJ. Methods for imaging the structure and function of living tissues and cells: 3. Confocal microscopy and micro-radiology. J Pathol. 2000; 191 (4):345–354

[30] Sankar T, Delaney PM, Ryan RW, et al. Miniaturized handheld confocal microscopy for neurosurgery: results in an experimental glioblastoma model. Neurosurgery. 2010; 66(2):410–417, discussion 417–418

[31] Guo YT, Li YQ, Yu T, et al. Diagnosis of gastric intestinal metaplasia with confocal laser endomicroscopy in vivo: a prospective study. Endoscopy. 2008; 40(7):547–553

[32] Giovannini M, Caillol F, Poizat F, et al. Feasibility of intratumoral confocal microscopy under endoscopic ultrasound guidance. Endosc Ultrasound. 2012; 1(2):80–83

[33] Shahid MW, Buchner A, Gomez V, et al. Diagnostic accuracy of probe-based confocal laser endomicroscopy and narrow band imaging in detection of dysplasia in duodenal polyps. J Clin Gastroenterol. 2012; 46(5):382–389

[34] Fuchs FS, Zirlik S, Hildner K, et al. Fluorescein-aided confocal laser endomicroscopy of the lung. Respiration. 2011; 81(1):32–38

[35] Wu K, Liu JJ, Adams W, et al. Dynamic real-time microscopy of the urinary tract using confocal laser endomicroscopy. Urology. 2011; 78(1):225–231

[36] Sharma P, Meining AR, Coron E, et al. Real-time increased detection of neoplastic tissue in Barrett's esophagus with probe-based confocal laser endomicroscopy: final results of an international multicenter, prospective, randomized, controlled trial. Gastrointest Endosc. 2011; 74(3):465–472

[37] Minsky M. Memoir on inventing the confocal scanning microscope. Scanning. 1988

[38] Ye X, McCluskey MD. Modular scanning confocal microscope with digital image processing. PLoS One. 2016; 11(11):e0166212

[39] Delaney PM, King RG, Lambert JR, Harris MR. Fibre optic confocal imaging (FOCI) for subsurface microscopy of the colon in vivo. J Anat. 1994; 184(Pt 1):157–160

[40] Flusberg BA, Cocker ED, Piyawattanametha W, Jung JC, Cheung EL, Schnitzer MJ. Fiber-optic fluorescence imaging. Nat Methods. 2005; 2(12):941–950

[41] Flusberg BA, Nimmerjahn A, Cocker ED, et al. High-speed, miniaturized fluorescence microscopy in freely moving mice. Nat Methods. 2008; 5(11): 935–938

[42] Helmchen F. Miniaturization of fluorescence microscopes using fibre optics. Exp Physiol. 2002; 87(6):737–745

[43] Hoffman A, Goetz M, Vieth M, Galle PR, Neurath MF, Kiesslich R. Confocal laser endomicroscopy: technical status and current indications. Endoscopy. 2006; 38(12):1275–1283

[44] Brezinski ME, Tearney GJ, Bouma B, et al. Optical biopsy with optical coherence tomography. Ann N Y Acad Sci. 1998; 838:68–74

[45] Bussau LJ, Vo LT, Delaney PM, Papworth GD, Barkla DH, King RG. Fibre optic confocal imaging (FOCI) of keratinocytes, blood vessels and nerves in hairless mouse skin in vivo. J Anat. 1998; 192(Pt 2):187–194

[46] Koenig F, Knittel J, Stepp H. Diagnosing cancer in vivo. Science. 2001; 292 (5520):1401–1403

[47] Papworth GD, Delaney PM, Bussau LJ, Vo LT, King RG. In vivo fibre optic confocal imaging of microvasculature and nerves in the rat vas deferens and colon. J Anat. 1998; 192(Pt 4):489–495

[48] Lopez A, Zlatev DV, Mach KE, et al. Intraoperative optical biopsy during robotic assisted radical prostatectomy using confocal endomicroscopy. J Urol. 2016; 195(4, Pt 1):1110–1117

[49] Grewe BF, Langer D, Kasper H, Kampa BM, Helmchen F. High-speed in vivo calcium imaging reveals neuronal network activity with near-millisecond precision. Nat Methods. 2010; 7(5):399–405

[50] Maitland KC, Gillenwater AM, Williams MD, El-Naggar AK, Descour MR, Richards-Kortum RR. In vivo imaging of oral neoplasia using a miniaturized fiber optic confocal reflectance microscope. Oral Oncol. 2008; 44(11):1059–1066

[51] Tanbakuchi AA, Rouse AR, Udovich JA, Hatch KD, Gmitro AF. Clinical confocal microlaparoscope for real-time in vivo optical biopsies. J Biomed Opt. 2009; 14(4):044030

[52] Liu JTC, Mandella MJ, Loewke NO, et al. Micromirror-scanned dual-axis confocal microscope utilizing a gradient-index relay lens for image guidance during brain surgery. J Biomed Opt. 2010; 15(2):026029

[53] Bozinovic N, Ventalon C, Ford T, Mertz J. Fluorescence endomicroscopy with structured illumination. Opt Express. 2008; 16(11):8016–8025

[54] Neil MA, Juskaitis R, Wilson T. Method of obtaining optical sectioning by using structured light in a conventional microscope. Opt Lett. 1997; 22(24): 1905–1907

[55] Lim D, Ford TN, Chu KK, Mertz J. Optically sectioned in vivo imaging with speckle illumination HiLo microscopy. J Biomed Opt. 2011; 16(1):016014

[56] Carlson K, Chidley M, Sung K-B, et al. In vivo fiber-optic confocal reflectance microscope with an injection-molded plastic miniature objective lens. Appl Opt. 2005; 44(10):1792–1797

[57] Jean F, Bourg-Heckly G, Viellerobe B. Fibered confocal spectroscopy and multicolor imaging system for in vivo fluorescence analysis. Opt Express. 2007; 15(7):4008–4017

[58] Laemmel E, Genet M, Le Goualher G, Perchant A, Le Gargasson J-F, Vicaut E. Fibered confocal fluorescence microscopy (Cell-viZio) facilitates extended imaging in the field of microcirculation. A comparison with intravital microscopy. J Vasc Res. 2004; 41(5):400–411

[59] Liang C, Sung K-B, Richards-Kortum RR, Descour MR. Design of a high-numerical-aperture miniature microscope objective for an endoscopic fiber confocal reflectance microscope. Appl Opt. 2002; 41(22):4603–4610

[60] Makhlouf H, Gmitro AF, Tanbakuchi AA, Udovich JA, Rouse AR. Multispectral confocal microendoscope for in vivo and in situ imaging. J Biomed Opt. 2008; 13(4):044016

[61] Muldoon TJ, Pierce MC, Nida DL, Williams MD, Gillenwater A, Richards-Kortum R. Subcellular-resolution molecular imaging within living tissue by fiber microendoscopy. Opt Express. 2007; 15(25):16413–16423

[62] Sabharwal YS, Rouse AR, Donaldson L, Hopkins MF, Gmitro AF. Slit-scanning confocal microendoscope for high-resolution in vivo imaging. Appl Opt. 1999; 38(34):7133–7144

[63] Sun Y, Phipps J, Elson DS, et al. Fluorescence lifetime imaging microscopy: in vivo application to diagnosis of oral carcinoma. Opt Lett. 2009; 34(13):2081–2083

[64] Sung KB, Liang C, Descour M, et al. Near real time in vivo fibre optic confocal microscopy: sub-cellular structure resolved. J Microsc. 2002; 207(Pt 2):137–145

[65] Wang TD, Friedland S, Sahbaie P, et al. Functional imaging of colonic mucosa with a fibered confocal microscope for real-time in vivo pathology. Clin Gastroenterol Hepatol. 2007; 5(11):1300–1305

[66] Flusberg BA, Jung JC, Cocker ED, Anderson EP, Schnitzer MJ. In vivo brain imaging using a portable 3.9 gram two-photon fluorescence microendoscope. Opt Lett. 2005; 30(17):2272–2274

[67] Helmchen F, Fee MS, Tank DW, Denk W. A miniature head-mounted two-photon microscope. high-resolution brain imaging in freely moving animals. Neuron. 2001; 31(6):903–912

[68] Lee CM, Engelbrecht CJ, Soper TD, Helmchen F, Seibel EJ. Scanning fiber endoscopy with highly flexible, 1 mm catheterscopes for wide-field, full-color imaging. J Biophotonics. 2010; 3(5–6):385–407

[69] Ota T, Fukuyama H, Ishihara Y, Tanaka H, Takamatsu T. In situ fluorescence imaging of organs through compact scanning head for confocal laser microscopy. J Biomed Opt. 2005; 10(2):024010

[70] Seibel EJ, Smithwick QYJ. Unique features of optical scanning, single fiber endoscopy. Lasers Surg Med. 2002; 30(3):177–183

[71] Dickensheets DL, Kino GS. Micromachined scanning confocal optical microscope. Opt Lett. 1996; 21(10):764–766

[72] Piyawattanametha W, Barretto RPJ, Ko TH, et al. Fast-scanning two-photon fluorescence imaging based on a microelectromechanical systems two-dimensional scanning mirror. Opt Lett. 2006; 31(13):2018–2020

[73] Pan Y, Xie H, Fedder GK. Endoscopic optical coherence tomography based on a microelectromechanical mirror. Opt Lett. 2001; 26(24):1966–1968

[74] Ren H, Waltzer WC, Bhalla R, et al. Diagnosis of bladder cancer with microelectromechanical systems-based cystoscopic optical coherence tomography. Urology. 2009; 74(6):1351–1357

[75] Kumar K, Avritscher R, Wang Y, et al. Handheld histology-equivalent sectioning laser-scanning confocal optical microscope for interventional imaging. Biomed Microdevices. 2010; 12(2):223–233

[76] Ra H, Piyawattanametha W, Mandella MJ, et al. Three-dimensional in vivo imaging by a handheld dual-axes confocal microscope. Opt Express. 2008; 16(10):7224–7232

[77] Shin H-J, Pierce MC, Lee D, Ra H, Solgaard O, Richards-Kortum R. Fiber-optic confocal microscope using a MEMS scanner and miniature objective lens. Opt Express. 2007; 15(15):9113–9122

[78] Fu L, Jain A, Cranfield C, Xie H, Gu M. Three-dimensional nonlinear optical endoscopy. J Biomed Opt. 2007; 12(4):040501

[79] Zehri AH, Ramey W, Georges JF, et al. Neurosurgical confocal endomicroscopy: a review of contrast agents, confocal systems, and future imaging modalities. Surg Neurol Int. 2014; 5:60

[80] Belykh E, Martirosyan NL, Yagmurlu K, et al. Intraoperative fluorescence imaging for personalized brain tumor resection: current state and future directions. Front Surg. 2016; 3:55

[81] Eschbacher J, Martirosyan NL, Nakaji P, et al. In vivo intraoperative confocal microscopy for real-time histopathological imaging of brain tumors. J Neurosurg. 2012; 116(4):854–860

[82] Sanai N, Eschbacher J, Hattendorf G, et al. Intraoperative confocal microscopy for brain tumors: a feasibility analysis in humans. Neurosurgery. 2011; 68(2) suppl operative:282–290, discussion 290

[83] Rouse AR, Gmitro AF. Multispectral imaging with a confocal microendoscope. Opt Lett. 2000; 25(23):1708–1710

[84] Udovich JA, Kirkpatrick ND, Kano A, Tanbakuchi A, Utzinger U, Gmitro AF. Spectral background and transmission characteristics of fiber optic imaging bundles. Appl Opt. 2008; 47(25):4560–4568

[85] Breuskin D, Szczygielski J, Urbschat S, Kim YJ, Oertel J. Confocal laser endomicroscopy in neurosurgery-an alternative to instantaneous sections? World Neurosurg. 2017; 100:180–185

[86] Dwyer PJ, DiMarzio CA, Rajadhyaksha M. Confocal theta line-scanning microscope for imaging human tissues. Appl Opt. 2007; 46(10):1843–1851

[87] Dwyer PJ, DiMarzio CA, Zavislan JM, Fox WJ, Rajadhyaksha M. Confocal reflectance theta line scanning microscope for imaging human skin in vivo. Opt Lett. 2006; 31(7):942–944

[88] Gareau DS, Abeytunge S, Rajadhyaksha M. Line-scanning reflectance confocal microscopy of human skin: comparison of full-pupil and divided-pupil configurations. Opt Lett. 2009; 34(20):3235–3237

[89] Koester CJ, Khanna SM, Rosskothen HD, Tackaberry RB, Ulfendahl M. Confocal slit divided-aperture microscope: applications in ear research. Appl Opt. 1994; 33(4):702–708

[90] Leigh SY, Liu JTC. Multi-color miniature dual-axis confocal microscope for point-of-care pathology. Opt Lett. 2012; 37(12):2430–2432

[91] Liu JTC, Mandella MJ, Crawford JM, Contag CH, Wang TD, Kino GS. Efficient rejection of scattered light enables deep optical sectioning in turbid media with low-numerical-aperture optics in a dual-axis confocal architecture. J Biomed Opt. 2008; 13(3):034020

[92] Liu JTC, Mandella MJ, Ra H, et al. Miniature near-infrared dual-axes confocal microscope utilizing a two-dimensional microelectromechanical systems scanner. Opt Lett. 2007; 32(3):256–258

[93] Liu JTC, Mandella MJ, Friedland S, et al. Dual-axes confocal reflectance microscope for distinguishing colonic neoplasia. J Biomed Opt. 2006; 11(5):054019

[94] Chen Y, Wang D, Liu JTC. Assessing the tissue-imaging performance of confocal microscope architectures via Monte Carlo simulations. Opt Lett. 2012; 37(21):4495–4497

[95] Wong LK, Mandella MJ, Kino GS, Wang TD. Improved rejection of multiply scattered photons in confocal microscopy using dual-axes architecture. Opt Lett. 2007; 32(12):1674–1676

[96] Piyawattanametha W, Ra H, Qiu Z, et al. In vivo near-infrared dual-axis confocal microendoscopy in the human lower gastrointestinal tract. J Biomed Opt. 2012; 17(2):021102

[97] Martirosyan NL, Eschbacher JM, Kalani MY, et al. Prospective evaluation of the utility of intraoperative confocal laser endomicroscopy in patients with brain neoplasms using fluorescein sodium: experience with 74 cases. Neurosurg Focus. 2016; 40(3):E11

[98] Charalampaki P, Javed M, Daali S, Heiroth HJ, Igressa A, Weber F. Confocal laser endomicroscopy for real-time histomorphological diagnosis: our clinical experience with 150 brain and spinal tumor cases. Neurosurgery. 2015; 62 suppl 1:171–176

[99] Guyotat J. Prise en charge chirugicale des glioblastomes: les evolutions technologiques. E-memoires de Academic Nationale de Chirugie.. 2013; 12(2):67–72

[100] xCharalampaki C. Confocal Laser Endomicroscopy (CLE) during Medically Induced Neurosurgery in Craniobasal and Glioma Tumours (Cleopatra). Available at: https://clinicaltrials.gov/ct2/show/NCT02491827?term=NCT02491827&rank=12015

[101] Song L, Hennink EJ, Young IT, Tanke HJ. Photobleaching kinetics of fluorescein in quantitative fluorescence microscopy. Biophys J. 1995; 68(6):2588–2600

[102] Lim DA, Cha S, Mayo MC, et al. Relationship of glioblastoma multiforme to neural stem cell regions predicts invasive and multifocal tumor phenotype. Neuro-oncol. 2007; 9(4):424–429

[103] Sanai N, Alvarez-Buylla A, Berger MS. Neural stem cells and the origin of gliomas. N Engl J Med. 2005; 353(8):811–822

# 16 Fluorescence-Guided Surgery, Intraoperative Imaging, and Brain Mapping (iMRI, DTI, and Cortical Mapping)

*Jan Coburger and Philippe Schucht*

## Abstract

Intraoperative MRI (iMRI) and intraoperative mapping/monitoring (IOM) have synergistic effects on fluorescence-guided surgery (FGS). iMRI has been shown to increase the extent of resection (EOR) of brain tumors, particularly high-grade gliomas. In combination with FGS, iMRI may identify tumor tissue undetected by FGS, with tumor tissue hidden in a surgical operculum or behind a nonfluorescent tissue layer. Diffusion tenser imaging helps estimate the location of essential tracts, such as the arcuate fascicle or the corticospinal tract, which is of particular interest in FGS as 5-aminolevulinic acid (5-ALA) induced fluorescence does not differentiate between eloquent and noneloquent areas. Ultimately, IOM have become an indispensable part of surgery, especially in FGS. Due to the higher sensitivity of 5-ALA-induced fluorescence compared to MRI gadolinium contrast enhancement, FGS can lead to tumor resections beyond the preoperative gadolinium-enhanced T1 imaging, bringing presumed-eloquent structures into harm's way. By clarifying whether these presumed eloquent, fluorescent tissue remnants actually harbor eloquent function, IOM, in the hands of the experienced neurosurgeon, can be used to safely increase the EOR in addition to protecting neurological function. Combining safety- and resection-enhancing intraoperative technologies (IOM and FGS) has been shown to result in more extensive resections, leading to a higher success rate of gross total resections, while simultaneously improving neurological outcome. Continuous dynamic mapping has evolved as a safe, ergonomic, and time-efficient strategy of IOM and hence has become the new benchmark of intraoperative function protection.

*Keywords:* intraoperative imaging, iMRI, DTI, IOM, motor mapping, continuous dynamic mapping

## 16.1 Fluorescence-Guided Surgery and Intraoperative MRI

Many authors refer to intraoperative magnetic resonance imaging (iMRI) as the "gold standard" of intraoperative imaging techniques in brain tumor surgery since it allows for a classical tomographical image of the whole brain during surgery. iMRI shows a detailed depiction of soft tissue. Further, additionally available sequences similar to standard diagnostic MRI host a broad range of indications from intra- and extra-axial lesions up to vascular malformations and functional imaging.

### 16.1.1 Principles of Intraoperative MRI

The basic idea for development of iMRI was the issue of intraoperative brain shift due to cerebrospinal fluid loss, tumor resection, and tissue edema leading to an increasing error of neuronavigation during surgery.[1,2] The first iMRI systems were so-called open scanners or double donut scanners (▶ Fig. 16.1).[3] Surgeons were operating in between the magnetic coils. Based on this configuration, it was only feasible to perform surgery using low magnetic field strength significantly below 1 T. Pre- and postoperative imaging, however, is routinely performed on a 1.5 or even 3-T magnet usually referred to as high-field MRIs. Thus, based on the low field strength, image quality was not

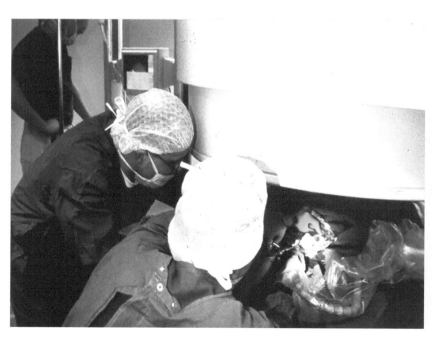

**Fig. 16.1** Magnetom open (0.2-T) installation: the surgeons are performing the case inside the isocenter of the scanner. (Reproduced with permission from Hlavac M, Konig R, Halatsch M, Wirtz CR. Intraoperative magnetic resonance imaging. Fifteen years' experience in the neurosurgical hybrid operating suite. [in German] Unfallchirurg. 2012;115(2):121–124.)

comparable to standard diagnostic imaging. Scanning time is long and the number of available sequences is limited on a low-field iMRI. Nevertheless, early data from low-field iMRI-assisted surgeries showed a safe application and a significant benefit of extent of resection (EOR) based on the chance of an intraoperative scan especially for glioma patients.[4,5,6,7] Using a low-field iMRI as well, Senft et al performed a randomized controlled trial (RCT) assessing iMRI assisted versus conventional microsurgical resection in patients with glioblastoma (GBM) tumors eligible for a gross total resection (GTR). The authors showed a significantly increased rate of GTR in the iMRI group leading to an increased progression-free survival (PFS) for those patients.[8] The data are monocentric and show a considerably lower case number as in the 5-aminolevulinic acid (5-ALA) trial by Stummer et al.[9] However, Senft et al provide the first study with

level-one evidence supporting the benefit of iMRI. Additionally, the importance of GTR as a crucial prognostic factor was emphasized. High-field iMRI systems require dedicated operating rooms (OR) with magnetic shielding and a 5-Gauss safety zone around the scanner (▶ Fig. 16.2). For an intraoperative scan, the patient is positioned in a dedicated head coil that allows for a sharp fixation of the patient's head using three or more pins (▶ Fig. 16.3). Most available head holders are flexible. However, patient positioning is limited when using high-field iMRI. Certain standard positions like park bench or sitting/semi-sitting positions are not possible. For high-field intraoperative MRI, most standard radiological diagnostic MRI scanners are used inside the OR. Thus, in contrast to low-field iMRI due to the significantly higher magnetic field, the surgery has to be performed distant from the magnet and a scan during surgery

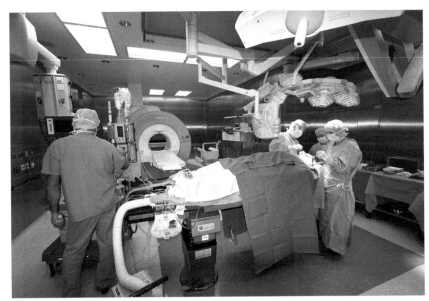

**Fig. 16.2** Hybrid operating room (Brainsuite by Brainlab, Feldkirchen, Germany) during an intracranial procedure at the University of Ulm, Campus Günzburg, Germany. The patient is fixed in a dedicated head holder. For an intraoperative scan, the OR table can be turned 90 degrees and the patient can be slid into the MRI bore. (Reproduced with permission from Hlavac M, Konig R, Halatsch M, Wirtz CR. Intraoperative magnetic resonance imaging. Fifteen years' experience in the neurosurgical hybrid operating suite. [in German] Unfallchirurg. 2012;115 (2):121–124.)

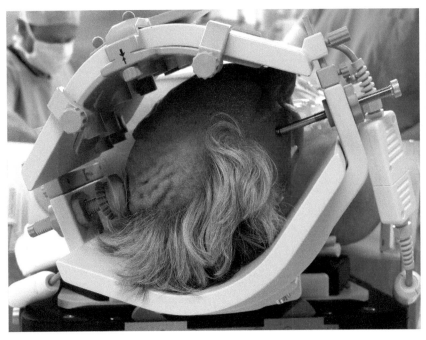

**Fig. 16.3** Patient fixated in a two-part eight-channel head coil integrated in a dedicated holder for automatic intraoperative registration (Noras MRI Products, Höchberg, Germany). For an intraoperative scan, the upper part of the coil is mounted. During surgery, this part is removed.

requires a transfer of the patient into the scanner as shown in ▸ Fig. 16.4. Due to the increased image acquisition speed in the high-field MRI, the overall workflow is improved compared to low-field iMRI.[10] Some centers even use the intraoperative MRI in a two-room solution for routine diagnostic imaging and intraoperative imaging for brain tumors (▸ Fig. 16.5).[11]

The development of high-field iMRI (1.5 and 3.0 T) allows for comparable image quality and similar available sequences as in routine diagnostic MRI. Tumor depiction is similar to preoperative imaging. ▸ Fig. 16.6 shows a T1 MPRAGE sequence with contrast from an intraoperative scan with the skull open. Assessment of images is simplified, and better depiction of residual tumor is possible due to increased image resolution during glioma and pituitary surgery when compared to low-field imaging.[10] The rate of GTR in low-grade gliomas was found to be increased in a retrospective multicenter series when a high-field iMRI was used instead of a low-field iMRI.[12] Further,

advances in diagnostic imaging can usually be translated to intraoperative use.

## 16.1.2 Intraoperative Diffusion Tenser Imaging and Its Clinical Implications

During glioma surgery, high-field iMRI allows for intraoperative functional imaging sequences that can be of high surgical value. Especially relevant in this regard is the acquisition of diffusion tenser imaging (DTI) data.[13] Based on this MRI sequence, a probabilistic or deterministic fiber tracking of functional relevant cerebral tracts like the corticospinal tract (CST), arcuate fascicle, or optic radiation can be performed preoperatively and integrated in the neuronavigation system.[14,15] Using high-field iMRI, these data can be updated intraoperatively. It has been shown that due to intraoperative brain shift, a significant

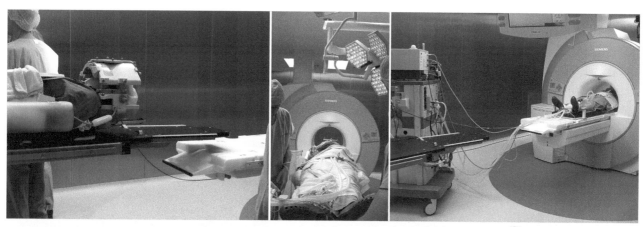

**Fig. 16.4** Transfer of the patient from OR table to MRI table and insight into the MRI scanner (from left to right).

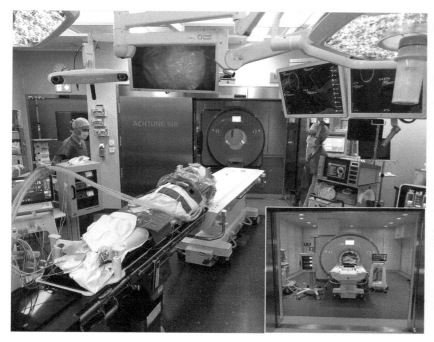

**Fig. 16.5** Two-room solution of a 1.5-T installation at the Department of Neurosurgery, Bern, Switzerland.

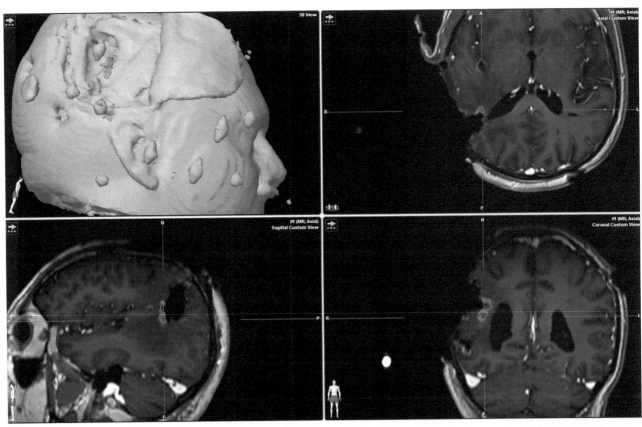

**Fig. 16.6** Screenshot of the navigation system (Iplan 3.0, Brainlab, Germany) demonstrating the intraoperative MRI scan (T1 MPRAGE with Gd-DTPA on a Simens Espree 1.5-T scanner; Erlangen, Germany) with open skull depicting residual faint contrast enhancement after microsurgical resection of the solid part of a glioblastoma. Residual enhancement was segmented in the navigation system (red object) and resected. It revealed tumor in all sections.

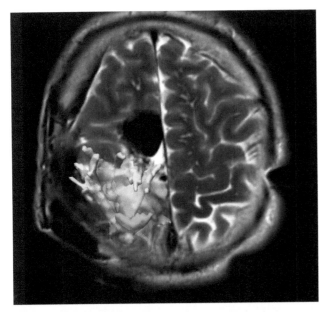

**Fig. 16.7** Significant shift of the corticospinal tract (CST) during resection of a diffuse astrocytoma. Green shows the CST in preoperative fiber tracking and yellow shows the intraoperative data. A significant shift of the CST anteriorly toward the resection cavity was noticed, which could be replicated by subcortical mapping during surgery.

change of the position of crucial tracts like the CST can occur.[16] ▶ Fig. 16.7 shows an intraoperative example of shift of the CST that was verified by intraoperative subcortical mapping. iMRI-based intraoperative tractography shows a high sensitivity localizing the CST.[17] However, intraoperative DTI imaging data can be disturbed by artifacts surgeons should be aware of. Especially in superficial locations or in resection cavities that cannot be filled with saline properly during the iMRI scan, the air to brain interface can distort DTI images significantly.[18] Thus, a combined use of subcortical mapping of the CST and an intraoperative update of DTI images using iMRI is the method of choice to maximize safety for patients.

### 16.1.3 Intraoperative Functional Imaging

Additional MRI sequences beyond gadolinium-diethylenetri-amine pentaacetic acid (Gd-DTPA) enhanced T1, T2, FLAIR, and diffusion-weighted imaging (DWI) are perfusion-weighted imaging (PWI) and MRI spectroscopy. Both methods are of significant value in diagnostic imaging but can also be used to detect residual tumor intraoperatively.[19,20] ▶ Fig. 16.8 shows an example of intraoperative PWI compared to preoperative diagnostic imaging and amino acid PET (AA-PET) imaging. Even resting state connectivity networks were assessed intraoperatively in a first pilot

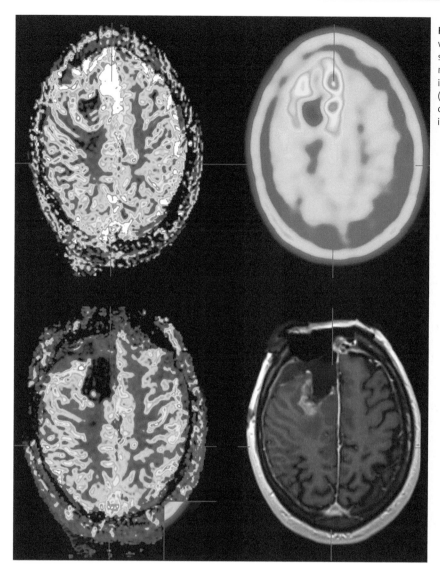

**Fig. 16.8** Comparison of preoperative perfusion-weighted imaging (cerebral blood volume sequence) (upper left) and preoperative methionine PET-CT (upper right) and intraoperative perfusion-weighted imaging (lower left) and intraoperative T1 gadolinium-diethylenetriamine pentaacetic acid enhanced images (lower right).

study during general anesthesia, proving very interesting future perspective for functional imaging in patients with eloquent gliomas.[21]

## 16.1.4 Limitations of Intraoperative MRI

Concerning surgical workflow, an intraoperative MRI scan is time consuming, especially if additional diagnostic sequences beyond the routine are performed. Further, repetitive administration of Gd-DTPA leads to a nonspecific parenchymal enhancement. Surgical induced changes in T2 might further lead to a decrease of specificity after repetitive scans.[22] Thus, while theoretically a GTR should be possible using iMRI as the gold standard of intraoperative imaging in all eligible cases, several practical constraints might hamper a GTR also when using iMRI. In the literature, EOR with iMRI in a patient in whom a GTR was feasible is reported to be around 97%.[8,23,24] Additionally to the interruption of surgical workflow, constructional requirements and high primary costs hamper the distribution of the technique. A central issue in the assessment of a method for accuracy of tumor detection is the definition of a lesion in the typical imaging techniques. In GBM, typically contrast-enhanced T1 imaging is used to define the borders of the solid tumor. Based on AA-PET and histopathological studies, it is well known that the tumor extends well beyond the borders of the contrast enhancement.[25,26,27,28] Thus, high-field iMRI-based resection is limited by the general interpretation of MRI data by surgeons and the respective conclusions and strategies derived from it.

## 16.1.5 Combined Use of 5-ALA and Intraoperative MRI

Other intraoperative imaging or visualization techniques like 5-ALA provide a different depiction of tumor tissue based on the technique itself. Due to the direct metabolism of 5-ALA to fluorescent protoporphyrin IX (PpIX), 5-ALA provides better detection of solid and invasive tumor compared to intraoperative Gd-DTPA enhancement alone during iMRI.[29] However, a single center retrospective analysis shows a potential advantage concerning rate of GTR of iMRI-assisted resection compared to 5-ALA-based surgery alone.[24] This might be due to the

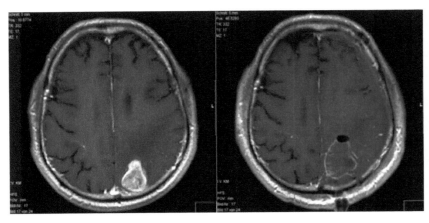

**Fig. 16.9** Gadolinium-enhanced T1-weighted MR sequences before and after fluorescence-guided surgery of a glioblastoma. The resection cavity (right side, postoperative) appears larger than the preoperative contrast-enhancing tumor (left side): resection based on 5-aminolevulinic acid fluorescence went further than gadolinium enhancement. (Reproduced with permission from Schucht et al.[33])

intraoperative update of navigation data and the excellent overview of the resection cavity using an intraoperative MRI. Further, potential satellite lesions can be detected with iMRI that might be missed using 5-ALA.

Based on the different ways of tumor detection, there is a high potential for a combined use of 5-ALA and iMRI. Ideally, the tumor resection is performed using 5-ALA and intraoperative continuous monitoring. After complete resection of fluorescent tissue, iMRI may identify tumor tissue undetected by FGS, either because the tissue resides behind a nonfluorescent tissue layer or in a "surgical operculum." Typical spots may be below a cottonoid, a retractor, or in a part of the resection cavity that cannot be visualized directly with the fluorescence-emitting light. Further, intraoperative DTI helps estimate the location of essential tracts, such as the arcuate fascicle or the CST, which is of particular interest in FGS as 5-ALA fluorescence does not differentiate between eloquent and noneloquent areas. A prospective study comparing the combined use of iMRI and 5-ALA with use of iMRI only showed a significant increase of EOR with increasing neurological deficits. However, no benefit of PFS or OS could be shown so far.[23] Hence, the synergistic use of FGS with intraoperative MRI and continuous intraoperative mapping/monitoring (IOM) may be the ideal strategy in high-grade glioma (HGG) surgery.

## 16.2 Fluorescence-Guided Surgery and Brain Mapping

### 16.2.1 Influence of FGS on the Extent of Tumor Resection

The use of 5-ALA FGS as an intraoperative method of optical imaging has become increasingly popular in the wake of the milestone RCT by Stummer et al.[9] But which part of the infiltrating glioma does 5-ALA fluorescence detect? Different from gadolinium-based MRI, which largely shows the degree of disruption of the blood–brain barrier, 5-ALA-induced fluorescence is a metabolic marker that also depends on a variety of other factors, mainly the oncometabolism of the glioma cell and the altered microenvironment.[30] To believe that these two imaging modalities—gadolinium-enhanced T1 MRI and 5-ALA-induced fluorescence—show the same volume of the diffusely

infiltrating glioma would be a bold and potentially dangerous assumption.

Various investigations have revealed that 5-ALA-induced fluorescence has a higher sensitivity for coalescent glioma than gadolinium-enhanced T1 MRI.[31,32] Given the known high specificity of 5-ALA-induced fluorescence for detecting glioma tissue, we must assume that FGS is more efficient in detecting and guiding glioma resection than relying only on MRI.[31] This implies that performing a 5-ALA complete resection of the contrast-enhancing tumor ultimately leads to a larger resection volume than the surgeon anticipated based on preoperative gadolinium-enhanced T1 imaging. In fact, a volumetric analysis revealed that 5-ALA FGS complete resections significantly extend beyond the volume of corresponding preoperative gadolinium-enhancing compartments on MRI and that this effect is often obscured by the shift of peritumoral tissue into the resection cavity after glioma resection (▶ Fig. 16.9).[33]

### 16.2.2 Risks of Neurological Deficits in Fluorescence-Guided Surgery

The increased volume of resection in FGS could lead to an increased rate of neurological deficits if eloquent brain tissue that appears to be outside of the gadolinium-enhancing tumor bulk on preoperative (or intraoperative) MRI reveals fluorescence and is subsequently resected. This hypothesis is supported by findings of Stummer's RCT, in which the rate of postoperative neurological deficits was higher in patients undergoing 5-ALA FGS compared to white-light surgery (26.2 and 14.5% after 48 hours, and 17.1 and 11.3% after 6 weeks, for FGS and white-light surgery, respectively).[34] It is worth mentioning that the rate of complete resection of the contrast enhancing tumor in this trial was increased from roughly 36 to 65% of cases, and not to nearly 100%, as one might have hoped given the higher sensitivity of 5-ALA-induced tumor fluorescence. As a matter of fact, surgeons were aware of residual tumor being left behind based on concerns for function in 30% of cases. Sophisticated mapping and monitoring techniques were rarely used in that study at the time. Surgeons' concerns for neurological deficits was the most important factor limiting resection. This emphasizes how an unclear functional border at a later stage of resection represents a risk factor for both neurological deficits and incomplete resection.

## 16.2.3 Brain Mapping and Fluorescence-Guided Surgery

### Does Brain Mapping Limit the Benefits of FGS?

If a glioma appears to be safely resectable based on preoperative imaging, it does not automatically imply that a 5-ALA complete resection is safely feasible. As a rule of thumb, a rim of 1 cm around the enhancing glioma should be regarded as tissue at risk of being potentially targeted by 5-ALA FGS.[33] Clarifying whether an area of presumed eloquence actually is eloquent by means of intraoperative electrophysiology becomes a decisive necessity of surgery, and has a significant protective effect on neurological function.[35] Does this benefit of maintaining neurological integrity (and thus, quality of life) come at the price of a smaller extent of tumor resection resulting in an inferior oncological benefit of surgery? Is there a fixed trade-off between neurological integrity and the oncological benefit of surgery? Or is it possible that IOM even increases the extent of HGG resection since it identifies the exact borders of resection, permitting the surgeon to resect a glioma right up to areas of eloquence without safety margins? A trial on 53 consecutive patients with gliomas amenable to a complete resection of enhancing tumor (CRET; criteria identical to the Stummer RCT) evaluated the influence of combining FGS with IOM and reported a 96% rate of CRET with a 7.5% rate of neurological deficits,[36] which compares favorably to the FGS cohort of the Stummer RCT, which did not undergo IOM. One reason why the FGS cohort in the Stummer RCT had a rate of (only) 65% complete resections despite using fluorescence was that the surgeons did in fact fear that they were approaching eloquent areas during resection. The increased rate of postoperative neurological deficits (17%) suggests that their fear was at least partially justified. Adding IOM might have clarified in which areas surgery should have been continued and in which it should have been stopped.

### Synergistic Effects of Brain Mapping and FGS

Hence, IOM does not restrict the EOR but rather allows resection beyond a safety margin and up to the real functional boundary of a tumor. This is of particular importance in 5-ALA FGS, since fluorescence can be visualized beyond the MRI gadolinium contrast enhancement, extending resections closer to eloquent structures than a surgeon might have assumed based on the preoperative MRI. In conclusion, mapping and monitoring of motor function not only helps avoid permanent motor deficits, but also indirectly increases the success rate of radical resection by clarifying the functional relevance of a presumably eloquent area. Combining safety- and resection-enhancing intraoperative technologies (IOM and FGS) does indeed allow for more extensive resections and improves neurological outcome at the same time.

## 16.2.4 Modalities of Intraoperative Mapping/Monitoring

### Cortical and Subcortical Mapping

Cortical mapping of motor and speech function is crucial in the initial stages of surgery,[37] as it clarifies whether a certain area can be resected or used as an entry point to a deep-seated lesion. However, the biggest challenge often looms toward the end of surgery, when neuronavigation has gradually lost its accuracy and tumor decompression has shifted eloquent structures into the resection cavity and into harm's way. The oncological advantage of a more radical resection may now be counterweighed by an increasing risk of neurological deficits: removal of the last 1 to 2% of the contrast-enhancing (or fluorescent) glioma not only has the greatest survival impact from an oncological point of view, but also carries the greatest risk for neurological impairment.[38,39,40]

### Motor Mapping for Identification of Function; MEP Monitoring to Check for Functional Integrity

Monitoring of motor evoked potentials (MEPs) by direct cortical stimulation using a strip electrode provides a continuous real-time assessment of the functional integrity of the CST.[41,42] Although MEPs are a useful predictor of postoperative motor deficits, their actual stand-alone value during surgery is limited because signal alterations may be abrupt and irreversible as the damage may already be complete by the time MEP monitoring warns the surgeon.

Motor mapping has drawbacks as well. Even though it provides reliable information on the functional relevance of an area prior to resection,[43] damage proximal to the stimulation site may go unnoticed by mapping since it only verifies the functional integrity from the site of stimulation toward the spinal cord and fails to detect damage of the CST proximal to the stimulation site. Combining mapping with monitoring abrogates this risk. MEP monitoring confirms the functional integrity of the primary motor system, while mapping informs of the functional relevance of the tissue visualized during surgery.[44]

### Continuous Dynamic Mapping Keeps Neurological Deficits at Bay in FGS

Continuous dynamic mapping is a strategy that uses high-frequency train stimulation on a monopolar probe that has been integrated into the surgeon's resection tools, preferably the suction device.[45] High-frequency short train stimulation is associated with a lower incidence of intraoperative seizures, allowing continuous stimulation. Integrating the monopolar probe into the suction device abrogates the need to switch back and forth between resection instruments and the mapping probe (▶ Fig. 16.10). In addition, motor thresholds can be used to analyze the current-to-distance relationship, not only informing the surgeon of the function of the tissue in sight, but also giving the surgeon an estimate of the remaining distance to the CST. As part of this strategy, motor mapping becomes a radarlike, real-time information system on the spatial relationship of the resection site and eloquent motor structures, instead of being a time-consuming interruption of resection. Synchronized with tumor removal, continuous dynamic mapping overcomes the temporal and spatial limitations of classic subcortical mapping of the CST and has been shown to keep neurological deficits very low, even during surgery within primary motor areas (▶ Fig. 16.11).[46]

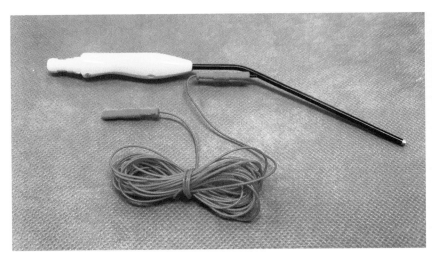

**Fig. 16.10** Continuous dynamic mapping device. The suction is electrically isolated up to its tip. Thanks to a connection beneath the handle, the suction device can be used as a stimulation probe.

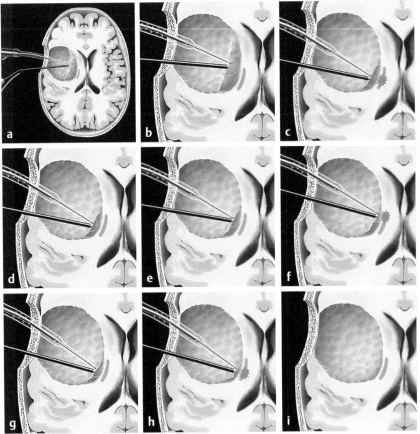

**Fig. 16.11** Strategy of continuous dynamic mapping. The device is used as a suction device parallel to the resection tool. Once an estimated distance of 10 to 15 mm to the corticospinal tract (CST) is reached, the device is activated (**a**). An initial stimulation intensity of 10 to 15 mA is used, corresponding to an estimated distance of 10 to 15 mm (**b**). The instant a motor evoked potential (MEP) is triggered the surgeon is warned by a switch from the high-pitch negative control sound to a low-pitch alert sound (**c**). The stimulation intensity is then reduced by 2 mA, and the resection is continued at sites negative for the set current (**d,e**), until again the change from the negative control to the alert sound warns the surgeon that the next motor threshold has been reached (**f**). This stepwise approach is continued until a minimal threshold is reached (**g–i**). Pink indicates tumor tissue, blue indicates CST fibers, and green indicates the electrical field that elicits an MEP and triggers the alert sound if it reaches the CST (*red star*). (Reproduced from Schucht et al[43] with permission. (c) Inselspital Bern.)

# References

[1] Trantakis C, Tittgemeyer M, Schneider JP, et al. Investigation of time-dependency of intracranial brain shift and its relation to the extent of tumor removal using intra-operative MRI. Neurol Res. 2003; 25(1):9–12

[2] Nimsky C, Ganslandt O, Cerny S, Hastreiter P, Greiner G, Fahlbusch R. Quantification of, visualization of, and compensation for brain shift using intraoperative magnetic resonance imaging. Neurosurgery. 2000; 47(5):1070–1079, discussion 1079–1080

[3] Albert FK, et al. Intraoperative diagnostic and interventional MRI. In: Hellwig D, Bauer B, eds. Neurosurgery: First Experience with an "Open MR" System, in Minimally Invasive Techniques for Neurosurgery. Berlin: Springer; 1998:229–235

[4] Wirtz CR, Knauth M, Staubert A, et al. Clinical evaluation and follow-up results for intraoperative magnetic resonance imaging in neurosurgery. Neurosurgery. 2000; 46(5):1112–1120, discussion 1120–1122

[5] Nimsky C, Fujita A, Ganslandt O, Von Keller B, Fahlbusch R. Volumetric assessment of glioma removal by intraoperative high-field magnetic resonance imaging. Neurosurgery. 2004; 55(2):358–370, discussion 370–371

[6] Black PM, Alexander E, III, Martin C, et al. Craniotomy for tumor treatment in an intraoperative magnetic resonance imaging unit. Neurosurgery. 1999; 45(3):423–431, discussion 431–433

[7] Nabavi A, Mamisch CT, Gering DT, et al. Image-guided therapy and intraoperative MRI in neurosurgery. Minim Invasive Ther Allied Technol. 2000; 9(3)(4):277–286

[8] Senft C, Bink A, Franz K, Vatter H, Gasser T, Seifert V. Intraoperative MRI guidance and extent of resection in glioma surgery: a randomised, controlled trial. Lancet Oncol. 2011; 12(11):997–1003

[9] Stummer W, Pichlmeier U, Meinel T, Wiestler OD, Zanella F, Reulen HJ, ALA-Glioma Study Group. Fluorescence-guided surgery with 5-aminolevulinic acid for resection of malignant glioma: a randomised controlled multicentre phase III trial. Lancet Oncol. 2006; 7(5):392–401

[10] Nimsky C, Ganslandt O, Fahlbusch R. Comparing 0.2 tesla with 1.5 tesla intraoperative magnetic resonance imaging analysis of setup, workflow, and efficiency. Acad Radiol. 2005; 12(9):1065–1079

[11] Pamir MN, Ozduman K, Dinçer A, Yildiz E, Peker S, Ozek MM. First intraoperative, shared-resource, ultrahigh-field 3-Tesla magnetic resonance imaging system and its application in low-grade glioma resection. J Neurosurg. 2010; 112(1):57–69

[12] Coburger J, Merkel A, Scherer M, et al. Low-grade glioma surgery in intraoperative magnetic resonance imaging: results of a multicenter retrospective assessment of the German study group for intraoperative magnetic resonance imaging. Neurosurgery. 2016; 78(6):775–786

[13] Basser PJ, Mattiello J, LeBihan D. MR diffusion tensor spectroscopy and imaging. Biophys J. 1994; 66(1):259–267

[14] Nimsky C, Ganslandt O, Fahlbusch R. Implementation of fiber tract navigation. Neurosurgery. 2006; 58(4) suppl 2:292–303, discussion 303–304

[15] Kuhnt D, Bauer MH, Becker A, et al. Intraoperative visualization of fiber tracking based reconstruction of language pathways in glioma surgery. Neurosurgery. 2012; 70(4):911–919, discussion 919–920

[16] Nimsky C, Ganslandt O, Hastreiter P, et al. Preoperative and intraoperative diffusion tensor imaging-based fiber tracking in glioma surgery. Neurosurgery. 2005; 56(1):130–137, discussion 138

[17] Javadi SA, et al. Evaluation of diffusion tensor imaging-based tractography of the corticospinal tract: a correlative study with intraoperative magnetic resonance imaging and direct electrical subcortical stimulation. Neurosurgery. 2016

[18] Ostrý S, Belšan T, Otáhal J, Beneš V, Netuka D. Is intraoperative diffusion tensor imaging at 3.0 T comparable to subcortical corticospinal tract mapping? Neurosurgery. 2013; 73(5):797–807, discussion 806–807

[19] Roder C, Skardelly M, Ramina KF, et al. Spectroscopy imaging in intraoperative MR suite: tissue characterization and optimization of tumor resection. Int J CARS. 2014; 9(4):551–559

[20] Roder C, et al. Intraoperative visualization of residual tumor: the role of perfusion-weighted imaging in a high-field intraoperative MR scanner. Neurosurgery. 2012

[21] Roder C, Charyasz-Leks E, Breitkopf M, et al. Resting-state functional MRI in an intraoperative MRI setting: proof of feasibility and correlation to clinical outcome of patients. J Neurosurg. 2016; 125(2):401–409

[22] Knauth M, Aras N, Wirtz CR, Dörfler A, Engelhorn T, Sartor K. Surgically induced intracranial contrast enhancement: potential source of diagnostic error in intraoperative MR imaging. AJNR Am J Neuroradiol. 1999; 20(8):1547–1553

[23] Coburger J, Hagel V, Wirtz CR, König R. Surgery for glioblastoma: impact of the combined use of 5-aminolevulinic acid and intraoperative MRI on extent of resection and survival. PLoS One. 2015; 10(6):e0131872

[24] Roder C, Bisdas S, Ebner FH, et al. Maximizing the extent of resection and survival benefit of patients in glioblastoma surgery: high-field iMRI versus conventional and 5-ALA-assisted surgery. Eur J Surg Oncol. 2014; 40(3):297–304

[25] Yamahara T, Numa Y, Oishi T, et al. Morphological and flow cytometric analysis of cell infiltration in glioblastoma: a comparison of autopsy brain and neuroimaging. Brain Tumor Pathol. 2010; 27(2):81–87

[26] Pirotte BJ, Levivier M, Goldman S, et al. Positron emission tomography-guided volumetric resection of supratentorial high-grade gliomas: a survival analysis in 66 consecutive patients. Neurosurgery. 2009; 64(3):471–481, discussion 481

[27] Stockhammer F, Misch M, Horn P, Koch A, Fonyuy N, Plotkin M. Association of F18-fluoro-ethyl-tyrosin uptake and 5-aminolevulinic acid-induced fluorescence in gliomas. Acta Neurochir (Wien). 2009; 151(11):1377–1383

[28] Arbizu J, Tejada S, Marti-Climent JM, et al. Quantitative volumetric analysis of gliomas with sequential MRI and 11C-methionine PET assessment: patterns of integration in therapy planning. Eur J Nucl Med Mol Imaging. 2012; 39(5):771–781

[29] Coburger J, Engelke J, Scheuerle A, et al. Tumor detection with 5-aminolevulinic acid fluorescence and Gd-DTPA-enhanced intraoperative MRI at the border of contrast-enhancing lesions: a prospective study based on histopathological assessment. Neurosurg Focus. 2014; 36(2):E3

[30] Collaud S, Juzeniene A, Moan J, Lange N. On the selectivity of 5-aminolevulinic acid-induced protoporphyrin IX formation. Curr Med Chem Anticancer Agents. 2004; 4(3):301–316

[31] Stummer W, Novotny A, Stepp H, Goetz C, Bise K, Reulen HJ. Fluorescence-guided resection of glioblastoma multiforme by using 5-aminolevulinic acid-induced porphyrins: a prospective study in 52 consecutive patients. J Neurosurg. 2000; 93(6):1003–1013

[32] Stummer W, Reulen HJ, Meinel T, et al. ALA-Glioma Study Group. Extent of resection and survival in glioblastoma multiforme: identification of and adjustment for bias. Neurosurgery. 2008; 62(3):564–576, discussion 564–576

[33] Schucht P, Knittel S, Slotboom J, et al. 5-ALA complete resections go beyond MR contrast enhancement: shift corrected volumetric analysis of the extent of resection in surgery for glioblastoma. Acta Neurochir (Wien). 2014; 156(2):305–312, discussion 312

[34] Stummer W, Tonn JC, Mehdorn HM, et al. ALA-Glioma Study Group. Counterbalancing risks and gains from extended resections in malignant glioma surgery: a supplemental analysis from the randomized 5-aminolevulinic acid glioma resection study. Clinical article. J Neurosurg. 2011; 114(3):613–623

[35] De Witt Hamer PC, Robles SG, Zwinderman AH, Duffau H, Berger MS. Impact of intraoperative stimulation brain mapping on glioma surgery outcome: a meta-analysis. J Clin Oncol. 2012; 30(20):2559–2565

[36] Schucht P, Beck J, Abu-Isa J, et al. Gross total resection rates in contemporary glioblastoma surgery: results of an institutional protocol combining 5-aminolevulinic acid intraoperative fluorescence imaging and brain mapping. Neurosurgery. 2012; 71(5):927–935, discussion 935–936

[37] Berger MS, Kincaid J, Ojemann GA, Lettich E. Brain mapping techniques to maximize resection, safety, and seizure control in children with brain tumors. Neurosurgery. 1989; 25(5):786–792

[38] Kreth FW, Thon N, Simon M, et al. German Glioma Network. Gross total but not incomplete resection of glioblastoma prolongs survival in the era of radiochemotherapy. Ann Oncol. 2013; 24(12):3117–3123

[39] Stummer W, van den Bent MJ, Westphal M. Cytoreductive surgery of glioblastoma as the key to successful adjuvant therapies: new arguments in an old discussion. Acta Neurochir (Wien). 2011; 153(6):1211–1218

[40] Stupp R, Mason WP, van den Bent MJ, et al. European Organisation for Research and Treatment, of Cancer Brain Tumor and Radiotherapy Groups, National Cancer Institute of Canada Clinical Trials Group. Radiotherapy plus concomitant and adjuvant temozolomide for glioblastoma. N Engl J Med. 2005; 352(10):987–996

[41] Neuloh G, Pechstein U, Cedzich C, Schramm J. Motor evoked potential monitoring with supratentorial surgery. Neurosurgery. 2004; 54(5):1061–1070, discussion 1070–1072

[42]  Sala F, Lanteri P. Brain surgery in motor areas: the invaluable assistance of intraoperative neurophysiological monitoring. J Neurosurg Sci. 2003; 47(2): 79–88

[43]  Schucht P, Seidel K, Beck J, et al. Intraoperative monopolar mapping during 5-ALA-guided resections of glioblastomas adjacent to motor eloquent areas: evaluation of resection rates and neurological outcome. Neurosurg Focus. 2014; 37(6):E16

[44]  Seidel K, Beck J, Stieglitz L, Schucht P, Raabe A. The warning-sign hierarchy between quantitative subcortical motor mapping and continuous motor evoked potential monitoring during resection of supratentorial brain tumors. J Neurosurg. 2013; 118:287–296

[45]  Seidel K, Beck J, Stieglitz L, Schucht P, Raabe A. Low-threshold monopolar motor mapping for resection of primary motor cortex tumors. Neurosurg. 2012; 71(1 Suppl Operative):104–115

[46]  Raabe A, Beck J, Schucht P, Seidel K. Continuous dynamic mapping of the corticospinal tract during surgery of motor eloquent brain tumors: evaluation of a new method. J Neurosurg. 2014; 120(5):1015–1024

# 17  Raman Spectroscopy and Brain Tumors

*Todd C. Hollon, Steven N. Kalkanis, and Daniel A. Orringer*

## Abstract

Label-free imaging techniques rely on the intrinsic biochemical properties of tissues to generate image contrast and identify tumor infiltration. Spontaneous and coherent Raman scattering techniques allow for chemical characterization of the underlying tissue. Raman spectroscopy can detect variations in water, lipid, protein, and cholesterol content of normal versus brain tumor tissue. Raman spectra analysis allows neurosurgeons to reliably differentiate normal tissue, necrotic, and viable tumor in fresh and frozen surgical specimens. By focusing on specific regions of the Raman spectra, coherent Raman scattering microscopy can be used to rapidly generate histologic images. Stimulated Raman scattering (SRS) microscopy can detect brain tumor infiltration with high (> 90%) accuracy. Advances in fiber-laser technology have allowed for the development of a clinical SRS microscope for intraoperative brain tumor diagnosis. In stimulated Raman histology, a hematoxylin and eosin color scheme is applied to SRS data, yielding a label-free intraoperative pathology method, enabling rapid and accurate brain tumor diagnosis. In this chapter, we review how Raman-based techniques can improve the surgical management of brain tumor patients by detecting tumor infiltration, guiding tumor biopsy/resection, and providing label-free images for accurate histopathologic diagnosis.

*Keywords:* Raman spectroscopy, hyperspectral Raman microscopy, coherent Raman imaging, stimulated Raman scattering microscopy, stimulated Raman histology, coherent anti-Stokes Raman scattering microscopy, label-free histology, intraoperative pathology

## 17.1  Introduction

Image-guided neurosurgery for the treatment of central nervous system (CNS) tumors has resulted in greater extent of resection and improved patient outcomes.[1,2,3] Intraoperative imaging techniques allow neurosurgeons to evaluate residual tumor burden that would have otherwise gone undetected.[4,5] Fluorescence-guided neurosurgery represents a major advancement for the surgical treatment of CNS tumors in the 21st century. Wide-field fluorescence imaging using 5-aminolevulinic acid (5-ALA) in high-grade gliomas enables more complete tumor resections, thereby improving progression-free survival. However, any imaging method that relies on labeling agents will face the challenge of nonspecific or nonsensitive tumor detection in the operative setting.[6]

Label-free methods rely on the intrinsic biochemical properties of normal and lesional tissue to provide image contrast. Raman-based imaging modalities have emerged as promising label-free methods for the detection and diagnosis of primary and metastatic CNS tumors.[7,8,9] Spontaneous Raman spectroscopy and coherent Raman scattering (CRS) microscopy have both found applications in image-guided neurosurgery with promising results. Here, we provide a brief description of spontaneous and CRS. We then detail the applications of Raman-based modalities to image-guided neurosurgery.

## 17.2  Overview of Spontaneous Raman Scattering

Elastic photon scattering (i.e., Rayleigh's scattering) occurs when an incident photon has the same wavelength as the scattered photon after interacting with a media or tissue. The majority of photons in the visible spectrum (380–750 nm) are scattered elastically. A small proportion of photons transfer energy to (red-shift, Stokes scattering) or absorb energy from (blue-shift, anti-Stokes scattering) the object being imaged. This transfer of energy results in inelastic scattering and is called the Raman effect, discovered in 1930.[10] The energy difference between the incident and scattered photon is called the Raman shift and is measured in wavenumbers (waves per centimeter). The Raman effect is weak relative to elastic scattering. However, using narrowband laser excitation and a sensitive spectrometer, Raman scattering can be detected and measured to generate spectra from the incident tissue.

Raman spectroscopy has wide applications in chemistry and biology for its ability to characterize individual molecules and biological tissues. The Raman spectrum of a molecule can be determined by measuring the Raman shifts caused by interactions with each of its constituent chemical bonds. Raman spectral peaks correspond to specific vibrational modes (e.g., stretching, bending, or scissoring) produced by the chemical bond. For example, the –CH2 symmetric stretching mode plays an essential role in characterizing biological tissues using Raman spectroscopy due to its high concentration in fatty acids. Raman spectra can therefore be used as a means to quantify the chemical composition of biological tissues. The vibrational fingerprint of biological tissues is a product of its composition of macromolecules (i.e., nucleic acids, protein, and lipids) and the sum of the vibrational spectra of the tissue constituents. Investigators hypothesized that the chemical differences between normal tissue and tumor may produce sufficiently distinct Raman spectra to allow accurate detection of brain tumor infiltration.

### 17.2.1  Raman Spectroscopy for Brain Tumor Detection

Early investigations using spontaneous Raman spectroscopy to characterize brain tissue were conducted in the 1990s and involved distinguishing normal versus edematous brain.[11] A strong 3,390/cm Raman peak corresponding the O–H stretching mode identified greater water content in edematous brain. Krafft and colleagues were instrumental in performing influential early studies on the applications of Raman spectroscopy in neuro-oncology.[12] After performing a detailed spectral analysis of 12 major brain lipids,[12] they were able to differentiate glioblastoma tissue from healthy brain tissue using lipid and water content and they confirmed these differences using mass spectroscopy.[13] The same group performed a landmark proof-of-concept study employing Raman spectroscopy to detect intracerebral tumors in vivo by brain surface mapping.[14] In a murine metastatic brain tumor model, hyperspectral Raman spectroscopy covering $3.6 \times 3.2$ mm of cortical surface was able to detect melanotic tumors in the murine brain. The Raman spectra of the metastatic tumors display additional Raman shifts near 597, 976, 1,404, and 1,595/cm due to melanin pigment contribution.

Several studies have investigated using Raman spectroscopy for intraoperative brain tumor biopsy guidance. Identifying regions of vital tumor in glioblastoma increases the diagnostic yield of biopsy specimens. Necrotic specimens from brain tumor biopsies show a prominent Raman peak at 1,739/cm, consistent with significantly higher concentration of cholesterol and cholesteryl esters.[15] Using linear discriminant analysis of specimen spectral data, accuracy for discriminating necrotic versus vital tumor approaches 100% (► Fig. 17.1). Leveraging these spectral differences, Kalkanis and colleagues were able to differentiate normal brain, necrosis, and glioblastoma tissue in frozen brain tumor sections with an accuracy of 97.8%.[8] In a subsequent investigation, five frozen sections (normal, necrosis, dense glioblastoma, and two infiltrating glioblastoma) were mapped at five Raman shift wavenumbers across the entire specimen in 300 μm² step sizes.[16] Tissue maps were able to identify boundaries between gray and white matter, necrosis, glioblastoma, and infiltrating tumor. Further narrowing to three key Raman spectral regions allowed for the development of a virtual red, green, and blue (RGB) color scheme.[17] Red (1,004/cm channel), green (1,300:1,344/cm channel), and blue (1,600/cm channel) color scales were assigned to Raman peak intensities and fused for multichannel imaging (► Fig. 17.2). The multichannel color maps were used to discriminate white matter, gray matter, and tumor tissue with diagnostic accuracy of approximately 90% on a cross-validation.

Improvements in fiber-laser technology have allowed for the development of a Raman spectroscopy probe system for in vivo intraoperative brain tissue classification.[18] In a recent clinical study, a handheld fiberoptic probe was placed in direct contact with the brain in the resection cavities of 17 patients with gliomas (low and high grade; ► Fig. 17.3).[19] Time to image acquisition was 0.2 seconds for each area interrogated and measured 0.5 mm in diameter; sampling depth of the probe was 1 mm. Using a boosted tree method to analyze intraoperative Raman spectra, the investigators were able to distinguish normal brain from tumor-invaded brain (> 15% tumor cell invasion) with an

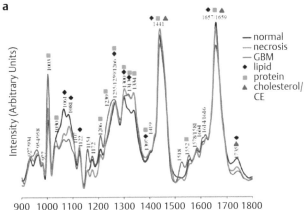

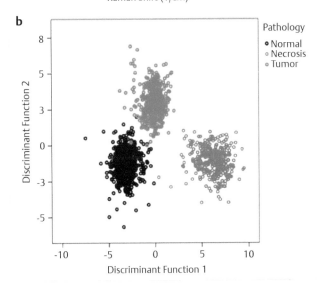

**Fig. 17.1** Raman spectroscopy for discriminating normal brain, necrosis, and tumor tissue. **(a)** Mean spectrum of normal, necrosis, and tumor from training data, with visible Raman peaks labeled. **(b)** Plot of discriminant function analysis scores for training data. (Reproduced with permission from Kalkanis et al.[8])

accuracy of 92% (sensitivity = 93%; specificity = 91%). Both low- and high-grade gliomas were able to be detected with similar accuracy. These results represent a promising step forward toward translating Raman spectroscopy to real-time intraoperative use and brain tumor resection guidance.

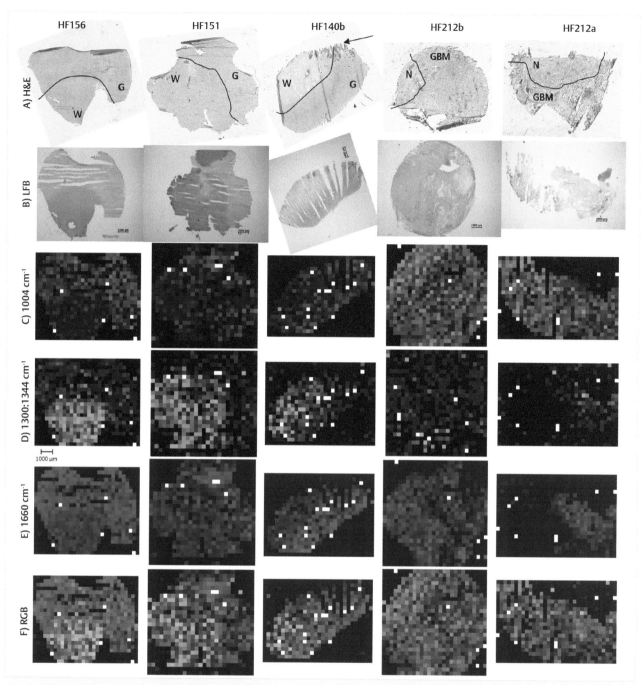

**Fig. 17.2** Correlating hematoxylin and eosin (H&E) and Raman images for five representative tissues. **(a)** Standard H&E histology, **(b)** LFB staining, **(c)** concentration of phenylalanine (1,004/cm) on red channel, **(d)** ratio of 1,300:1,344/cm shows approximate lipid:protein ratio on green channel, **(e)** concentration of 1,660/cm on blue channel, and **(f)** combined red, green, and blue images. W, white matter; G, gray matter; N, necrosis; GBM, glioblastoma; each Raman image pixel represents an area of 300 μm x 300 μm. Note: The upper left area of tissue HF140B, identified as white matter on histology review, exhibited pallor on both LFB and H&E staining, which appears to be artifactual, potentially due to tissue freezing or edema. (Reproduced with permission from Kast et al.[17])

**a**

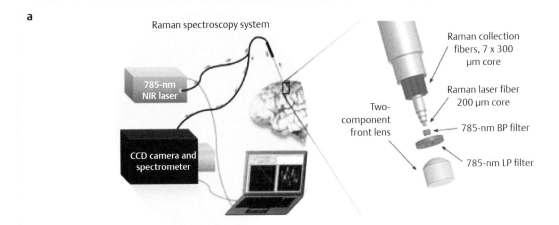

**b**

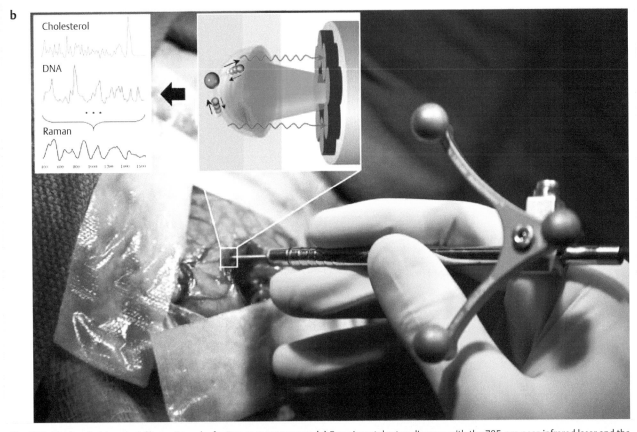

Fig. 17.3 The handheld contact fiberoptic probe for Raman spectroscopy. (a) Experimental setup diagram with the 785-nm near-infrared laser and the high-resolution charged-couple device spectroscopic detector used with the Raman fiberoptic probe. The core material was fused silica. BP, bandpass; LP, long-pass. (b) The probe (Emvision, LLC) was used to interrogate brain tissue during surgery. A schematic diagram illustrates the excitation of different molecular species, such as cholesterol and DNA, to produce the Raman spectra of cancer versus normal brain tissue. The spectral differences occur owing to the vibrational modes of various molecular species. A simple molecular vibrational mode is conceptually depicted (individual atoms in blue and green) inter-acting with the laser light (in red) to produce Raman scattering (in purple). (Reproduced with permission from Jermyn et al.[19])

## 17.3 Overview of Coherent Raman Scattering Microscopy

The shortcoming of spontaneous Raman scattering and the major limitation for translating Raman spectroscopy to the clinical setting is the poor signal-to-noise ratio. The vast majority of incident photons ($10^8$) are scattered elastically, necessitating long exposure times and advanced statistical/machine learning algorithms (e.g., principal component analysis, support vector machines, decision tree models) to detect spectral differences. CRS microscopy was developed to improve the signal-to-noise ratio; rather than obtaining a broadband Raman spectra across a range of Raman shift wavenumbers, CRS increases signal intensity by targeting a specific wavenumber (narrowband) using a second excitation beam to coherently drive the vibrational frequency of Raman active chemical bonds. CRS can produce histologic images of biological tissues because the Raman signal is multiple orders of magnitude greater (> 10,000-fold) than that of spontaneous Raman scattering. Because Raman signal is a product of the biochemical composition of tissues, image contrast can be generated without the need for labels or dyes. Label-free CRS microscopy eliminates the need for extensive tissue preparation, making the technique a potentially ideal candidate for intraoperative brain tumor imaging. The two major methods of CRS are coherent anti-Stokes Raman scattering (CARS) microscopy and stimulated Raman scattering (SRS) microscopy.

### 17.3.1 Coherent Anti-Stokes Raman Scattering Microscopy

CARS microscopy was used by Evans and colleagues to image fresh unfixed and unstained ex vivo samples from an orthotopic human astrocytoma mouse model.[20,21] High-resolution mosaic images of a mouse brain in coronal sections were obtained using $700 \times 700$ µm fields of view. Histoarchitectural features shown in CARS images were comparable to standard hematoxylin and eosin (H&E) histology. Imaging depth ranged from 25 to 80 µm depending on tissue type and wavelength. CARS microscopy was capable of generating chemically selective images of lipid (2,845/cm, $CH_2$ symmetric stretching) and proteins ($CH_3$ stretch, 2,920/cm; amide I vibration, 2,960/cm) within samples. Focusing on different peaks of the Raman spectra easily differentiated lipid-rich myelin or protein-rich cell bodies. The chemical selectivity of CARS imaging allowed for brain tumor margin delineation in the mouse model. Another investigation tuned CARS imaging to probe C–H molecular vibrations in different brain tumors (glioblastoma, melanoma, and breast cancer metastasis) to assess lipid content compared to normal brain tissue.[22] All tumor types were found to have a lower CARS signal intensity than normal parenchyma, reflecting decreased lipid/protein ratio within malignant tissues. The morphochemical contrast between normal brain and tumor enabled CARS images to delineate tumor tissue irrespective of tumor type.

A broadband CARS technique has been developed that uses greater spectral breadth within the fingerprint region of the Raman spectra without compromising imaging speed or sensitivity.[23] The biologically relevant Raman window (500–3.500/cm)

was used to image a xenograft glioblastoma mouse model at high resolution (< 10/cm). Pseudocolor three-channel broadband CARS microscopy was able to identify interfaces between xenograft brain tumors and the surrounding healthy brain matter (▶ Fig. 17.4).

### 17.3.2 Stimulated Raman Scattering Microscopy

Developed in 2008, SRS microscopy provides superior nuclear contrast compared to CARS, a linear relationship between signal intensity and chemical concentration, and a nondistorted spectrum nearly identical to spontaneous Raman scattering. Freudiger and colleagues published a landmark paper on SRS microscopy for label-free biomedical imaging.[24] Subsequent innovations enhancing the collection of the backscattered signal and increasing the imaging speed by three orders of magnitude to video rate.[25] This approach allowed label-free in vivo imaging of biological tissues and the potential for clinical translation.

Ji and colleagues described the use of SRS microscopy for differentiating healthy human and mouse brain tissue from tumor-infiltrated brain based on histoarchitectural and biochemical differences.[26] Two-color SRS microscopy with green assigned to 2,845/cm wavenumber and blue to 2,930 to 2,845/cm wavenumber highlighted the contrast between lipid and protein, respectively. Overlay of the two channels provided a blue–green histologic image. During a simulated tumor resection using a xenograft mouse model, SRS microscopy was able to reveal tumor margins that were undetectable under standard operative conditions (▶ Fig. 17.5). In order to quantify the degree of tumor infiltration in SRS images, a classifier system based on tissue cellularity, axonal density, and protein/lipid ratio was developed.[27] The SRS image classifier system was able to detect tumor infiltration with 97.5% sensitivity and 98.5% specificity. Quantitative SRS microscopy detected tumor infiltration in grossly normal brain, providing evidence that this technique could improve tumor detection during brain tumor surgery.

In addition to detecting brain tumor infiltration, SRS microscopy can serve as a method for rapid intraoperative histology of unprocessed surgical specimens. Current intraoperative H&E histology requires extensive tissue processing, which is both time and labor intensive.[28] Utilizing recent breakthroughs in fiber-laser technology,[29] a clinical SRS microscope has been engineered and deployed in our operating rooms.[9] Stimulated Raman histology (SRH), which utilized SRS images to create a virtual H&E image akin to standard intraoperative pathology, reveals the key diagnostic features of human brain tumor specimens (▶ Fig. 17.6). In a simulation of intraoperative pathologic consultation in 30 patients, we found near-perfect concordance of SRH and conventional H&E histology for predicting diagnosis (Cohen's kappa, κ > 0.89), with accuracy exceeding 92%. Because SRH provides intraoperative digital images, they can be used in real time for automated machine learning-based diagnosis. A validated multilayer perceptron neural network was able to predict brain tumor subtype with 90% accuracy. SRH has the potential to improve the care of brain tumor patients by eliminating the need for tissue processing, expediting brain tumor diagnosis, and guiding brain tumor resections.

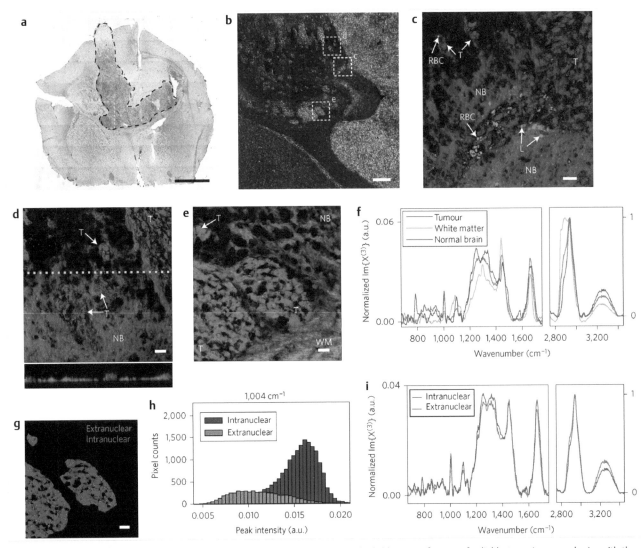

**Fig. 17.4** Histopathology using broadband coherent Raman imaging (CRI). **(a)** Bright-field image of xenograft glioblastoma in mouse brain, with the tumor hard boundary outlined (*black dashed line*). The cyan dashed box indicates a region of interest (ROI). Scale bar: 2 mm. **(b)** Phase contrast micrograph of broadband coherent anti-Stokes Raman scattering (BCARS) ROIs with boxes and associated subfigure labels. Scale bar: 200 μm. **(c)** Pseudocolor BCARS image of tumor and normal brain tissue, with nuclei highlighted in blue, lipid content in red, and red blood cells in green. **(d)** BCARS image and axial scan with nuclei highlighted in blue and lipid content in red. **(e)** BCARS image with nuclei highlighted in blue, lipid content in red, and $CH_3$ stretch–$CH_2$ stretch in green. NB, normal brain; T, tumor cells; RBC, red blood cells; L, lipid bodies; WM, white matter. **(f)** Single-pixel spectra. **(g)** Spectrally segmented image of internuclear (*blue*) and extranuclear (*red*) tumoral spaces. **(h)** Histogram analysis of phenylalanine content. **(i)** Mean spectra from within a tumor mass. (**c**–**e** and **g**; scale bars: 20 μm.) (Reproduced with permission from Camp et al.[23])

# 17.4 Future Directions

Future directions for Raman spectroscopy and CRS microscopy include stereotactic brain tumor biopsy guidance. Obtaining high-yield diagnostic specimens is essential during brain tumor biopsy procedures. As a nondestructive optical imaging technique, specimens imaged intraoperatively can be used to establish final pathologic diagnosis. During tumor resections, CRS microscopy can be used to assess residual tumor burden with tumor resection cavities. Microscopy-guided surgery with CRS may increase extent of resection and better delineate the brain tumor margin. Current CRS microscopy techniques focus on the C–H spectral region, which reflects the concentration of lipid and protein macromolecules. Future studies can explore the Raman fingerprint region (700–1,700/cm), where more specific biochemical information can be gleaned. Real-time detection of oncometabolites and downstream metabolic aberrations has implications for intraoperative molecular diagnosis, tumor-cell-specific CRS microscopy, and in vivo investigation of brain tumor biology. Finally, the application of machine learning techniques to Raman-based imaging presents an opportunity to combine powerful computational tools to digital microscopy images that contain an abundance of biochemical data. Deep learning architectures and computer vision techniques that analyze subtle, but clinically significant biochemical information and image features, may result in better diagnostic classification and prognostication.

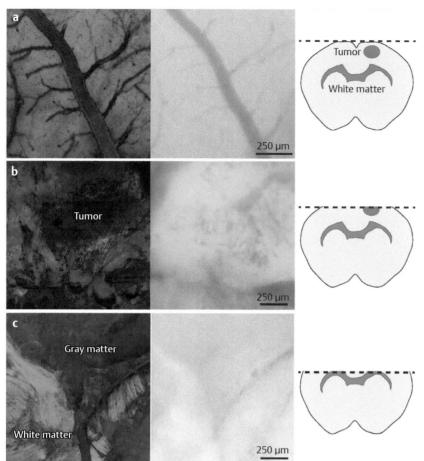

**Fig. 17.5** Stimulated Raman scattering (SRS) imaging during simulated tumor resection on mouse brain. En face, epi-SRS images were obtained in vivo during various stages of a simulated tumor removal. The cartoons on the right show the depth of imaging. **(a)** In a tumor located beneath the cortical surface, there is no obvious abnormality in SRS (*left*) or bright-field images (*middle*) when imaging the cortical surface. **(b)** After a portion of the cortex has been removed, the tumor is revealed. Blood was present on the dissected surface but did not adversely affect the distinction of tumor-infiltrated regions from noninfiltrated regions. **(c)** Because dissection was carried deep past the tumor, the normal appearance of white matter and cortex was again visible. (Reproduced with permission from Ji et al.[27])

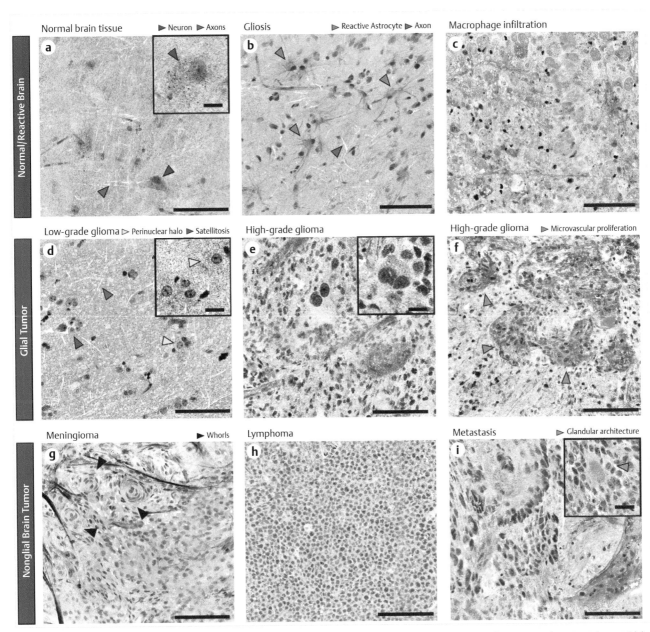

**Fig. 17.6** Imaging of key diagnostic histoarchitectural features with stimulated Raman histology (SRH). **(a)** Normal cortex reveals scattered pyramidal neurons (*blue arrowheads*) with angulated boundaries and lipofuscin granules, which appear red. White linear structures are axons (*green arrowheads*). **(b)** Gliotic tissue contains reactive astrocytes with radially directed fine protein-rich processes (*red arrowheads*) and axons (*green arrowheads*). **(c)** A macrophage infiltrate near the edge of a glioblastoma reveals round, swollen cells with lipid-rich phagosomes. **(d)** SRH reveals scattered "fried egg" tumor cells with round nuclei, ample cytoplasm, perinuclear halos (*inset and yellow arrowheads*) and neuronal satellitosis (*purple arrowhead*) in a diffuse 1p19q-co-deleted low-grade oligodendroglioma. Axons (*green arrowhead*) are apparent in this tumor-infiltrated cortex as well. **(e)** SRH demonstrates hypercellularity, anaplasia, and cellular and nuclear pleomorphism (*inset*) in a glioblastoma. A large binucleated tumor cell is shown (*inset*) in contrast to smaller adjacent tumor cells. **(f)** SRH of another glioblastoma reveals microvascular proliferation (*orange arrowheads*) with protein-rich basement membranes of angiogenic vasculature appearing purple. **(g,i)** SRH reveals the whorled architecture of meningioma (*black arrowheads*, **g**); monomorphic cells of lymphoma with high nuclear:cytoplasmic ratio **(h)** and the glandular architecture (*inset; gray arrowhead*) of a metastatic colorectal adenocarcinoma **(i)**. Insets are magnified images from the same specimens. Large-image scale bars: 100 µm; inset-image scale bars: 20 µm. (Reproduced with permission from Orringer et al.[9])

# References

[1] Barone DG, Lawrie TA, Hart MG. Image guided surgery for the resection of brain tumours. Cochrane Database Syst Rev. 2014(1):CD009685

[2] Senft C, Bink A, Franz K, Vatter H, Gasser T, Seifert V. Intraoperative MRI guidance and extent of resection in glioma surgery: a randomised, controlled trial. Lancet Oncol. 2011; 12(11):997–1003

[3] Stummer W, Pichlmeier U, Meinel T, Wiestler OD, Zanella F, Reulen HJ, ALA-Glioma Study Group. Fluorescence-guided surgery with 5-aminolevulinic acid for resection of malignant glioma: a randomised controlled multicentre phase III trial. Lancet Oncol. 2006; 7(5):392–401

[4] Orringer D, Lau D, Khatri S, et al. Extent of resection in patients with glioblastoma: limiting factors, perception of resectability, and effect on survival. J Neurosurg. 2012; 117(5):851–859

[5] Albert FK, Forsting M, Sartor K, Adams HP, Kunze S. Early postoperative magnetic resonance imaging after resection of malignant glioma: objective evaluation of residual tumor and its influence on regrowth and prognosis. Neurosurgery. 1994; 34(1):45–60, discussion 60–61

[6] Lau D, Hervey-Jumper SL, Chang S, et al. A prospective phase II clinical trial of 5-aminolevulinic acid to assess the correlation of intraoperative fluorescence intensity and degree of histologic cellularity during resection of high-grade gliomas. J Neurosurg. 2016; 124(5):1300–1309

[7] Hollon T, Lewis S, Freudiger CW, Sunney Xie X, Orringer DA. Improving the accuracy of brain tumor surgery via Raman-based technology. Neurosurg Focus. 2016; 40(3):E9

[8] Kalkanis SN, Kast RE, Rosenblum ML, et al. Raman spectroscopy to distinguish grey matter, necrosis, and glioblastoma multiforme in frozen tissue sections. J Neurooncol. 2014; 116(3):477–485

[9] Orringer DA, Pandian B, Niknafs YS, Hollon TC, Boyle J, et al. Rapid intraoperative histology of unprocessed surgical specimens via fibre-laser-based stimulated Raman scattering microscopy. Nat Biomed Eng. 2017; 1:0027

[10] Raman CV, Krishnan KS. A new type of secondary radiation. Nature. 1928; 121(3048):501–502

[11] Tashibu K. Analysis of water content in rat brain using Raman spectroscopy. No To Shinkei. 1990; 42(10):999–1004

[12] Krafft C, Neudert L, Simat T, Salzer R. Near infrared Raman spectra of human brain lipids. Spectrochim Acta A Mol Biomol Spectrosc. 2005; 61(7):1529–1535

[13] Köhler M, Machill S, Salzer R, Krafft C. Characterization of lipid extracts from brain tissue and tumors using Raman spectroscopy and mass spectrometry. Anal Bioanal Chem. 2009; 393(5):1513–1520

[14] Kirsch M, Schackert G, Salzer R, Krafft C. Raman spectroscopic imaging for in vivo detection of cerebral brain metastases. Anal Bioanal Chem. 2010; 398(4):1707–1713

[15] Koljenović S, Choo-Smith LP, Bakker Schut TC, Kros JM, van den Berge HJ, Puppels GJ. Discriminating vital tumor from necrotic tissue in human glioblastoma tissue samples by Raman spectroscopy. Lab Invest. 2002; 82(10):1265–1277

[16] Kast RE, Auner GW, Rosenblum ML, et al. Raman molecular imaging of brain frozen tissue sections. J Neurooncol. 2014; 120(1):55–62

[17] Kast R, Auner G, Yurgelevic S, et al. Identification of regions of normal grey matter and white matter from pathologic glioblastoma and necrosis in frozen sections using Raman imaging. J Neurooncol. 2015; 125(2):287–295

[18] Desroches J, Jermyn M, Mok K, et al. Characterization of a Raman spectroscopy probe system for intraoperative brain tissue classification. Biomed Opt Express. 2015; 6(7):2380–2397

[19] Jermyn M, Mok K, Mercier J, et al. Intraoperative brain cancer detection with Raman spectroscopy in humans. Sci Transl Med. 2015; 7(274):274ra19

[20] Evans CL, Xu X, Kesari S, Xie XS, Wong ST, Young GS. Chemically-selective imaging of brain structures with CARS microscopy. Opt Express. 2007; 15(19):12076–12087

[21] Evans CL, Xie XS. Coherent anti-stokes Raman scattering microscopy: chemical imaging for biology and medicine. Annu Rev Anal Chem (Palo Alto, Calif). 2008; 1:883–909

[22] Uckermann O, Galli R, Tamosaityte S, et al. Label-free delineation of brain tumors by coherent anti-Stokes Raman scattering microscopy in an orthotopic mouse model and human glioblastoma. PLoS One. 2014; 9(9):e107115

[23] Camp CH, Jr, Lee YJ, Heddleston JM, et al. High-speed coherent Raman fingerprint imaging of biological tissues. Nat Photonics. 2014; 8:627–634

[24] Freudiger CW, Min W, Saar BG, et al. Label-free biomedical imaging with high sensitivity by stimulated Raman scattering microscopy. Science. 2008; 322(5909):1857–1861

[25] Saar BG, Freudiger CW, Reichman J, Stanley CM, Holtom GR, Xie XS. Video-rate molecular imaging in vivo with stimulated Raman scattering. Science. 2010; 330(6009):1368–1370

[26] Ji M, Orringer DA, Freudiger CW, et al. Rapid, label-free detection of brain tumors with stimulated Raman scattering microscopy. Sci Transl Med. 2013; 5(201):201ra119

[27] Ji M, Lewis S, Camelo-Piragua S, et al. Detection of human brain tumor infiltration with quantitative stimulated Raman scattering microscopy. Sci Transl Med. 2015; 7(309):309ra163

[28] Somerset HL, Kleinschmidt-DeMasters BK. Approach to the intraoperative consultation for neurosurgical specimens. Adv Anat Pathol. 2011; 18(6):446–449

[29] Freudiger CW, Yang W, Holtom GR, Peyghambarian N, Xie XS, Kieu KQ. Stimulated Raman scattering microscopy with a robust fibre laser source. Nat Photonics. 2014; 8(2):153–159

# 18 Indocyanine Green and Cerebral Aneurysms

*David Bervini and Andreas Raabe*

**Abstract**

When performing aneurysm clipping, the surgeon has to ensure that the aneurysm is completely obliterated and the parent, branching, and perforating vessels are patent. Several techniques are available for assessing whether aneurysm clipping has been done correctly. However, disadvantages such as their invasiveness, incomplete effectiveness, and spatial and temporal limitations, as well as their costs, are causes of concern for both patients and surgeons. Indocyanine green (ICG) videoangiography is a reliable, fast, repeatable, noninvasive, and cost-effective technique that allows real-time intraoperative assessment of vascular anatomy and analysis of flow dynamics. This chapter describes the principles of ICG videoangiography and its value in aneurysm surgery, and presents a critical appraisal of the validity and limitations of intraoperative ICG videoangiography. The focus is on practical aspects helpful during aneurysm surgery. ICG videoangiography represents a technical innovation meeting an important need in the microsurgical management of aneurysms, and it should be part of the state-of-the-art neurosurgical armory.

*Keywords:* indocyanine green, intraoperative technique, intracranial aneurysm, surgery

## 18.1 Introduction

Surgical clip ligation is a reliable treatment modality for intracranial aneurysms. The effectiveness of surgery depends on the clip(s) position, which needs to occlude the aneurysm and maintain blood flow in parent, branching, and perforating arteries. Several techniques are available for determining whether these goals have been achieved. Their value has to be balanced against their invasiveness, spatial and temporal limitations, as well as their costs. Indocyanine green (ICG) videoangiography has become a useful way to allow real-time assessment of intraoperative vascular anatomy and analysis of flow dynamics.

### 18.1.1 Surgical Clipping of Intracranial Aneurysms

Intracranial aneurysms are the most frequently diagnosed and increasingly common cerebrovascular malformation with a prevalence of 2 to 3% in the overall population.[1,2] Aneurysm rupture has an incidence of about 9 per 100,000, accounting for approximately 5% of all strokes,[3,4] and has a high case fatality and morbidity rate. Due to its occurrence at a young age[3,5,6] and its poor outcome, the loss of productive life-years in the general population as a result of aneurysmal subarachnoid hemorrhage is as large as that from ischemic cerebral infarction, the most common type of stroke.[4,7,8,9,10,11]

Surgical clip ligation is a validated treatment modality for intracranial aneurysms. Approximately 90% of such aneurysms are smaller than 10 mm[1] and surgery is routinely performed under microscope magnification. The technique consists of the dissection of the brain and vessels and the placement of one or more metallic clips in order to occlude and exclude the aneurysm from the normal arterial blood circulation of the brain.[12,13] The size, shape, number, and arrangement of clips depend on each patient's unique vascular anatomy. Aneurysms have a close anatomical relationship to their parent vessels and to branching or perforating arteries. Surgical manipulation and aneurysm clipping put these vessels at risk for stenosis, occlusion, or insult, potentially leading to brain ischemia and infarction.[14,15,16,17] These risks can be minimized by the surgeon only by error avoidance and prompt error correction. As a rule of thumb, neurosurgeons consider that there is a time limit of 8 to 10 minutes before an ischemic event becomes irreversible.

Proven aneurysm remnants may regrow and lead to recurrent symptoms of hemorrhage or mass effect.[18,19,20,21] Together with the need for retreatment, this has a negative impact on the postoperative natural history.

When routinely performing postoperative angiography after clipping, the incidence of residual aneurysm filling reportedly ranges from 4 to 19%,[22,23,24,25,26,27] and the incidence of parent or branching arteries ranges from 0.3 to 12%.[22,23,24,25,26] Most of these findings (~10% combined incidence) are unexpected by the surgeon.

To lower this rate, diagnostic imaging of the vascular anatomy has to be made available in the operating room to allow assessment of clip position and to improve surgical results when suboptimal or wrong clip placement is detected. In light of the above-mentioned challenges faced during surgery, the ability to immediately evaluate and correct an imperfectly placed clip and/or cerebrovascular flow obstruction is highly desirable.

### 18.1.2 Techniques in Cerebrovascular Neurosurgery

#### Surgical Microscopy

The availability of the apochromatic optic, the zoom, the varioscopic focus, and direct surgical field illumination allows the surgeon to work with high-contrast and sharp images. The smooth device handling via touchscreen, handgrips, mouth switch, and wireless foot control panel help the surgeon to obtain a sharp focus on cerebrovascular structures and the surrounding brain. In specific circumstances, the surgeon can detect arterial blood turbulence and flow. However, this information alone is not sufficient to judge on correct vessel patency or complete aneurysm occlusion by clipping. Moreover, some compression maneuvers can be performed using bipolar forceps to stretch an arterial segment to empty it of blood and observe refilling.

#### Intraoperative Digital Subtraction Angiography

Due to its high-quality image definition, the multiple angles of view, and the three-dimensional vascular reconstruction modalities, rotational digital subtraction angiography (DSA) has been considered the gold standard diagnostic modality for cerebrovascular pathologies. Assessment is not limited to exposed vessels and the absence of subtraction artifacts from surgical metallic clips allows detailed vascular assessment.

Various authors have reported correction of an imperfectly positioned clip leading to improvement of the surgical procedure in 7 to 34% of selected cases.[28] However, several drawbacks are associated with intraoperative DSA. These include the reduced image quality in the operating theater, the limited ability to visualize small perforating arteries, the rather long setup times (15–60 minutes), the possibility of brain ischemia in the case of artery occlusion, the invasiveness (direct puncture, exposure to ionizing radiation, dye injection), the required continuing use, experience, and resource consumption, and the high financial costs. Its rate of severe complications, which include stroke, arterial dissection, and retroperitoneal hemorrhage, has been reported to be up to 3.5%.[29,30,31,32,33] Therefore, although intraoperative DSA may be considered the gold standard, its drawbacks have kept it from becoming a "standard of care." In most sites, its application is limited to selected cases and only a few centers around the world have the capability to use it as a routine intraoperative tool.

### Microvascular Doppler

The microvascular Doppler (MVD) system has become a standard piece of equipment that is routinely used during aneurysm clipping, available on the operating table and ready for use. It is inexpensive, easy to use, fast, and noninvasive.[34,35] The MVD easily diagnoses occlusion of parent or branching arteries and incomplete clipping provided that there is high flow filling of the aneurysm dome.[36] However, MVD requires direct vessel contact and mostly fails in perforating arteries.[36] Observing the signal curve or judging the change in noise is always subjective, and a hemodynamically critical stenosis can rarely be reliably identified. Low flow filling of the aneurysm sac after incomplete clipping and small caliber vessel flow can also often be missed.[35,36] The newly developed Charbel–Doppler flow probe measures blood flow quantitatively.[37] Although this new flow probe improves the diagnostic accuracy of the Doppler, especially in assessing vessel stenosis, it has the disadvantage of being somewhat bulky in some situations and, like MVD, fails in perforating arteries. However, it is a technological innovation that has overcome some of the limitations of MVD.

## 18.2 Indocyanine Green Angiography

### 18.2.1 Principles of Indocyanine Green Videoangiography

ICG is a near-infrared (NIR) fluorescent tricarbocyanine dye that was approved by the U.S. Food and Drug Administration in 1956 for diagnostic use in disorders of cardiocirculatory and liver function. Supplemental U.S. FDA approval for ophthalmic angiography was granted in 1975. After intravenous bolus injection, ICG is bound within 1 to 2 seconds, mainly to globulins (α1-lipoproteins), and remains intravascular with normal vascular permeability. ICG is not metabolized in the body and is excreted exclusively by the liver, with a plasma half-life of 3 to 4 minutes. It is not reabsorbed from the intestine and does not undergo enterohepatic recirculation. The recommended dose for ICG videoangiography is 0.2 to 0.5 mg/kg; the maximal daily dose should not exceed 5 mg/kg.

ICG absorption and emission peaks lie within the "optical window" of tissue, where absorption attributable to endogenous chromophores is low. NIR light can therefore penetrate tissue to depths from several millimeters to a few centimeters. The operative field is illuminated by a light source with a wavelength covering part of the ICG absorption band (range 700–850 nm, maximum 805 nm). Once the dye solution reaches the vessels of the NIR light–illuminated field of interest, ICG fluorescence is induced. The fluorescence (range 780–950 nm, maximum 835 nm) is recorded by a nonintensified video camera. An optical filter blocks both ambient and excitation light so that only ICG-induced fluorescence is visualized. Thus, arterial, capillary, and venous angiographic images can be observed on the video screen in real time. The latest generations of microscopes integrate ICG videoangiography technology, enabling high-resolution and high-contrast NIR images to be obtained. The setup allows high-resolution NIR images based on ICG fluorescence to be visualized and stored without eliminating visible light during the investigation (i.e., without moving the microscope from the surgical field or needing to interrupt the operation).

## 18.2.2 ICG Videoangiography and Aneurysm Surgery

ICG videoangiography was first introduced in neurosurgery in 2003[38] as a new method to visualize flow in vessels exposed in the surgical field. The clinical benefit of ICG in cerebrovascular neurosurgery was reported in 2005,[28] after adding NIR imaging to surgical microscopes and comparing it with intraoperative or postoperative DSA. ICG videoangiography was able to identify a suboptimal or wrong clip position in 8% of a total of 10%, and the 9% rate of relevant information provided by ICG angiography for the surgical procedure was compatible with the reported rates associated with intraoperative DSA.[28] Its value in influencing the intraoperative decision to correct the aneurysm clip has since been reported as being in the range of 1.8 to 38%[28,35,36,39,40,41,42,43,44,45,46,47,48,49,50,51,52,53,54,55] (▶ Table 18.1).

The strength of ICG videoangiography is its high image quality, especially in small vessels, and the ease of clinical use in routine situations. The procedure can be performed at any time during surgery, and repeated administration is possible after a time interval of 5 to 15 minutes to allow some clearance of the dye. ICG videoangiography allows the surgeon to examine and manipulate the cerebrovascular anatomy, for instance the clipped aneurysm, in a manner that is not possible with intraoperative DSA.

ICG videoangiography has been validated as a reliable technique for the distinct visualization and flow assessment of perforating arteries and inframillimetric vessels exposed during surgery. This is otherwise rarely achievable with other intraoperative techniques, including intraoperative DSA.[36,39] This is relevant given the rate of perforating vessel occlusion of up to 8% of all postclipping cases.[56]

The incidence of adverse reactions to the ICG dye is similar to that for other types of contrast media: ranging from 0.05% for

**Table 18.1** Summary of findings of studies on the use of indocyanine green (ICG) videoangiography during intracranial aneurysm surgery

| Author | Year | No. of patients | No. of aneurysms | ICG influenced surgery (%) | ICG false-negative outcome (%) |
|---|---|---|---|---|---|
| Raabe et al[28] | 2005 | 114 | 124 | 8.8 | 10.0 |
| de Oliveira et al[39] | 2007 | 60 | 64 | 2.8 | 5.6 |
| Imizu et al[40] | 2008 | 13 | 13 | 38.0 | NA |
| Dashti et al[62] | 2009 | 190 | 239 | NA | 12.1 |
| Li et al[41] | 2009 | 120 | 148 | 9.3 | 6.5 |
| Ma et al[42] | 2009 | 45 | 45 | 17.8 | 2.3 |
| Jing et al[43] | 2010 | 42 | 42 | 11.9 | 0 |
| Khurana et al[44] | 2010 | 27 | 27 | 22.2 | 0 |
| Fischer et al[36] | 2010 | 40 | 50 | 8.0 | 10.0 |
| Oda et al[59] | 2011 | 39 | 43 | 10.3 | NA |
| Gruber et al[35] | 2011 | 104 | 123 | 6.5 | 2.4 |
| Wang et al[46] | 2011 | 129 | 152 | 2.1 | 0.7 |
| Washington et al[47] | 2013 | 155 | 59 | 4.1 | 14.3 |
| Moon et al[48] | 2013 | 119 | 127 | 6.3 | 0.8 |
| Della Puppa et al[49] | 2013 | 26 | 34 | 8.8 | 5.6 |
| Özgiray et al[50] | 2013 | 86 | 109 | 1.8 | 1.8 |
| Caplan et al[51] | 2014 | 37 | 47 | 8.1 | 10.8 |
| Hardesty et al[52] | 2014 | 100 | 122 | 4.0 | 1.0 |
| Lai et al[53] | 2014 | 91 | 100 | 15.0 | 2.0 |
| Roessler et al[54] | 2014 | 232 | 295 | 13.4 | 9.1 |
| Sharma et al[55] | 2014 | 112 | 126 | 8.9 | 4.5 |
| Mean, % (95% CI) | | | | 8.7 (7.4–10) | 5.3 (4.4–6.6) |

Abbreviations: 95% CI = 95% confidence interval; NA, not available.

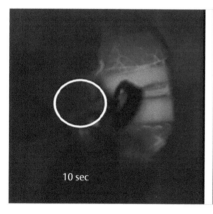
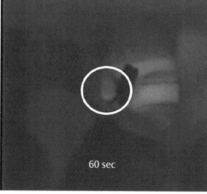

**Fig. 18.1** Indocyanine green videoangiography images: 10 seconds (*left image*) and 60 seconds (*right image*) after dye injection, showing incomplete clip occlusion and delayed dye filling of the aneurysm (*right image, circled*).

severe side effects (hypotension, arrhythmia, or, more rarely, anaphylactic shock) to 0.2% for moderate or mild side effects (nausea, pruritus, syncope, or skin eruption),[38] and it can therefore be considered a safe intraoperative tool.

### 18.2.3 Limitations of ICG Videoangiography and Technical Tips

#### Residual Aneurysm Filling

In most cases of incomplete clipping, only a small communication is left between the vessel and the aneurysm. Therefore, the concentration of ICG dye inside the aneurysm increases only slowly. This leads to the observation that in the first seconds after ICG injection, the aneurysm seems to be occluded, but after 30 to 60 seconds, the aneurysm becomes brighter because of the increasing dye inflow (▶ Fig. 18.1).

### Occlusion of Parent, Branching, or Perforating Arteries

The high-quality imaging of small vessels is one of the most valuable features of ICG angiography, but large vessels also show excellent contrast, provided that no major calcification or thrombosis is present. For assessing patency, the first 1 to 3 seconds of the ICG angiography are the most important. Stenosis or occlusion can only be diagnosed in the early phase of arterial filling. Backflow will often illuminate the vessel, and assessing it after the first inflow increases the rate of false-negative findings, that is, missing the stenosis or occlusion.

There is one particular feature of the microscope that we regard as indispensable for ICG angiography: the loop function. Often the surgeon is busy maintaining the view through the microscope and opening the surgical field for optimal illumination and exposure during ICG angiography, and cannot watch the original video in real time. The loop automatically repeats the first 3 to 5 seconds and the surgeon can observe the critical moment of the first inflow as many times as needed. The loop function is a simple and quick feature that is integrated into the microscope and available within a few seconds. This is the best method to diagnose a delay in filling, which always has to be considered unsatisfactory. As no reliable quantitative measurement method exists, any delay should trigger a correction of the clip position. In the case of a branch occlusion, either a contrast breakoff or a pulsating level can be observed, with visible backflow filling (▶ Fig. 18.2).

## Stenosis

The diagnosis of a hemodynamically relevant stenosis with ICG videoangiography is very difficult and depends on the length of the exposed segment of the vessel. When only a short segment is exposed, such as A2 after clipping of an anterior communicating artery aneurysm, it is almost impossible to see a delay in inflow (▶ Fig. 18.3). When a longer segment is exposed, as in middle cerebral artery aneurysms (▶ Fig. 18.4), the chances are better. Again, the short loop of the inflow video is the best tool for providing the critical information that there is a delay in filling, which should raise the suspicion of a hemodynamically relevant stenosis and should suggest clip repositioning. The same holds true for perforating arteries, where ICG videoangiography can be considered the gold standard of intraoperative imaging (▶ Fig. 18.5).

## Situations of Reduced Image Quality

Image quality may be reduced in the deep surgical fields due to the weak NIR illumination and the requirement for a line of sight directly onto the structure. This is particularly true for deeply located aneurysms.[35,43] Areas on the reverse side of the aneurysm, and typically aneurysm neck remnants, can be obscured by the clips or by other anatomy and hence may be difficult to visualize using ICG videoangiography. The same applies to thrombosed or heavily calcified aneurysms and vessels, due to insufficient transillumination of these tissues, and in acute cases with coagulation disorders and constant microbleeding, where

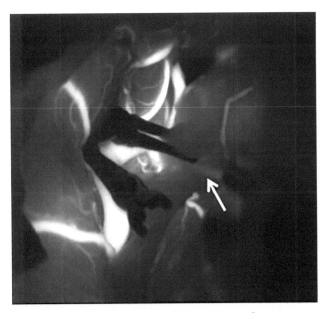

**Fig. 18.2** Indocyanine green videoangiography image after aneurysm clipping and dye injection, showing arterial branch occlusion (*arrow*).

**Fig. 18.3** Indocyanine green videoangiography image of a clipped anterior communicating artery aneurysm. Because of the short exposure, the narrow surgical field, and the short length of the arterial segments involved, the existence of a branch artery stenosis cannot be assessed.

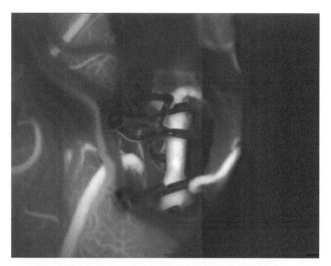

**Fig. 18.4** Indocyanine green videoangiography image showing sufficient vessel exposure to rule out branch stenosis in a middle cerebral artery aneurysm.

ICG dye effusion makes the evaluation difficult.[36] These drawbacks can be partly minimized with experience, by employing additional techniques like endoscope-integrated ICG technology[57,58] or by using additional software functions for reviewing the video and interpreting the findings.[59] The FLOW 800 (Carl Zeiss, Oberkochen, Germany) is a microscope-integrated additional software tool for instant color-coded visualization and analysis of the temporal distribution dynamics of the fluorescence ICG dye.[59] The emission signal of the fluorescence light is recorded and color-coded transit maps are generated by the software for visualization of macrocirculatory flow and microcirculatory perfusion. The FLOW 800–generated color-coded maps can be considered an adjunct to the short loop of the ICG inflow video in visualizing occlusion or stenosis of parent, branching, or perforating arteries and has been reported to be useful in detecting cerebral flow direction[60] (▶ Fig. 18.6).

The likelihood of false-negative results, or missed findings, of ICG videoangiography confirmed by intra- or postoperative DSA varies between 0 and 14%, with an average of 5% of cases[47] (▶ Table 18.1). From larger studies, a branch occlusion rate of 6

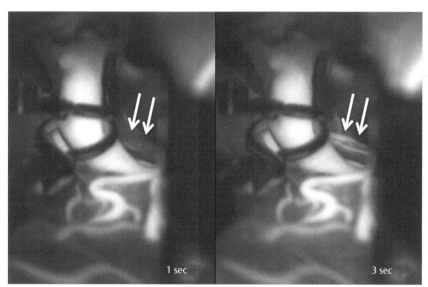

**Fig. 18.5** Indocyanine green videoangiography image showing perforating artery stenosis and delayed dye filling (*arrows*).

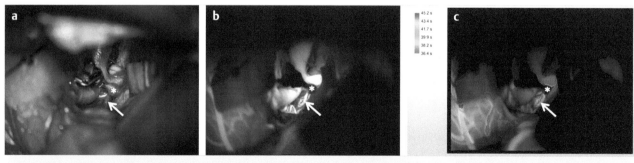

**Fig. 18.6** Intraoperative images of a left intracranial aneurysm (ICA) bifurcation aneurysm clipping. **(a)** Magnified microscopic image showing the main branching arteries, the aneurysm (*asterisk*), and the ICA perforating arteries (*arrow*). **(b)** Indocyanine green videoangiography image showing complete aneurysm occlusion (*asterisk*) and perforating arteries patency (*arrow*). **(c)** FLOW 800–generated color-coded maps, confirming aneurysm complete occlusion (*asterisk*) and normal flow in the perforating arteries (*arrow*).

to 7.3% has been reported.[28,61] However, because of the anticipation of intraoperative imaging feedback—mostly DSA—these results should be interpreted with caution.[28,47,51] Nevertheless, these numbers compare well with recent series assessing the accuracy of intraoperative DSA demonstrating 5 to 9% rates of false-negative findings and accuracy rates of 88 to 95%.[33,62,63]

Overall, in about 9% of cases and studies reported in the literature (range 2–38%), ICG prompted clip adjustment; this underlines the clinical value of the method.

## 18.3 Conclusion

Because no intraoperative method is absolutely reliable, the use of ICG videoangiography should be considered as one valuable tool among others, to be used in association with other intraoperative techniques like visual inspection, intraoperative MVD, intraoperative neuromonitoring, and, in specific circumstances, intraoperative DSA. This combination of complementary techniques offers the best approach to reducing the morbidity related to aneurysm clipping, reserving the use of intraoperative DSA for particular cases where the limitations of the alternative techniques have to be expected.

ICG videoangiography offers a new reliable, fast, repeatable, noninvasive, and cost-effective technique allowing real-time intraoperative assessment of vascular anatomy and analysis of flow dynamics. It represents a technical innovation, meeting an important need in the microsurgical management of aneurysms and because of its ease of use, it is becoming a safe first-line intraoperative modality.

## References

[1] Vlak MH, Algra A, Brandenburg R, Rinkel GJ. Prevalence of unruptured intracranial aneurysms, with emphasis on sex, age, comorbidity, country, and time period: a systematic review and meta-analysis. Lancet Neurol. 2011; 10 (7):626–636

[2] Vernooij MW, Ikram MA, Tanghe HL, et al. Incidental findings on brain MRI in the general population. N Engl J Med. 2007; 357(18):1821–1828

[3] de Rooij NK, Linn FHH, van der Plas JA, Algra A, Rinkel GJE. Incidence of subarachnoid haemorrhage: a systematic review with emphasis on region, age, gender and time trends. J Neurol Neurosurg Psychiatry. 2007; 78(12): 1365–1372

[4] Feigin VL, Lawes CM, Bennett DA, Barker-Collo SL, Parag V. Worldwide stroke incidence and early case fatality reported in 56 population-based studies: a systematic review. Lancet Neurol. 2009; 8(4):355–369

[5] van Gijn J, Kerr RS, Rinkel GJE. Subarachnoid haemorrhage. Lancet. 2007; 369 (9558):306–318

[6] Nieuwkamp DJ, Setz LE, Algra A, Linn FH, de Rooij NK, Rinkel GJ. Changes in case fatality of aneurysmal subarachnoid haemorrhage over time, according to age, sex, and region: a meta-analysis. Lancet Neurol. 2009; 8(7):635–642

[7] Hop JW, Rinkel GJ, Algra A, van Gijn J. Quality of life in patients and partners after aneurysmal subarachnoid hemorrhage. Stroke. 1998; 29(4):798–804

[8] Johnston SC, Selvin S, Gress DR. The burden, trends, and demographics of mortality from subarachnoid hemorrhage. Neurology. 1998; 50(5):1413–1418

[9] Wermer MJH, Kool H, Albrecht KW, Rinkel GJE. Subarachnoid hemorrhage treated with clipping. Neurosurgery. 2007; 60(1):91–97

[10] Al-Khindi T, Macdonald RL, Schweizer TA. Cognitive and functional outcome after aneurysmal subarachnoid hemorrhage. Stroke. 2010; 41(8):e519–e536

[11] Springer MV, Schmidt JM, Wartenberg KE, Frontera JA, Badjatia N, Mayer SA. Predictors of global cognitive impairment 1 year after subarachnoid hemorrhage. Neurosurgery. 2009; 65(6):1043–1050, discussion 1050–1051

[12] Spetzler RF, Zabramski JM, McDougall CG, et al. Analysis of saccular aneurysms in the Barrow Ruptured Aneurysm Trial. J Neurosurg. 2018; 128 (1):120–125

[13] Molyneux AJ, Kerr RS, Yu L-M, et al. International Subarachnoid Aneurysm Trial (ISAT) Collaborative Group. International subarachnoid aneurysm trial (ISAT) of neurosurgical clipping versus endovascular coiling in 2143 patients with ruptured intracranial aneurysms: a randomised comparison of effects on survival, dependency, seizures, rebleeding, subgroups, and aneurysm occlusion. Lancet. 2005; 366(9488):809–817

[14] Bekelis K, Missios S, MacKenzie TA, et al. Predicting inpatient complications from cerebral aneurysm clipping: the Nationwide Inpatient Sample 2005–2009. J Neurosurg. 2014; 120(3):591–598

[15] Bruneau M, Amin-Hanjani S, Koroknay-Pal P, et al. Surgical clipping of very small unruptured intracranial aneurysms: a multicenter international study. Neurosurgery. 2016; 78(1):47–52

[16] Bulters DO, Santarius T, Chia HL, et al. Causes of neurological deficits following clipping of 200 consecutive ruptured aneurysms in patients with good-grade aneurysmal subarachnoid haemorrhage. Acta Neurochir (Wien). 2011; 153(2):295–303

[17] Le Roux PD, Elliott JP, Eskridge JM, Cohen W, Winn HR. Risks and benefits of diagnostic angiography after aneurysm surgery: a retrospective analysis of 597 studies. Neurosurgery. 1998; 42(6):1248–1254, discussion 1254–1255

[18] Lin T, Fox AJ, Drake CG. Regrowth of aneurysm sacs from residual neck following aneurysm clipping. J Neurosurg. 1989; 70(4):556–560

[19] Drake CG, Vanderlinden RG. The late consequences of incomplete surgical treatment of cerebral aneurysms. J Neurosurg. 1967; 27(3):226–238

[20] Feuerberg I, Lindquist C, Lindqvist M, Steiner L. Natural history of postoperative aneurysm rests. J Neurosurg. 1987; 66(1):30–34

[21] Johnston SC, Dowd CF, Higashida RT, Lawton MT, Duckwiler GR, Gress DR, CARAT Investigators. Predictors of rehemorrhage after treatment of ruptured intracranial aneurysms: the Cerebral Aneurysm Rerupture After Treatment (CARAT) study. Stroke. 2008; 39(1):120–125

[22] Alexander TD, Macdonald RL, Weir B, Kowalczuk A. Intraoperative angiography in cerebral aneurysm surgery: a prospective study of 100 craniotomies. Neurosurgery. 1996; 39(1):10–17, discussion 17–18

[23] Drake CG, Allcock JM. Postoperative angiography and the "slipped" clip. J Neurosurg. 1973; 39(6):683–689

[24] Macdonald RL, Wallace MC, Kestle JRW. Role of angiography following aneurysm surgery. J Neurosurg. 1993; 79(6):826–832

[25] Proust F, Hannequin D, Langlois O, Freger P, Creissard P. Causes of morbidity and mortality after ruptured aneurysm surgery in a series of 230 patients. The importance of control angiography. Stroke. 1995; 26(9):1553–1557

[26] Rauzzino MJ, Quinn CM, Fisher WS, III. Angiography after aneurysm surgery: indications for "selective" angiography. Surg Neurol. 1998; 49(1):32–40, discussion 40–41

[27] Suzuki J, Kwak R, Katakura R. Review of incompletely occluded surgically treated cerebral aneurysms. Surg Neurol. 1980; 13(4):306–310

[28] Raabe A, Nakaji P, Beck J, et al. Prospective evaluation of surgical microscope-integrated intraoperative near-infrared indocyanine green videoangiography during aneurysm surgery. J Neurosurg. 2005; 103(6):982–989

[29] Chiang VL, Gailloud P, Murphy KJ, Rigamonti D, Tamargo RJ. Routine intraoperative angiography during aneurysm surgery. J Neurosurg. 2002; 96 (6):988–992

[30] Katz JM, Gologorsky Y, Tsiouris AJ, et al. Is routine intraoperative angiography in the surgical treatment of cerebral aneurysms justified? A consecutive series of 147 aneurysms. Neurosurgery. 2006; 58(4):719–727, discussion 719–727

[31] Klopfenstein JD, Spetzler RF, Kim LJ, et al. Comparison of routine and selective use of intraoperative angiography during aneurysm surgery: a prospective assessment. J Neurosurg. 2004; 100(2):230–235

[32] Martin N, Doberstein C, Bentson J, Vinuela F, Dion J, Becker D. Intraoperative angiography in cerebrovascular surgery. Clin Neurosurg. 1991; 37:312–331

[33] Tang G, Cawley CM, Dion JE, Barrow DL. Intraoperative angiography during aneurysm surgery: a prospective evaluation of efficacy. J Neurosurg. 2002; 96 (6):993–999

[34] Bailes JE, Tantuwaya LS, Fukushima T, Schurman GW, Davis D. Intraoperative microvascular Doppler sonography in aneurysm surgery. Neurosurgery. 1997; 40(5):965–970, discussion 970–972

[35] Gruber A, Dorfer C, Standhardt H, Bavinzski G, Knosp E. Prospective comparison of intraoperative vascular monitoring technologies during cerebral aneurysm surgery. Neurosurgery. 2011; 68(3):657–673, discussion 673

[36] Fischer G, Stadie A, Oertel JMK. Near-infrared indocyanine green videoangiography versus microvascular Doppler sonography in aneurysm surgery. Acta Neurochir (Wien). 2010; 152(9):1519–1525

[37] Amin-Hanjani S, Meglio G, Gatto R, Bauer A, Charbel FT. The utility of intraoperative blood flow measurement during aneurysm surgery using an

ultrasonic perivascular flow probe. Neurosurgery. 2006; 58(4) suppl 2:305–312, discussion 312

[38] Raabe A, Beck J, Gerlach R, Zimmermann M, Seifert V. Near-infrared indocyanine green video angiography: a new method for intraoperative assessment of vascular flow. Neurosurgery. 2003; 52(1):132–139, discussion 139

[39] de Oliveira JG, Beck J, Seifert V, Teixeira MJ, Raabe A. Assessment of flow in perforating arteries during intracranial aneurysm surgery using intraoperative near-infrared indocyanine green videoangiography. Neurosurgery. 2007; 61(3) suppl:63–72, discussion 72–73

[40] Imizu S, Kato Y, Sangli A, Oguri D, Sano H. Assessment of incomplete clipping of aneurysms intraoperatively by a near-infrared indocyanine green-video angiography (NIICG-VA) integrated microscope. Minim Invasive Neurosurg. 2008; 51(4):199–203

[41] Li J, Lan Z, He M, You C. Assessment of microscope-integrated indocyanine green angiography during intracranial aneurysm surgery: a retrospective study of 120 patients. Neurol India. 2009; 57(4):453–459

[42] Ma C-Y, Shi J-X, Wang H-D, Hang C-H, Cheng H-L, Wu W. Intraoperative indocyanine green angiography in intracranial aneurysm surgery: microsurgical clipping and revascularization. Clin Neurol Neurosurg. 2009; 111(10):840–846

[43] Jing Z, Ou S, Ban Y, Tong Z, Wang Y. Intraoperative assessment of anterior circulation aneurysms using the indocyanine green video angiography technique. J Clin Neurosci. 2010; 17(1):26–28

[44] Khurana VG, Seow K, Duke D. Intuitiveness, quality and utility of intraoperative fluorescence videoangiography: Australian neurosurgical experience. Br J Neurosurg. 2010; 24(2):163–172

[45] Oda J, Kato Y, Chen SF, et al. Intraoperative near-infrared indocyanine green-videoangiography (ICG-VA) and graphic analysis of fluorescence intensity in cerebral aneurysm surgery. J Clin Neurosci. 2011; 18(8):1097–1100

[46] Wang S, Liu L, Zhao Y, Zhang D, Yang M, Zhao J. Evaluation of surgical microscope-integrated intraoperative near-infrared indocyanine green videoangiography during aneurysm surgery. Neurosurg Rev. 2010; 34(2):209–215

[47] Washington CW, Zipfel GJ, Chicoine MR, et al. Comparing indocyanine green videoangiography to the gold standard of intraoperative digital subtraction angiography used in aneurysm surgery. J Neurosurg. 2013; 118(2):420–427

[48] Moon H-S, Joo S-P, Seo B-R, Jang J-W, Kim J-H, Kim T-S. Value of indocyanine green videoangiography in deciding the completeness of cerebrovascular surgery. J Korean Neurosurg Soc. 2013; 53(6):349–355

[49] Della Puppa A, Volpin F, Gioffre G, Rustemi O, Troncon I, Scienza R. Microsurgical clipping of intracranial aneurysms assisted by green indocyanine videoangiography (ICGV) and ultrasonic perivascular microflow probe measurement. Clin Neurol Neurosurg. 2014; 116:35–40

[50] Özgiray E, Aktüre E, Patel N, et al. How reliable and accurate is indocyanine green video angiography in the evaluation of aneurysm obliteration? Clin Neurol Neurosurg. 2013; 115(7):870–878

[51] Caplan JM, Sankey E, Yang W, et al. Impact of indocyanine green videoangiography on rate of clip adjustments following intraoperative angiography. Neurosurgery. 2014; 75(4):437–443, 444

[52] Hardesty DA, Thind H, Zabramski JM, Spetzler RF, Nakaji P. Safety, efficacy, and cost of intraoperative indocyanine green angiography compared to intraoperative catheter angiography in cerebral aneurysm surgery. J Clin Neurosci. 2014; 21(8):1377–1382

[53] Lai LT, Morgan MK. Use of indocyanine green videoangiography during intracranial aneurysm surgery reduces the incidence of postoperative ischaemic complications. J Clin Neurosci. 2014; 21(1):67–72

[54] Roessler K, Krawagna M, Dörfler A, Buchfelder M, Ganslandt O. Essentials in intraoperative indocyanine green videoangiography assessment for intracranial aneurysm surgery: conclusions from 295 consecutively clipped aneurysms and review of the literature. Neurosurg Focus. 2014; 36(2):E7

[55] Sharma M, Ambekar S, Ahmed O, et al. The utility and limitations of intraoperative near-infrared indocyanine green videoangiography in aneurysm surgery. World Neurosurg. 2014; 82(5):e607–e613

[56] Hoh BL, Curry WT, Jr, Carter BS, Ogilvy CS. Computed tomographic demonstrated infarcts after surgical and endovascular treatment of aneurysmal subarachnoid hemorrhage. Acta Neurochir (Wien). 2004; 146 (11):1177–1183

[57] Bruneau M, Appelboom G, Rynkowski M, Van Cutsem N, Mine B, De Witte O. Endoscope-integrated ICG technology: first application during intracranial aneurysm surgery. Neurosurg Rev. 2013; 36(1):77–84, discussion 84–85

[58] Nishiyama Y, Kinouchi H, Senbokuya N, et al. Endoscopic indocyanine green video angiography in aneurysm surgery: an innovative method for intraoperative assessment of blood flow in vasculature hidden from microscopic view. J Neurosurg. 2012; 117(2):302–308

[59] Kamp MA, Slotty P, Turowski B, et al. Microscope-integrated quantitative analysis of intraoperative indocyanine green fluorescence angiography for blood flow assessment: first experience in 30 patients. Neurosurgery. 2012; 70(1) suppl operative:65–73, discussion 73–74

[60] Murai Y, Nakagawa S, Matano F, Shirokane K, Teramoto A, Morita A. The feasibility of detecting cerebral blood flow direction using the indocyanine green video angiography. Neurosurg Rev. 2016; 39(4):685–690

[61] Dashti R, Laakso A, Niemelä M, Porras M, Hernesniemi J. Microscope-integrated near-infrared indocyanine green videoangiography during surgery of intracranial aneurysms: the Helsinki experience. Surg Neurol. 2009; 71(5):543–550, discussion 550

[62] Barrow DL, Boyer KL, Joseph GJ. Intraoperative angiography in the management of neurovascular disorders. Neurosurgery. 1992; 30(2):153–159

[63] Popadić A, Witzmann A, Amann T, et al. The value of intraoperative angiography in surgery of intracranial aneurysms: a prospective study in 126 patients. Neuroradiology. 2001; 43(6):466–471

# 19 Indocyanine Green Videoangiography and Arteriovenous Malformations

*Justin R. Mascitelli, Jan-Karl Burkhardt, and Michael T. Lawton*

## Abstract

Indocyanine green videoangiography (ICG-VA) is a useful intra-operative tool for outlining the anatomy and assessing extent of resection of intracranial arteriovenous malformations (AVMs). ICG is a dye that can be injected intravenously and then can be seen with the operative microscope using an optical filter that allows only fluorescence in the ICG emission wavelength to pass through and be detected by infrared cameras. ICG-VA can be performed prior to, during, and following AVM resection. Benefits include safety, ease of use, and ability to distinguish AVM vessels from normal vessels. Limitations include that it can only visualize vessels that can be seen directly by the microscope and therefore poorly visualizes obscured anatomy, deep lesions, and deep venous drainage, as well as vessels covered by brain parenchyma or hematoma. In a published series, postresection ICG-VA fails to identify residual AVM in up to 12.5% of cases. Therefore, ICG-VA should be used as an adjunct to, but not as a replacement of, intraoperative or postoperative digital subtraction angiography. FLOW 800 software provides quantitative measurements of flow and may enhance ICG-VA during intracranial AVM resection, but has not been proven to impact intraoperative decision-making or patient outcome. ICG-VA is also particularly useful in the treatment of intracranial and spinal dural arteriovenous fistulas, in which the dye can readily identify the fistulous point and subsequent disconnection.

*Keywords:* indocyanine green videoangiography, arteriovenous malformation, arteriovenous fistula, fluorescence

## 19.1 Introduction

The goal of cerebral arteriovenous malformation (AVM) surgery is complete AVM resection with preservation of normal vascular and neural tissue. Accomplishing this goal, however, can be quite challenging. AVMs can abut or frankly involve eloquent brain tissue, they frequently receive arterial supply from en passage arteries that go on to supply vital brain structures, and their complete obliteration is not always obvious to the naked eye. Throughout AVM surgery, the surgeon is constantly walking the fine line between the AVM and normal brain structures. Inevitably, this delicate balance translates to a percentage of incomplete AVM resections.

The postoperative digital subtraction angiogram (DSA) is the gold standard for assessing the extent of AVM resection. This test, however, is performed after the surgery has been completed and, in turn, after there is an opportunity to resect residual AVM, if present. To address this problem, a number of intraoperative techniques have been developed over time to assess the extent of resection well before the postoperative angiogram and allow the surgeon to perform further resection, if needed, without having to perform a second operation. These techniques include the use of microvascular Doppler and flow probe measurements, intraoperative DSA, and indocyanine green videoangiography (ICG-VA).

## 19.2 Intraoperative Digital Subtraction Angiography

Intraoperative DSA has been used since the 1960s during cerebrovascular surgery[1,2] and is the standard by which all other intraoperative modalities are assessed. Despite its long-standing use, its routine application has been debated. Issues such as safety, efficacy, and practicality have been brought into question. Additionally, its usefulness has also been reconsidered given the more widespread use of ICG videoangiography as well as the trend of more complex cerebrovascular cases being treated by endovascular means. In a review of over 1,000 patients undergoing cerebrovascular surgery, including over 100 patients undergoing AVM resection, Chalouhi et al found that complications were all minor and transient and occurred in less than 1% of cases.[3] In this series, the rate of detection of residual AVM by intraoperative DSA was 9.8%, which falls in the previously reported range of 3.7 to 27.3%.[4] The practicality of using intraoperative DSA is institution specific. Certain drawbacks include the need for an interventional radiologist (if the neurosurgeon performing the surgery is not dual trained), poorer quality images using a mobile fluoroscopic unit, and increased operative time. Increased availability of hybrid operating rooms has the potential to mitigate the practicality issue.[5]

## 19.3 Indocyanine Green Videoangiography

ICG is a fluorescent molecule that can be used to view the cerebral vasculature. The dye is administered via a peripheral venous line by the anesthesiologist (typically 25 mg in 10 mL of saline) and can be seen within the cerebral arteries 3 to 12 seconds after injection. Intra-arterial administration of ICG has also been described, but is not the common route.[6] After administration, the molecule is immediately bound by globulins and remains in the intravascular space until excretion by the liver. It has absorption and emission peaks of 805 and 835 nm, respectively. The microscope records in real time with an optical filter that allows only fluorescence in the ICG emission wavelength. The dye rapidly passes into capillaries and then veins. Arterialized veins fluoresce in the late arterial phase. Therefore, the ICG-VA can be used to assess both physiological and pathological states, such as cerebral AVMs. Importantly, only vessels in the operative field that are directly visible by the microscope will be visualized with ICG-VA.[4]

Fluorescence-based angiography has been used for decades to assess the retinal vasculature during ophthalmological procedures. Although the use of fluorescence for viewing cerebral vasculature was reported as early as the 1960s,[7] the application of ICG-VA was first introduced into neurosurgery in the early 2000s.[8,9] ICG-VA was first employed during aneurysm[10] and bypass surgery,[11] and then subsequently in AVM surgery.[4]

### 19.3.1 Indocyanine Green Videoangiography for Intracranial AVMs

ICG-VA can be performed prior to, during, and following AVM resection. Typically, the dye is injected once the dura is open and vessels directly visualized. It can be performed prior to dural opening, however, to help visualize vessels through the dura and improve the safety of dural opening.[12] ICG-VA can be performed before, during, and after AVM resection and is most useful for superficial AVMs with anatomy that can be directly viewed (▶ Fig. 19.1 and ▶ Fig. 19.2; Video 19.1). The initial ICG-VA should focus on fully understanding the AVM anatomy by identifying feeding arteries, nidal arteries, and draining veins. The surgeon must distinguish pathological and normal vessels (▶ Fig. 19.3), which may include primary and secondary veins, terminal feeding arteries, transit (or en passage) arteries, and bystander arteries.[13] Special attention should be paid to protecting the primary draining vein as well as identifying and

preserving transit and bystander arteries, both of which go on to supply normal brain. Visualization of deep vessels (deep veins, perforating arteries, and choroidal feeding arteries) will frequently not be possible with the initial ICG-VA as the AVM nidus and normal parenchyma will block the line of sight to these deep vessels (▶ Fig. 19.4).

▶ Table 19.1 summarizes the available series evaluating traditional ICG-VA for AVMs (not using FLOW 800 software, which is discussed later).[4,14,15,16,17,18,19,20] In 2009, Killory et al published the first series utilizing ICG angiography for 10 patients with intracranial AVMs.[4] The authors found it useful in 9 of 10 patients. Two patients had residual AVM on intraoperative DSA, one of which had an ICG-VA that was deemed negative at the time but positive in retrospect. ICG also helped identify a small residual nidus within a hematoma. The authors concluded that the limitations of ICG-VA use are deep-seated lesions or when AVM vessels are not on the surface. Hänggi et al reported its use in 17 patients (15 AVMs and 2 arteriovenous fistulas [AVFs]).[14] The surgical strategy was changed in two cases based on ICG findings. One patient had a false-negative ICG-VA that failed to demonstrate a small residual nidus that was seen on the postoperative DSA. Bilbao et al reported 37 patients with AVMs and compared ICG-VA to both intraoperative and postoperative DSA.[18] Residual AVM was identified on intraoperative DSA in

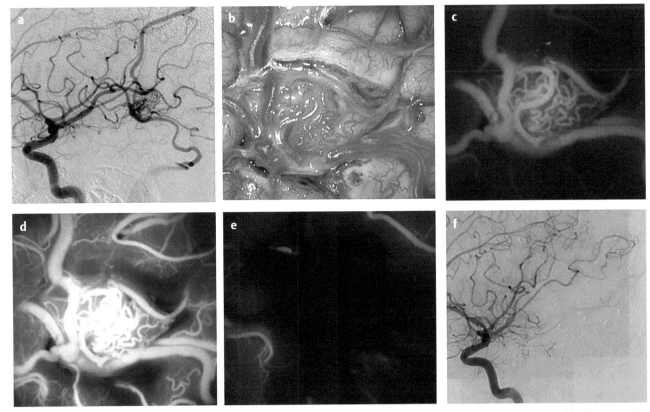

Fig. 19.1 Indocyanine green videoangiography (ICG-VA) before and after arteriovenous malformation (AVM) resection. A 53-year-old male presented with seizures secondary to a small, compact, unruptured right temporal AVM (Spetzler–Martin [SM] grade 1; supplemented SM grade 5) supplied by the inferior division of the right middle cerebral artery with superficial drainage into the superior sagittal and sigmoid sinuses (a). The patient was treated with surgical resection via a right temporal craniotomy (b). ICG-VA was performed prior to resection. Comparison of early arterial (c) and early venous (d) phases demonstrates the large early draining veins related to the AVM. The arterial feeders and AVM nidus can also be appreciated. Postresection ICG-VA (e) and DSA (f) demonstrated complete resection. This example demonstrates how ICG-VA is useful to evaluate AVM anatomy and confirm resection for simple, superficial AVMs.

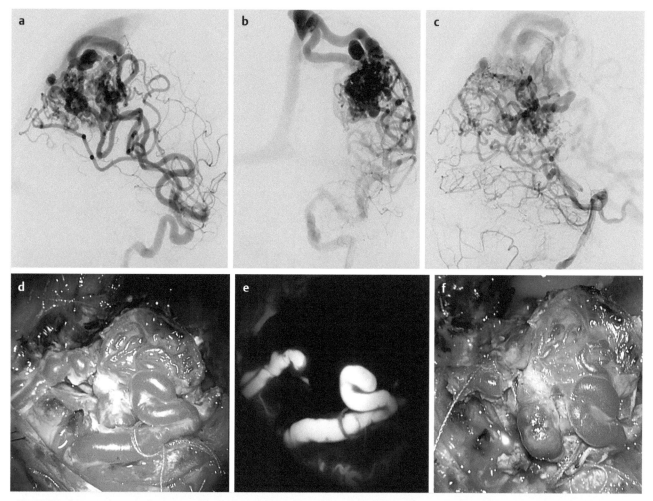

**Fig. 19.2** Indocyanine green videoangiography (ICG-VA) during arteriovenous malformation (AVM) resection. This 41-year-old female patient presented with a seizure and was diagnosed with an unruptured, medium-sized, compact, left frontal AVM (Spetzler–Martin [SM] grade 3; supplemented SM grade 7) mainly fed by the left middle cerebral artery **(a,b)** and posterior cerebral artery branches **(c)**. Venous drainage was superficial through two main draining veins into the superior sagittal sinus. ICG-VA was performed toward the end of resection and demonstrated residual flow through the large draining veins **(d)**. After complete resection of the AVM, the draining vein was divided and AVM removed **(e,f)**. This example demonstrates how ICG-VA can be used mid-resection to guide further resection.

two patients and postoperative DSA in one patient. The authors concluded that ICG-VA should only be used as an adjunct and that deep/high-grade AVMs were the most difficult to visualize.

In the largest series evaluating ICG-VA use for AVMs, Zaidi et al compared 56 ICG cases to 74 non-ICG cases with the goal of determining if it improves extent of resection or clinical outcomes (by identifying en passage vessels).[17] They found no difference in the reoperation rate (12.5 vs. 14.9%; $p = 0.8$) or change in modified Rankin scale (0.6 vs. 0.4; $p = 0.17$). Della Puppa et al described using ICG-VA in combination with flowmetry and temporary arterial clipping with neurophysiological monitoring.[20] They found that the combination of all three modalities gave the best intraoperative assessment of AVM resection but that flowmetry was better than ICG-VA at detecting residual nidus at the end of resection. In all published series, there were no adverse reactions to ICG administration.

In summary, the benefits of ICG-VA include safety, ease of use, and ability to distinguish AVM vessels from normal vessels. Its drawbacks include that it can only visualize vessels that can

be seen directly by the microscope and therefore poorly visualizes deep lesions and deep venous drainage, as well as those covered by parenchyma or hematoma. Therefore, ICG-VA should be used as an adjunct to, but not as a replacement of, intraoperative or postoperative DSA.

## 19.3.2 Indocyanine Green Videoangiography with FLOW 800

Conventional ICG-VA depends on the surgeon's subjective interpretation of the rate of filling of the arteries and veins. FLOW 800 (Carl Zeiss Meditec, Inc., Dublin, CA) is an analytical color visualization map that provides an objective evaluation of intraoperative ICG-VA. On this map, the vessels are labeled by different colors depending on the direction of blood flow. Red represents that initial blood inflow and then is followed by a gradient scale for subsequent flow giving a temporal resolution of flow dynamics. The map can help differentiate feeding

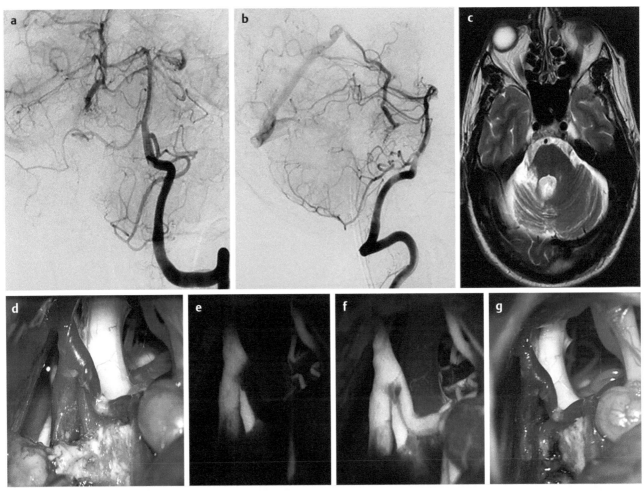

**Fig. 19.3** Indocyanine green videoangiography (ICG-VA) to differentiate normal and pathological anatomy. This 62-year-old man has a history of a severe headache 4 years ago and was diagnosed with ruptured right lateral pontine arteriovenous malformation (AVM). He underwent partial embolization of the malformation immediately, and then went on to have gamma knife radiosurgery 3 months later. Follow-up catheter angiography and MRI demonstrated a small residual right lateral pontine AVM with some surrounding radiosurgical scar. The nidus measures less than a centimeter and drains to a petrosal vein that connects to the vein of Galen (Spetzler–Martin [SM] grade 3; supplemented SM grade 6). **(a–c)** After a retrosigmoid craniotomy, the cerebellopontine angle was opened widely and the arterialized draining vein then could be identified just above the seventh and eighth nerves, and coursed to the petrosal vein. Intraoperative image confirmed the arterialized draining vein next to normal cerebellar draining veins **(d)**, which could be differentiated during early and late phases of ICG-VA **(e,f)** before dividing of the draining vein and resection of the AVM **(g)**. This example demonstrates how ICG-VA can be utilized to differentiate normal and pathological veins.

arteries, normal cortical arteries, and draining veins. Kato et al reported its initial use in 2011 and found that the FLOW 800 technology is easy to interpret, is highly reproducible, and gives real-time identification of feeding arteries and side-to-side comparison of the flow dynamics of AVM before and after clipping, increasing the safety of surgery.[22] In addition, as the AVM is progressively resected, repeated ICG injections with FLOW 800 can display a quantitative reduction in flow. FLOW 800 has the same limitation as ICG-VA in that it can only visualize vessels that can be seen by the microscope.

Since this initial publication, there have been other reports using FLOW 800 technology.[23,24,25] Ye et al reported its use in 87 patients, 25 of which were AVMs.[23] They found the maximum fluorescence intensity and the slope of the ICG curve to be higher in AVM feeding arteries and veins compared to normal vessels, the transit time was shorter through the AVM than in normal cortical vessels, and there was increased cerebral

flow after AVM resection. Fukuda et al reported on seven cases in which FLOW 800 was used.[25] The authors demonstrate how the color flow maps can quantify time intervals to reach maximal dye intensity, how subtle flow patterns within an AVM can be better assessed with FLOW 800, and how AVMs can alter normal perfusion in adjacent tissue. In response, however, Kalyvas and Spetzler remind us that FLOW 800 does not circumvent many of the limitations of traditional ICG-VA and that it has yet to be shown that FLOW 800 alters intraoperative decision-making or improves technical or clinical outcomes.[26]

## 19.3.3 Indocyanine Green Videoangiography for Intracranial AVFs

Although there has been a trend for many intracranial dural arteriovenous fistulas (dAVFs) to be treated with endovascular

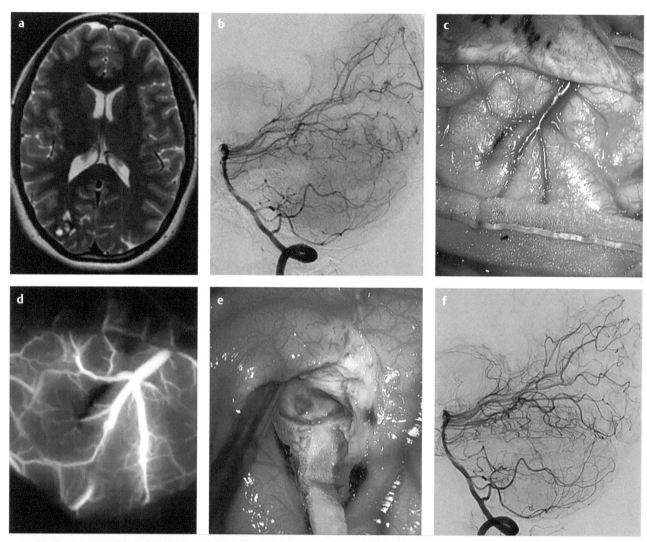

**Fig. 19.4** Indocyanine green videoangiography (ICG-VA) limitation in deep arteriovenous malformations (AVMs). A 26-year-old female presented initially with a small, compact, ruptured right occipital AVM that was treated acutely with embolization. MRI demonstrated the AVM nidus below the cortical surface **(a)**. Follow-up digital subtraction angiogram (DSA) demonstrated residual AVM filling with arterial supply from the right posterior cerebral artery and drainage medially to the superior sagittal sinus **(b)**. At the time of surgery, a normal vein can be seen on the surface of the brain by both normal inspection **(c)** and ICG-VA **(d)**. The AVM nidus and hemosiderin are found deep to the cortical surface **(e)**. Postresection repeat ICG-VA did not provide useful information once again, but conventional DSA confirmed AVM obliteration **(f)**. This example demonstrates a limitation of ICG-VA: it can only visualize vessels that can be seen directly by the microscope and therefore poorly visualizes obscured anatomy, such as AVMs below the cortical surface.

techniques, there is still a subset that requires microsurgery due to anatomical considerations and endovascular risk. ICG-VA can be used during the surgical treatment of intracranial dAVFs as well. Unlike AVMs that require systematic dissection and resection of feeding arteries, AVM nidus, and draining veins, many AVFs can be treated by simply clipping the fistulous point. Choosing the exact point is important, however. Occluding the AVF too proximally may incompletely treat the shunt and allow for future arterial recruitment. On the other hand, too distal an occlusion may sacrifice normal venous drainage of the brain and result in edema, seizures, hemorrhage, and/or stroke. Once the vessels have been exposed, ICG-VA can help identify the exact fistulous point and can be repeated following clipping to confirm complete disconnection (▶ Fig. 19.5).

In 2010, Schuette et al reported 25 patients with AVFs (13 cranial), in which ICG-VA was used.[27] ICG identified and confirmed disconnection of the fistula in all 13 cases. The cases included 7 tentorial, 3 anterior fossa, and 3 foramen magnum AVFs, all of which were high-risk locations for endovascular treatment.

### 19.3.4 ICG-VA for Spinal Vascular Malformations

Similar to cranial pathology, ICG-VA can be used during the surgical treatment of spinal vascular malformations as well (▶ Fig. 19.6). Once the laminectomy is performed and dura

**Table 19.1** Summary of literature evaluating indocyanine green (ICG) during arteriovenous malformation (AVM) surgery

| Author | N | False-negative rate | Benefits | Limitations |
|---|---|---|---|---|
| Killory et al[4] | 10 | 10.0% | • Distinguish normal vs. AVM | • Deep lesions |
| Hänggi et al[14] | 15 | 6.7% | • Fast, easy to perform, and safe<br>• Differentiate between arterial, early venous, capillary, and venous phases<br>• Adjust surgical strategy | • Deep lesions |
| Taddei et al[15] | 9 | 0.0% | • Easily performed<br>• Can confirm completeness of resection | • High-grade lesions<br>• Lesions covered by hematoma or parenchyma |
| Takagi et al[16] | 11 | 0.0% | • Effective in visualizing nidus, superficial draining veins, and changes in flow during resection | • AVMs covered by parenchyma<br>• Deep lesions |
| Zaidi et al[17] | 56 | 12.5% | • Quick and safe | • Deep lesions<br>• Does not improve identification of residual disease or clinical outcome |
| Bilbao et al[18] | 37 | 8.1% | • Helpful for small, superficial AVMs | • Detection of residual AVM<br>• Deep lesions |
| Oya et al[19] | 8[a] | 0.0% | • Localization of AV shunts of micro-AVMs with superficial drainage<br>• Confirming complete obliteration | • Lesions with deep venous drainage |
| Della Puppa et al[20] | 27 | 3.7% | • Multimodal flow-assessment approach can assist AVM surgery in different phases of resection | • Flowmetry was more reliable than ICG in detecting residual nidus missed at resection |

[a]Study only included "micro-AVMs."

opened, an initial ICG-VA can be performed to demonstrate the fistula. During this step, the precise fistula site can be determined as well as involvement from adjacent levels. Following clipping of the fistula, a repeat ICG-VA can be performed and should be notable for absence of arteriovenous shunting and delayed filling of the venous plexus surrounding the spinal cord. For more complex fistulas, ICG-VA can be repeated multiple times throughout the surgery to progressively demonstrate reduction in flow into the draining vein. ICG-VA is particularly useful for spinal pathology given that intraoperative DSA can be awkward in the prone position.

In 2010, Hanel et al reported its early use in six patients with spinal dural AVFs.[28] In all six cases, the fistula, feeding arteries, and draining veins were identified. In one case, additional supply from an adjacent level was ruled out with ICG-VA. The authors found ICG-VA the most useful in identifying the fistula site, which can sometimes be difficult to identify with the naked eye. All six patients had postoperative DSA that confirmed complete AVF disconnection. In the same year, Schuette et al reported 25 patients with AVFs (13 spinal), in which ICG was used.[27] ICG-VA identified and confirmed disconnection of the fistula in all 13 cases. In 2013, Walsh et al reported on 27 patients, of which 21 were type I dural AVFs, 2 were type II intramedullary AVMs, and 4 were type IV perimedullary AVFs.[29]

The authors comment on the ability of ICG-VA to enhance the understanding of the malformation beyond the preoperative DSA. For type I lesions, ICG-VA was most useful for low-flow fistulas, for which clipping does not result in a major change to the naked eye. In one of the two type II lesions, the ICG-VA failed to demonstrate residual nidus hidden within the spinal cord after resection. The authors found ICG-VA to be very helpful for the type IV lesions, especially since (for other reasons) these four patients had either inadequate or no preoperative DSA. In a series of over 100 spinal AVMs and AVFs, Rangel-Castilla et al found that ICG-VA was helpful in identifying arterial pedicles and early draining veins and that repeated ICG was helpful during AVM resection for identifying residual, early-filling pedicles that could then be obliterated.[30]

In summary, ICG-VA appears to be very useful for type I spinal dural AVFs. There have been fewer reports about its use in type II and IV malformations. Theoretical limitations include type II lesions that are hidden within the spinal cord and type IV lesions that are hidden ventral to the spinal cord and cannot be seen well from the dorsal approach. With that said, our personal experience using ICG-VA for type IV fistulas and conus AVMs, especially when using the occlusion-in-situ technique, is that repeated injections are very useful for demonstrating progressive occlusion of the fistula or AVM.

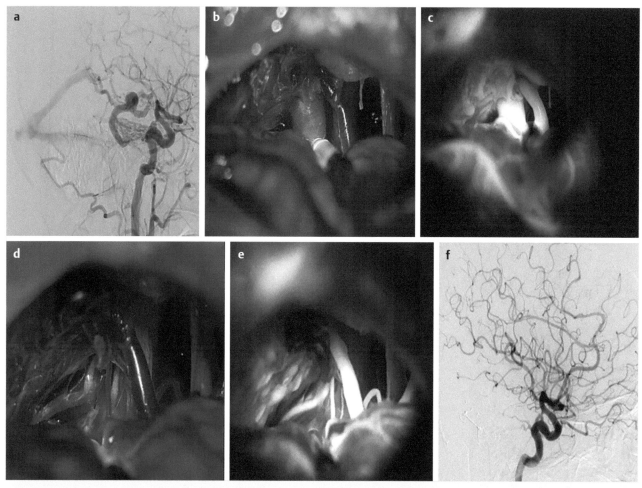

**Fig. 19.5** Indocyanine green videoangiography (ICG-VA) for intracranial dural arteriovenous fistulas (dAVFs). This 58-year-old male patient presented with headache and progressive gait disturbance and was diagnosed with a right-sided petrosal tentorial dAVF fed mainly by the internal carotid artery through branches of the meningohypophyseal trunk, specifically the tentorial artery of Bernasconi and Cassinari. Venous drainage was retrograde through a petrosal vein that connected to the basal vein of Rosenthal, with an associated venous varix compressing the brainstem (Borden type III, Cognard type IV, and tentorial dAVF type 51) **(a)**. Intraoperative image after an extended retrosigmoid craniotomy shows the arterialized draining vein from the fistula exiting the superior petrosal sinus **(b)**. ICG-VA confirmed early filling of the fistulous site **(c)** and the draining vein was occluded with a straight aneurysm clip, cauterized, and divided **(d)**. Repeated ICG-VA showed complete occlusion of the fistula without residual shunting into the draining vein as well as preservation of the normal petrosal vein **(e)**. Postoperative digital subtraction angiogram showed complete occlusion of the dAVF and venous varix **(f)**.

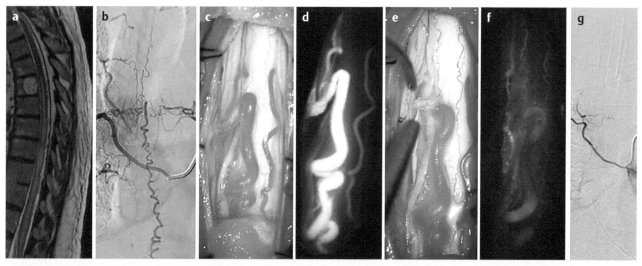

**Fig. 19.6** Indocyanine green videoangiography (ICG-VA) for spinal dural arteriovenous fistula (dAVF). A middle-aged male presented with progressive myelopathy secondary to a type 1 spinal dAVF fed primarily by the right T5 intercostal artery draining to a dorsal perimedullary vein **(a,b)**. The patient was taken for a laminectomy and dAVF disconnection. After dural opening, the fistula can be seen at the right T5 nerve sleeve with a prominent vein draining inferiorly **(c)**. ICG-VA confirmed the ultra-early filling of the draining vein **(d)**. The fistula was coagulated and cut **(e)**. ICG-VA confirmed stagnant flow in the draining vein **(f)** and postoperative digital subtraction angiogram confirmed complete occlusion of the fistula **(g)**.

# References

[1] Loop JW, Foltz EL. Applications of angiography during intracranial operation. Acta Radiol Diagn (Stockh). 1966; 5:363–367

[2] Bartal AD, Tirosh MS, Weinstein M. Angiographic control during total excision of a cerebral arteriovenous malformation. Technical note. J Neurosurg. 1968; 29(2):211–213

[3] Chalouhi N, Theofanis T, Jabbour P, et al. Safety and efficacy of intraoperative angiography in craniotomies for cerebral aneurysms and arteriovenous malformations: a review of 1093 consecutive cases. Neurosurgery. 2012; 71 (6):1162–1169

[4] Killory BD, Nakaji P, Gonzales LF, Ponce FA, Wait SD, Spetzler RF. Prospective evaluation of surgical microscope-integrated intraoperative near-infrared indocyanine green angiography during cerebral arteriovenous malformation surgery. Neurosurgery. 2009; 65(3):456–462, discussion 462

[5] Kotowski M, Sarrafzadeh A, Schatlo B, et al. Intraoperative angiography reloaded: a new hybrid operating theater for combined endovascular and surgical treatment of cerebral arteriovenous malformations: a pilot study on 25 patients. Acta Neurochir (Wien). 2013; 155(11):2071–2078

[6] Kono K, Uka A, Mori M, Haga S, Hamada Y, Nagata S. Intra-arterial injection of indocyanine green in cerebral arteriovenous malformation surgery. Turk Neurosurg. 2013; 23(5):676–679

[7] Feindel W, Yamamoto YL, Hodge CP. Intracarotid fluorescein angiography: a new method for examination of the epicerebral circulation in man. Can Med Assoc J. 1967; 96(1):1–7

[8] Kuroiwa T, Kajimoto Y, Ohta T. Development and clinical application of near-infrared surgical microscope: preliminary report. Minim Invasive Neurosurg. 2001; 44(4):240–242

[9] Raabe A, Beck J, Gerlach R, Zimmermann M, Seifert V. Near-infrared indocyanine green videoangiography: a new method for intraoperative assessment of vascular flow. Neurosurgery. 2003; 52(1):132–139, discussion 139

[10] Raabe A, Nakaji P, Beck J, et al. Prospective evaluation of surgical microscope-integrated intraoperative near-infrared indocyanine green videoangiography during aneurysm surgery. J Neurosurg. 2005; 103(6):982–989

[11] Woitzik J, Horn P, Vajkoczy P, Schmiedek P. Intraoperative control of extracranial-intracranial bypass patency by near-infrared indocyanine green videoangiography. J Neurosurg. 2005; 102(4):692–698

[12] Della Puppa A, Rustemi O, Gioffrè G, Causin F, Scienza R. Transdural indocyanine green videoangiography of vascular malformations. Acta Neurochir (Wien). 2014; 156(9):1761–1767

[13] Lawton MT, ed. Seven AVMs: Tenets and Techniques for Resection. New York, NY: Thieme; 2014

[14] Hänggi D, Etminan N, Steiger HJ. The impact of microscope-integrated intraoperative near-infrared indocyanine green videoangiography on surgery of arteriovenous malformations and dural arteriovenous fistulae. Neurosurgery. 2010; 67(4):1094–1103, discussion 1103–1104

[15] Taddei G, Tommasi CD, Ricci A, Galzio RJ. Arteriovenous malformations and intraoperative indocyanine green videoangiography: preliminary experience. Neurol India. 2011; 59(1):97–100

[16] Takagi Y, Sawamura K, Hashimoto N, Miyamoto S. Evaluation of serial intraoperative surgical microscope-integrated intraoperative near-infrared indocyanine green videoangiography in patients with cerebral arteriovenous malformations. Neurosurgery. 2012; 70(1) suppl operative:34–42, discussion 42–43

[17] Zaidi HA, Abla AA, Nakaji P, Chowdhry SA, Albuquerque FC, Spetzler RF. Indocyanine green angiography in the surgical management of cerebral arteriovenous malformations: lessons learned in 130 consecutive cases. Neurosurgery. 2014; 10 suppl 2:246–251, discussion 251

[18] Bilbao CJ, Bhalla T, Dalal S, Patel H, Dehdashti AR. Comparison of indocyanine green fluorescent angiography to digital subtraction angiography in brain arteriovenous malformation surgery. Acta Neurochir (Wien). 2015; 157(3): 351–359

[19] Oya S, Nejo T, Fujisawa N, et al. Usefulness of repetitive intraoperative indocyanine green-based videoangiography to confirm complete obliteration of micro-arteriovenous malformations. Surg Neurol Int. 2015; 6:85

[20] Della Puppa A, Scienza R. Multimodal flow-assisted resection of brain AVMs. Acta Neurochir Suppl (Wien). 2016; 123:141–145

[21] Ahn JH, Cho YD, Kang HS, et al. Endovascular treatment of ophthalmic artery aneurysms: assessing balloon test occlusion and preservation of vision in coil embolization. AJNR Am J Neuroradiol. 2014; 35(11):2146–2152

[22] Kato Y, Jhawar SS, Oda J, et al. Preliminary evaluation of the role of surgical microscope-integrated intraoperative FLOW 800 colored indocyanine fluorescence angiography in arteriovenous malformation surgery. Neurol India. 2011; 59(6):829–832

[23] Ye X, Liu XJ, Ma L, et al. Clinical values of intraoperative indocyanine green fluorescence video angiography with Flow 800 software in cerebrovascular surgery. Chin Med J (Engl). 2013; 126(22):4232–4237

[24] Ng YP, King NK, Wan KR, Wang E, Ng I. Uses and limitations of indocyanine green videoangiography for flow analysis in arteriovenous malformation surgery. J Clin Neurosci. 2013; 20(2):224–232

[25] Fukuda K, Kataoka H, Nakajima N, Masuoka J, Satow T, Iihara K. Efficacy of FLOW 800 with indocyanine green videoangiography for the quantitative assessment of flow dynamics in cerebral arteriovenous malformation surgery. World Neurosurg. 2015; 83(2):203–210

[26] Kalyvas J, Spetzler RF. Does FLOW 800 technology improve the utility of indocyanine green videoangiography in cerebral arteriovenous malformation surgery? World Neurosurg. 2015; 83(2):147–148

[27] Schuette AJ, Cawley CM, Barrow DL. Indocyanine green videoangiography in the management of dural arteriovenous fistulae. Neurosurgery. 2010; 67(3): 658–662, discussion 662

[28] Hanel RA, Nakaji P, Spetzler RF. Use of microscope-integrated near-infrared indocyanine green videoangiography in the surgical treatment of spinal dural arteriovenous fistulae. Neurosurgery. 2010; 66(5):978–984, discussion 984–985

[29] Walsh DC, Zebian B, Tolias CM, Gullan RW. Intraoperative indocyanine green videoangiography as an aid to the microsurgical treatment of spinal vascular malformations. Br J Neurosurg. 2014; 28(2):259–266

[30] Rangel-Castilla L, Russin JJ, Zaidi HA, et al. Contemporary management of spinal AVFs and AVMs: lessons learned from 110 cases. Neurosurg Focus. 2014; 37(3):E14

# 20 Indocyanine Green and Cerebral Revascularization

*Lars Wessels, Nils Hecht, and Peter Vajkoczy*

## Abstract

Maintenance of cerebral blood flow is essential to prevent cerebral ischemia. In 10% of ischemic stroke patients, cerebral bypass surgery may be considered to treat chronic occlusion of the cerebral vasculature due to arteriosclerosis or moyamoya vasculopathy. In other situations, grafting of an interposition bypass may be needed to treat complex intracranial aneurysms or skull base tumors that require sacrifice of the main vessels supplying blood to the brain. However, flow augmentation or flow replacement by grafting of an intracranial to intracranial (IC-IC) or extracranial to intracranial (EC-IC) bypass is naturally also associated with an intraoperative risk of ischemic stroke or bypass failure, which may result in neurological deficits or even death. For this reason, immediate intraoperative control of bypass patency and function is required. Besides intraoperative digital subtraction angiography as the gold standard for bypass patency control, simpler and safer methods for immediate intraoperative assessment of bypass patency have been developed and implemented in recent years. Here, indocyanine green videoangiography has been validated as a reliable, cost-effective, and easy-to-use tool for immediate real-time visualization of bypass patency and cerebrovascular hemodynamics.

*Keywords:* indocyanine green, bypass, cerebral revascularization, cerebral bypass surgery, cerebral aneurysm, moyamoya, chronic cerebral ischemia, cerebrovascular disease, stroke

## 20.1 Introduction

Mainly two general indications for direct cerebral revascularization exist: (1) chronic hemodynamic compromise with the need to augment cerebral blood flow and (2) the need to replace blood flow completely following sacrifice of vessels that maintain cerebral blood flow (CBF) for treatment of complex vascular lesions or tumors of the skull base.

In both cases, positive and certain intraoperative assessment of bypass patency is essential, particularly following sacrifice of large vessels where bypass occlusion would result in ischemic stroke. To prevent this complication, intraoperative visualization of the cerebral vasculature is crucial. Therefore, additional visual information is necessary regarding blood flow in the recipient vessel, bypass patency, and blood flow in the bypass to estimate its performance. The following chapter provides an overview about the history, pitfalls, and pearls of intraoperative angiography by indocyanine green videoangiography (ICG-VA) during cerebral revascularization.

## 20.2 ICG as a Tool for Quality Control in Cerebral Revascularization

ICG was first described in 1975 by Flower and Hochheimer as a tool for angiography of the retina in ophthalmology.[1] In 2003,

ICG-VA was then introduced in vascular neurosurgery for non-invasive, angiographic real-time visualization of blood flow in the superficial vasculature of the brain.[2] The first technological ICG-VA setup was relatively complex in handling and consisted of a separate camera. In addition, analysis of the transit time of the fluorescent dye within the vasculature had to be done manually. Despite this initial workflow limitation, however, ICG-VA was a great advantage over intraoperative digital subtraction angiogram, mostly due to its low risk profile, simple handling, cost and time efficiency, and the fact that the procedure could be performed and interpreted by the surgeon without the need for radiological and/or neuroradiological assistance. Meanwhile, workflow and handling were significantly improved by routine integration of ICG-VA into the surgical microscope and more recently, a new software tool named FLOW 800 was introduced that allows immediate color-coded visualization and pseudo-quantitative analysis of the temporal distribution dynamics of the fluorescent ICG dye.[3]

In general, ICG-VA and FLOW 800 are based on the fluorescent properties of ICG, allowing angiographic visualization of flow through the vasculature within the imaging field of the surgical microscope. After intravenous injection of the dye (0.3 mg/kg body weight [25 mg dissolved in 2.5 mL water]),[4] the ICG-VA filter is activated by pushing a button on the handle of the surgical microscope, which activates an infrared laser light illumination (780-nm wavelength) together with a registration of the emitted light by a camera with a specific filter for the ICG absorption and emission peaks of 805 and 835 nm, respectively. The obtained images are recorded in black and white as a movie and played back and projected into the visual field of the surgical microscope. The mean rise time of fluorescent intensity after injection is 5.2 seconds and time to peak is 9.4 seconds. The half-time fluorescent intensity is around 20 seconds but depends on the cardiac output and on the blood flow in the vessel.[5,6] The fluorescence of the ICG dye is nonlinear to its concentration and doubles when the concentration increases 10-fold. The ICG dye remains intravascularly if there is no vascular leakage.[7] The injection can be repeated during one operation after an interval of 15 minutes.[8] ICG is not metabolized in the body. After systemic administration, it binds to a transport protein (glutathione S-transferase) and has no known interactions or modifications before its excretion into the bile juice with a plasma half-life of 4 minutes.[9]

The ICG-VA technique is very easy to perform, but there are some pitfalls that need to be avoided. First, intravenous application should be performed with standard intravenous access. Central venous injection will lead to much faster distribution into the cerebral vessels. Furthermore, the speed of the injection and the amount of fluid administered after injection of the dye can lead to significant variations of the time-to-peak fluorescence during surgery. Due to its systemic application, the cardiac output has influence on the ICG dye distribution. Atrial fibrillation and cardiac insufficiency can prolong the time to signal. In case of a missing signal after injection, possible extravessel injection should be checked for and fresh dye should be re-injected due to its instability from light exposure.

Apart from visualizing the patency of perforating arteries following aneurysm clipping, confirmation of the patency of an extracranial to intracranial (EC-IC) or intracranial to intracranial (IC-IC) bypass remains one of the key indications for ICG-VA. Mainly, this is because ICG-VA ensures quality control and patient safety during bypass surgery through immediate visualization of intravascular blood flow, providing the vascular neurosurgeon with relevant information extending simple patency control.

With a superficial temporal artery to middle cerebral artery (STA-MCA) bypass, visualization of blood flow and semi-quantitative information about local cerebral perfusion and vessel diameter can help find the right target vessel in the sylvian fissure.[8,10,11] This together with a standardized approach based on anatomic landmarks can optimize postoperative results regarding bypass patency.[12] Further, ICG is not able to penetrate the intact blood–brain barrier (BBB). Due to this property, ICG-VA visualizes disrupted or impaired BBB in ischemic areas or surrounding pathological vessels, as demonstrated in patients with ischemic stroke.[7,8]

The FLOW 800 software provides color-coded visualization of hemodynamic parameters during surgery. This allows a comparative assessment of changes within the micro- and macrocirculation before and after revascularization (► Fig. 20.1).[6] However, it should be noted that several confounding factors exist that may influence the hemodynamic readout of FLOW 800, such as the speed and route of intravenous injection or the circulation time depending on the cardiac output.[5] Consequently, FLOW 800 is not intended to measure perfusion directly or in a continuous fashion and therefore, the ICG-VA-based semi-quantification of the mean transit time of the fluorescent dye should mainly be used for an arbitrary estimation of relative flow velocity, ideally in a before-and-after setting. To further ensure graft patency, quantitative information on flow within the bypass graft as well as semi-quantitative information on cortical tissue perfusion can be intraoperatively obtained by perivascular ultrasonic flow measurements[13] and laser speckle imaging.[14,15] However, the ICG-based analysis of blood flow

after revascularization can help estimate the specific risk for postoperative hyperperfusion syndrome and may help provide these patients with intensified blood pressure monitoring after surgery.[7] In addition, the diameter of the vessel wall can be estimated with ICG-VA, because ICG only fills the lumen of the vessel and this can be subtracted from the vessel diameter under white light, which may help determine the grade of atherosclerosis or find pathological thin areas in the vessel wall with increased risk for insufficient anastomosis.[16] Lastly, ICG before craniotomy can help visualize the frontal branches of the middle meningeal artery in one-third of moyamoya patients before STA-MCA bypass surgery and helps preserve these vessels, a potential benefit if additional indirect revascularization is planned.[17]

Still the most important role of ICG-VA in cerebral revascularization is control of bypass patency during surgery. ICG-VA provides direct control of bypass patency during surgery and enables the surgeon to directly revise the anastomosis if it shows no optimal patency. This helps prevent early graft failure and ICG-VA can help identify the point of occlusion (Video 20.1).[4,18] One problem with ICG-VA is the inability to visualize the surrounding tissue. The monochrome gives no information about surrounding structures, which may lead to difficulties, especially in challenging anatomical situations. A new technology might be helpful in solving this problem by using dual-image videoangiography in addition to conventional ICG-VA, providing the surgeon with a white-light picture overlaid by the ICG-VA signal. This allows direct integration of the fluorescent signal into the anatomical structures.

## 20.3 Indocyanine Green in Different Bypass Indications

The need for intraoperative visualization of bypass and brain vessels is essential for various bypass techniques, although different aspects are important among different techniques and indications.

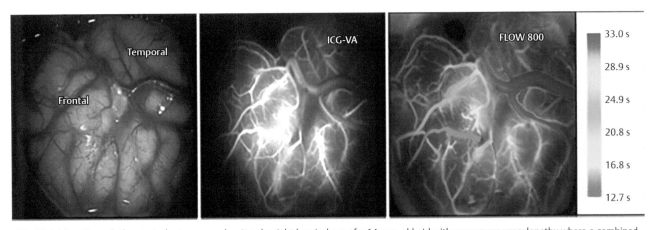

**Fig. 20.1** View through the surgical microscope showing the right hemisphere of a 14-year-old girl with moyamoya vasculopathy where a combined revascularization is planned. The color-coded FLOW 800 image after opening of the dura shows the mean transit time of the fluorescent indocyanine green dye in a color-coded blood flow map.

## 20.3.1 Cerebral Revascularization for Treatment of Chronic Hemodynamic Compromise

Chronic cerebral ischemia is responsible for up to 10% of all ischemic strokes and in patients with significantly reduced cerebrovascular reserve capacity (CVRC), stroke risk reaches up to 30%.[19,20] Chronic cerebral ischemia is often based on arteriosclerotic stenosis and occlusion due to endogenous changes of the vessel wall present in moyamoya disease or syndrome. Due to the chronic course of the occlusion, the reduction in cerebral perfusion pressure can be compensated to some degree by outgrowth of preformed collaterals at the level of the leptomeningeal anastomosis[7] and at the base of the brain via the anterior and posterior communicating arteries of the circle of Willis. The exhaustion of this system typically results in transitory ischemic attacks (TIAs), indicating that the endogenous compensation mechanism is not capable of maintaining a sufficient blood supply to the brain. Conservative treatment for prevention of stroke in affected patients consists of smoking withdrawal, optimizing blood pressure, administration of cholesterol-/lipid-lowering agents, and platelet inhibitors for both subgroups. However, despite best medical therapy, the problem remains that the chronically reduced cerebral perfusion is not adequately addressed. In such cases, bypass surgery for augmentation of collateral flow may be indicated. As a result of the randomized EC-IC bypass trial from 1985, where even acute and embolic ischemic strokes were considered for bypass revascularization,[21] hemodynamic failure has meanwhile been identified as the main prognostic variable that each patient needs to meet before an EC-IC bypass is considered as a treatment for prevention of ischemic stroke.[19,22,23] Thus, today there are strict criteria for patient evaluation for cerebral revascularization, such as angiographically diagnosed internal carotid artery (ICA) or MCA occlusion or high-grade stenosis, with recurrent TIAs and reduced CVRC proven by PET or xenon-CT with acetazolamide stimulation.

The typical revascularization technique for chronic cerebral ischemia is to perform a standard EC-IC bypass from the STA to a cortical branch of the MCA. Although failure of an STA-MCA bypass intended for flow augmentation will usually not directly result in failure-associated ischemia, the consequences of a failed bypass with the continuously high risk of hemodynamic stroke mandate a routine intraoperative assessment of bypass patency, so that—if needed—an immediate intraoperative revision can be performed. For this purpose, ICG-VA presents a valuable and routinely implemented tool with proven benefit to reduce the incidence of early bypass graft failure.[4] Further, ICG-VA can be helpful to identify an optimal recipient vessel for the bypass, and the newly introduced FLOW 800 software allows intraoperative color-coded visualization of the dynamic properties of the ICG dye, which within limits allows identification of improved or reduced hemodynamics in the downstream cortical region of the graft (▶ Fig. 20.1).[6] For the purpose of measuring cerebral perfusion within the parenchyma, however, optical imaging technologies for direct and continuous perfusion assessment, for example, noninvasive laser speckle imaging, are needed (▶ Fig. 20.2).[6,14]

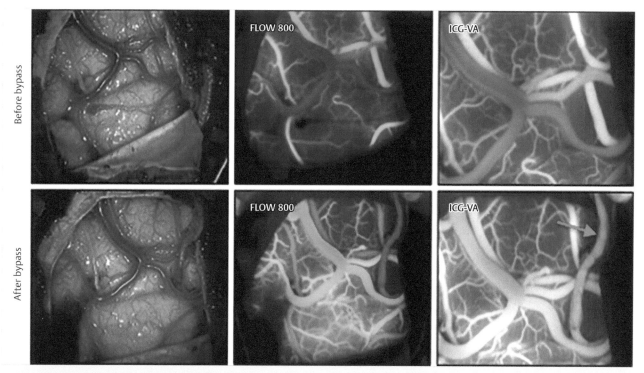

**Fig. 20.2** Cortical surface with intraoperative indocyanine green videoangiography and FLOW 800 images before (upper panels) and after (lower panels) grafting of a superficial temporal artery–middle cerebral artery bypass in a patient with hemodynamic compromise. The red arrow indicates the bypass graft. (Reproduced with permission from Prinz et al.[6])

## 20.3.2 Cerebral Revascularization for Treatment of Complex Aneurysms and Skull Base Tumors

Although most cerebral aneurysms can be treated by direct clip occlusion or endovascular treatment, certain aneurysms remain inaccessible for either direct clipping or coiling and require treatment by occlusion of the aneurysm harboring vessel segment following grafting of an EC-IC or IC-IC bypass for replacement of flow. The most common aneurysms requiring a combination of flow replacement and trapping are fusiform or dolichoectatic large (20–25 mm) or giant (> 25 mm) aneurysms, in which an entire vascular segment is diseased and perforating arteries are frequently involved. Next to their anatomical complexity, large and giant aneurysms are also associated with a significantly higher rupture rate than typical saccular aneurysms of smaller size.[4,15] Basically, three degrees of flow replacement are available:

- Standard-flow STA-MCA bypass.
- Intermediate-flow radial artery interposition bypass.
- High-flow saphenous vein interposition bypass.

Since each bypass also carries a risk profile that typically increases with the amount of flow that is provided, an exact preoperative evaluation of the required amount of flow substitution is mandatory with the goal to obtain information on the individual collateralization pattern and hemodynamic tolerance during test occlusion of the parent artery. The gold standard for these patients who typically present with aneurysms of the terminal ICA is a balloon occlusion test (BOT) with neurological assessment. In our institution, we additionally perform functional CBF monitoring with a thermal diffusion microprobe, which is implanted by local anaesthesia via a small burr hole prior to the BOT. During the occlusion, we perform an acetazolamide challenge to quantify the hemodynamic reserve measured invasively by the diffusion probe.[24] Depending on the results of BOT, the bypass type can be determined (▶ Table 20.1). In the best case, if no symptoms occur during the BOT together with a stable baseline perfusion and intact CVRC, the ICA can be primarily occluded without the need of a bypass.

In other cases, complete exclusion of the aneurysms from the circulation may require grafting of an IC-IC bypass, where essentially flow is not replaced by an extracranial source but redistributed between two intracranial ones.[25] The most frequent indication for this treatment are aneurysms involving the posterior inferior cerebellar artery (PICA), where a side-to-side anastomosis of both PICA loops is performed to allow sacrifice of the PICA and aneurysm distal to the anastomosis. It should be noted, however, that even in the most experienced hands, in situ bypass grafting is technically demanding due to the usually deep surgical field and a generally increased risk of perioperative ischemia, since grafting of the anastomosis requires temporary occlusion of two instead of one cerebral arteries and failure means loss of both vessels as the worst outcome. Finally, selected complex tumors of the skull base with involvement of the cerebral vasculature and the goal of radical tumor resection may also require sacrifice of the main blood supplying arteries with cerebral revascularization.[26] Nevertheless, an indication for vessel sacrifice for tumor resection is rare and particularly in malignant tumors the benefits and risks of bypass surgery and aggressive tumor resection should individually be weighed against overall oncological effectiveness of the interdisciplinary treatment strategy. Most importantly, cerebral revascularization for complex vascular lesions and skull base tumors should be performed in specialized centers with qualified personnel, not only regarding the neurosurgical team, but also with respect to dedicated anesthesiology, neuroradiology, neurological, and neurointensive care teams.

# References

[1] Flower RW, Hochheimer BF. A clinical technique and apparatus for simultaneous angiography of the separate retinal and choroidal circulations. Invest Ophthalmol. 1973; 12(4):248–261

[2] Raabe A, Beck J, Gerlach R, Zimmermann M, Seifert V. Near-infrared indocyanine green videoangiography: a new method for intraoperative assessment of vascular flow. Neurosurgery. 2003; 52(1):132–139, discussion 139

[3] Uchino H, Kazumata K, Ito M, Nakayama N, Kuroda S, Houkin K. Intraoperative assessment of cortical perfusion by indocyanine green videoangiography in surgical revascularization for moyamoya disease. Acta Neurochir (Wien). 2014; 156(9):1753–1760

[4] Woitzik J, Horn P, Vajkoczy P, Schmiedek P. Intraoperative control of extracranial-intracranial bypass patency by near-infrared indocyanine green videoangiography. J Neurosurg. 2005; 102(4):692–698

[5] Kamp MA, Slotty P, Turowski B, et al. Microscope-integrated quantitative analysis of intraoperative indocyanine green fluorescence angiography for blood flow assessment: first experience in 30 patients. Neurosurgery. 2012; 70(1) suppl operative:65–73, discussion 73–74

[6] Prinz V, Hecht N, Kato N, Vajkoczy P. FLOW 800 allows visualization of hemodynamic changes after extracranial-to-intracranial bypass surgery but not assessment of quantitative perfusion or flow. Neurosurgery. 2014; 10 suppl 2:231–238, discussion 238–239

[7] Awano T, Sakatani K, Yokose N, et al. EC-IC bypass function in moyamoya disease and non-moyamoya ischemic stroke evaluated by intraoperative indocyanine green fluorescence angiography. Adv Exp Med Biol. 2010; 662: 519–524

[8] Woitzik J, Peña-Tapia PG, Schneider UC, Vajkoczy P, Thomé C. Cortical perfusion measurement by indocyanine-green videoangiography in patients undergoing hemicraniectomy for malignant stroke. Stroke. 2006; 37(6): 1549–1551

[9] Alander JT, Kaartinen I, Laakso A, et al. A review of indocyanine green fluorescent imaging in surgery. Int J Biomed Imaging. 2012; 2012:940585

[10] Esposito G, Durand A, Van Doormaal T, Regli L. Selective-targeted extra-intracranial bypass surgery in complex middle cerebral artery aneurysms:

Table 20.1 Bypass types, blood flow, and hemodynamic criteria for choosing the different bypass types according to balloon occlusion test (BOT) results

| Bypass type | Blood flow (mL/min) | CBF decrease (%) | CVRC (%) | Clinical symptoms during BOT |
|---|---|---|---|---|
| Standard flow (i.e., STA-MCA) | 20–70 | < 30 | < 10 | No |
| Intermediate flow (radial artery graft) | 60–100 | 30–50 | – | No |
| High flow (saphenous vein graft) | 100–200 | > 50 | – | Yes |

Abbreviations: CBF, cerebral blood flow; CVRC, cerebrovascular reserve capacity; STA-MCA, superficial temporal artery–middle cerebral artery.

correctly identifying the recipient artery using indocyanine green videoangiography. Neurosurgery. 2012; 71(2) suppl operative: :274–284, discussion 284–285

[11] Rodríguez-Hernández A, Lawton MT. Flash fluorescence with indocyanine green videoangiography to identify the recipient artery for bypass with distal middle cerebral artery aneurysms: operative technique. Neurosurgery. 2012; 70:209–220

[12] Peña-Tapia PG, Kemmling A, Czabanka M, Vajkoczy P, Schmiedek P. Identification of the optimal cortical target point for extracranial-intracranial bypass surgery in patients with hemodynamic cerebrovascular insufficiency. J Neurosurg. 2008; 108(4):655–661

[13] Charbel FT, Hoffman WE, Misra M, Ostergren L. Ultrasonic perivascular flow probe: technique and application in neurosurgery. Neurol Res. 1998; 20(5): 439–442

[14] Hecht N, Woitzik J, Dreier JP, Vajkoczy P. Intraoperative monitoring of cerebral blood flow by laser speckle contrast analysis. Neurosurg Focus. 2009; 27(4):E11

[15] Hecht N, Woitzik J, König S, Horn P, Vajkoczy P. Laser speckle imaging allows real-time intraoperative blood flow assessment during neurosurgical procedures. J Cereb Blood Flow Metab. 2013; 33(7):1000–1007

[16] Nakagawa D, Shojima M, Yoshino M, et al. Wall-to-lumen ratio of intracranial arteries measured by indocyanine green angiography. Asian J Neurosurg. 2016; 11(4):361–364

[17] Tanabe N, Yamamoto S, Kashiwazaki D, et al. Indocyanine green visualization of middle meningeal artery before craniotomy during surgical revascularization for moyamoya disease. Acta Neurochir (Wien). 2017; 159 (3):567–575

[18] Januszewski J, Beecher JS, Chalif DJ, Dehdashti AR. Flow-based evaluation of cerebral revascularization using near-infrared indocyanine green videoangiography. Neurosurg Focus. 2014; 36(2):E14

[19] Grubb RL, Jr, Derdeyn CP, Fritsch SM, et al. Importance of hemodynamic factors in the prognosis of symptomatic carotid occlusion. JAMA. 1998; 280 (12):1055–1060

[20] Klijn CJ, Kappelle LJ, Tulleken CA, van Gijn J. Symptomatic carotid artery occlusion. A reappraisal of hemodynamic factors. Stroke. 1997; 28(10):2084–2093

[21] EC/IC Bypass Study Group. Failure of extracranial-intracranial arterial bypass to reduce the risk of ischemic stroke. Results of an international randomized trial. N Engl J Med. 1985; 313(19):1191–1200

[22] Schmiedek P, Piepgras A, Leinsinger G, Kirsch C-M, Einhäupl K. Improvement of cerebrovascular reserve capacity by EC-IC arterial bypass surgery in patients with ICA occlusion and hemodynamic cerebral ischemia. J Neurosurg. 1994; 81(2):236–244

[23] Powers WJ. Management of patients with atherosclerotic carotid occlusion. Curr Treat Options Neurol. 2011; 13(6):608–615

[24] Vajkoczy P, Roth H, Horn P, et al. Continuous monitoring of regional cerebral blood flow: experimental and clinical validation of a novel thermal diffusion microprobe. J Neurosurg. 2000; 93(2):265–274

[25] Lawton MT, Quiñones-Hinojosa A, Chang EF, Yu T. Thrombotic intracranial aneurysms: classification scheme and management strategies in 68 patients. Neurosurgery. 2005; 56(3):441–454, discussion 441–454

[26] Cornelius JF, George B, Kolb F. Combined use of a radial fore arm free flap for extra-intracranial bypass and for antero-lateral skull base reconstruction: a new technique and review of literature. Acta Neurochir (Wien). 2006; 148 (4):427–434

# Index

Note: Page numbers set **bold** or *italic* indicate headings or figures, respectively.